Educating Your Patient with Diabetes

CONTEMPORARY DIABETES

ARISTIDIS VEVES, MD
SERIES EDITOR

Educating Your Patient with Diabetes, edited by *Katie Weinger, EdD, RN and Catherine A. Carver, MS, APRN, BC, CDE, 2009*

The Diabetic Kidney, edited by *Pedro Cortes, MD and Carl Erik Mogensen, MD, 2006*

The Diabetic Foot, *Second Edition,* edited by *Aristidis Veves, MD, John M. Giurini, DPM, and Frank W. LoGerfo, MD, 2006*

Obesity and Diabetes, edited by *Chritos S. Mantzoros, MD, 2006*

Educating Your Patient with Diabetes

Edited by

Katie Weinger, EdD, RN

Joslin Diabetes Center, Boston, MA

Catherine A. Carver, MS, APRN, BC, CDE

Joslin Diabetes Center, Boston, MA

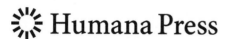 Humana Press

Editors
Katie Weinger
Joslin Diabetes Center
Boston, MA
katie.weinger@joslin.harvard.edu

Catherine A. Carver
Joslin Diabetes Center
Boston, MA
catherine.carver@joslin.harvard.edu

Series Editor
Aristidis Veves
Beth-Israel Deaconess Medical Center
Boston, MA

ISBN: 978-1-60327-207-0   e-ISBN: 978-1-60327-208-7
DOI 10.1007/978-1-60327-208-7

Library of Congress Control Number: 2008938924

Printed on acid-free paper

springer.com

PREFACE

Educating Your Patient with Diabetes

Those who provide diabetes education have a most important goal to support people as they struggle to normalize their lives with diabetes. Educators strive to help the person become an independent practitioner of diabetes, someone who can take advantage of community resources, make healthy lifestyle choices, and follow treatment recommendations and prescriptions. Of course, in reality, this dream is much too difficult for one person to achieve alone. Successful treatment of diabetes requires the coordinated efforts of the person with diabetes, the family, the community, and the multidisciplinary health-care team.

Diabetes is ever more prevalent with an estimated 24 million people in the United States suffering from diabetes, some of whom are unaware of their diagnosis. New medications and technology are available to help fight this disease. Yet the number of health-care professionals who are experts in the treatment and education of people with diabetes has not increased. Some may find meeting the challenges of treating diabetes daunting, although they encounter people with diabetes as part of their general practice, either in the community or in the hospital. We hope that this book will assist those experienced with the care of people with diabetes and those who are relatively new to their profession or who have only a handful of patients who need diabetes education. Diabetes can occur at any age, and the challenges it creates can differ across the lifespan. It touches not only those who have the diagnosis but family, friends, employers, and others. Because the experience of living with diabetes is individual and each person and family living with diabetes is unique, diabetes educators have come to expect the unexpected and have shared learning experiences with their patients as new technology provides interesting and innovative ways to combat diabetes, its complications, and side effects of its treatment.

In *Educating Your Patient with Diabetes*, we have tried to capture both the art and the science of diabetes self-management education and have tried to reflect the various patient experiences that health-care professionals who are serving as diabetes educators might meet during their clinical encounters. We hope that this book is a useful handbook that can serve to help these educators support their patients in their diabetes self-care efforts and to help them maximize the opportunities for patient learning whether that occurs in the hospital, the medical office, or in the community.

Ashley Leighton has been a significant contributor, not only as an author but also as an organized, thorough, and thoughtful administrator. We could not have done this without her. We appreciate the efforts of all the hardworking authors who were so willing to meet stringent deadlines in the midst of their busy clinical lives. We would also like to thank Paul Dolgert of Humana Press and Aristidis Veves, MD, the editor of the Contemporary Diabetes series at Humana Press, for their support of and interest in this book. We thank the clinicians and staff of the Joslin Diabetes Center for their patient-centered focus and their commitment to excellence. Most importantly, we would like to thank our patients who provided us with the valuable learning experiences upon which this book is based.

Katie Weinger, EdD, RN
Catherine A. Carver, MS, APRN, BC, CDE

CONTENTS

Preface v

Contributors.. ix

PART I: PRINCIPLES AND PRACTICES OF DIABETES EDUCATION

1. Living With Diabetes: The Role of Diabetes Education 3
   Katie Weinger and Ashley Leighton

2. Diabetes Mellitus Overview 15
   Catherine Carver and Martin Abrahamson

3. Models for Diabetes Education............................ 29
   Linda M. Siminerio

4. Diabetes Education Process............................... 45
   Amy P. Campbell and Elaine D. Sullivan

5. Making the Most of the Outpatient Visit 61
   Carolè Mensing and Deborah Hinnen

6. Meeting the Challenge of Inpatient Diabetes Education:
   An Interdisciplinary Approach 81
   Jane Seley and Marisa Wallace

7. Optimizing Self-Care with Diabetes Complications
   and Comorbidities...................................... 97
   Belinda P. Childs and Jolene Grothe

8. Role of Culture and Health Literacy in Diabetes Self-
   Management and Education 115
   Andreina Millan-Ferro and Enrique Caballero

9. Technology in Self-Care: Implications for
   Diabetes Education....................................135
   William C. Hsu and Howard A. Wolpert

10. Deciphering the Blood Glucose Puzzle with Pattern
    Management Skills....................................143
    Donna Tomky

11. Measuring Diabetes Outcomes and Measuring
    Behavior 159
    Malinda Peeples

12. Diabetes Education Program Evaluation: Ensuring Effective
    Operations 177
    Melinda D. Maryniuk and Judith E. Goodwin

PART II: EDUCATING SPECIFIC POPULATIONS

13. Working with Challenging Patients in Diabetes
    Treatment 197
    Marilyn D. Ritholz

14. Diabetes and Sexual Health 213
    Donna Rice, Janis Roszler, and Jo Anne B. Farrell

15. Diabetes in Pregnancy 235
    Elizabeth S. Halprin

16. Pediatric Diabetes Education: A Family Affair 251
    Arlene Smaldone and Margaret T. Lawlor

17. The Challenge of Weight and Diabetes Management in Clinical
    Practice 273
    *Ann E. Goebel-Fabbri, Gillian Grant Arathuzik,
    and Jacqueline I. Shahar*

18. Diabetes Education in Geriatric Populations 289
    Medha Munshi and Angela Botts

19. Prevention: Educating Those at Risk for Diabetes 309
    *Helena Duffy, Janet O. Brown-Friday,
    and Elizabeth A. Walker*

Index 321

CONTRIBUTORS

ABRAHAMSON, MARTIN, MD • *Joslin Diabetes Center, Boston, MA, USA*

ARATHUZIK, GILLIAN GRANT, RD, LDN, CDE • *Joslin Diabetes Center, Boston, MA, USA*

BOTTS, ANGELA, MD • *Beth Israel Deaconess Medical Center, Harvard Medical School, Boston, MA, USA*

BROWN-FRIDAY, JANET O., MSN, MPH, RN • *Albert Einstein College of Medicine, Bronx, NY, USA*

CARVER, CATHERINE, MS, APRN-BC, CDE • *Joslin Diabetes Center, Boston, MA, USA*

CAMPBELL, AMY, MS, RD, CDE • *Joslin Diabetes Center, Boston, MA, USA*

CABALLERO, ENRIQUE, MD • *Joslin Diabetes Center, Boston, MA, USA*

CHILDS, BELINDA, MN, ARNP, BC, CDE • *MidAmerica Diabetes Associates, PA, Wichita, KS, USA*

DUFFY, HELENA, APRN-BC, CDE • *Albert Einstein College of Medicine, Diabetes Clinical Trials Unit, Bronx, NY, USA*

FABBRI-GOEBEL, ANN, PhD • *Joslin Diabetes Center, Harvard Medical School, Boston, MA, USA*

FARRELL, JO ANNE B., BSN, RN, CDE • *Solvay Pharmaceuticals Inc., Pine Hill, NJ, USA*

GOODWIN, JUDITH E., MBA • *Joslin Diabetes Center, Boston, MA, USA*

GROTHE, JOLENE, BSN, RN, CDE • *MidAmerica Diabetes Associates, PA, Wichita, KS, USA*

HALPRIN, ELIZABETH, MD • *Joslin Diabetes Center, Harvard Medical School, Boston, MA, USA*

HINNEN, DEBORAH, ARNP, BC-ADM, CDE, FAAN • *Mid America Diabetes Associates, Wichita, KS, USA*

HSU, WILLIAM, MD • *Joslin Diabetes Center, Harvard Medical School, Boston, MA, USA*

LAWLOR, MARGARET T., MS, CDE • *Joslin Diabetes Center, Boston, MA, USA*

LEIGHTON, ASHLEY, BA • *Joslin Diabetes Center, Boston, MA, USA*

MARYNIUK, MELINDA, MEd, RD, CDE • *Joslin Diabetes Center, Boston, MA, USA*

MENSING, CAROLÈ, MA, RN, CDE • *Joslin Diabetes Center, Boston, MA, USA*

MILLAN-FERRO, ANDREINA • *Licentiate in Nutrition and Dietetics, Joslin Diabetes Center, Boston, MA, USA*

MUNSHI, MEDHA, MD • *Beth Israel Deaconess Medical Center, Joslin Diabetes Center, Harvard Medical School, Boston, MA, USA*

PEEPLES, MALINDA, MS, RN, CDE • *WellDoc Communications, Baltimore, MD, USA*

RICE, DONNA, MBA, BSN, RN, CDE • *Botsford Center for Lifestyle Management, Novi, MI, USA*

RITHOLZ, MARILYN, PhD • *Joslin Diabetes Center, Harvard Medical School, Boston, MA, USA*

ROSZLER, JANIS, RD, CDE, LD/N • *Diabetes Directions, LLC, Miami, FL*

SELEY, JANE, GNP, MPH, MSN, CDE • *New York Presbyterian/Weill Cornell Medical Center, New York, NY, USA*

SHAHAR, JACQUELINE I., M.ED., RCEP, CDE • *Joslin Diabetes Center, Boston, MA, USA*

SIMINERIO, LINDA, PhD, RN, CDE • *University of Pittsburgh Diabetes Institute, Pittsburgh, PA, USA*

SMALDONE, ARLENE, DNSc, CPNP, CDE • *Columbia University School of Nursing, New York, NY, USA*

SULLIVAN, ELAINE D., MS, RN, CDE • *Joslin Diabetes Center, Boston, MA, USA*

TOMKY, DONNA, MSN, RN, C-ANP, CDE • *ABQ Health Partners, Albuquerque, NM, USA*

WALKER, ELIZABETH A., PhD, RN, CDE • *The Diabetes Research and Training Center, Albert Einstein College of Medicine, Bronx, NY, USA*

WALLACE, MARISA, MS, FNP • *Naomi Berrie Diabetes Center, Columbia University Medical Center, New York, NY, USA*

WEINGER, KATIE, EdD, RN • *Joslin Diabetes Center, Harvard Medical School, Boston, MA, USA*

WOLPERT, HOWARD, MD • *Joslin Diabetes Center, Harvard Medical School, Boston, MA, USA*

I

Principles and Practices of Diabetes Education

1

Living With Diabetes: The Role of Diabetes Education

Katie Weinger, EdD, RN
and Ashley Leighton, BA

CONTENTS

BRIEF HISTORY OF DIABETES EDUCATION
DIABETES EDUCATION TODAY
MODEL OF SELF-CARE
PHASES OF LIVING WITH DIABETES
DIABETES DIAGNOSIS
PREVENTION PERIOD
WORRY ABOUT
  COMPLICATIONS/EARLY COMPLICATIONS
SEVERE COMPLICATIONS
DOES DIABETES EDUCATION WORK?
CONCLUSION
ACKNOWLEDGMENTS
REFERENCES

ABSTRACT

Living with diabetes can be challenging. The treatment is complex with significant lifestyle demands and fearsome acute and chronic complications. Both the disease and its treatment can impact the family as well as the person with diabetes. Many physicians, other health care professionals, and payors recognize the

From: *Contemporary Diabetes: Educating Your Patient with Diabetes*
Edited by: K. Weinger and C. A. Carver, DOI 10.1007/978-1-60327-208-7_1,
© Humana Press, a part of Springer Science+Business Media, LLC 2009

importance of diabetes education in supporting people in the efforts to realize treatment targets, yet the efficacy of diabetes education is still debated. This chapter will define diabetes education, briefly describe its origins, discuss factors that impact self-care, and address the question "does diabetes education work?"

Key Words: Education, Self-Care, Prevention, Diagnosis, Complications.

Some health professionals believe that health education is the provision of information or knowledge to the person afflicted. Diabetes education is much more. Diabetes education is the process of helping people, both patients and families, use information and skills in order to live better with this disease. This chapter provides an overview of diabetes self-care and of self-management education, briefly discusses the history of diabetes education, and provides evidence for its efficacy.

BRIEF HISTORY OF DIABETES EDUCATION

Eliot P. Joslin, MD, was the first champion of diabetes education, long before the discovery of insulin. He began his medical practice in 1898 and focused on diabetes early in his medical career *(1)*. To ensure appropriate care in the hospital and in his clinic, Dr. Joslin trained nurses in the treatment of people with diabetes. In a medical textbook published in 1917, Joslin described the importance of educating people with diabetes and documented the role of the nurses who helped with this education process *(2)*. He wrote many medical texts for physicians, and in 1918, he wrote the first of many educational manuals for patients and physicians that detailed how to live with diabetes, which foods to eat, how to exercise and test urine glucose, as well as other important topics to prolong life in a time when no medications were available *(3)*. Dr. Joslin understood that information alone was not enough. Not only did he teach patients individually and in groups, but he also trained nurses to become highly skilled in the care of people with diabetes.

Ms. Harriet MacKay was a graduate of the New England Deaconess Hospital School of Nursing class of 1922 *(1)*. She and her colleagues became the predecessors of Dr. Joslin's "wandering" nurse program. As a private duty nurse specially trained in diabetes care by Dr. Joslin, Ms. Mackay would live in patients' homes and help families learn how to live with diabetes. After insulin became commercially available in 1924, the wandering nurse program became formalized and expanded to be accessible to more than just a few wealthy families. Nurses would visit homes to help families deal with the complexities of diabetes treatment *(3)*. As time went on, others joined physicians and nurses on the diabetes education team: nutritionists, exercise physiologists, psychologists and social workers, podiatrists, pharmacists, optometrists, and others now all help in the care and education of those with diabetes.

In 1984, a group of organizations focusing on diabetes convened a group of health professionals who were charged with the task of developing national standards for diabetes education *(4)*. These standards are regularly updated *(4–7)* and serve as the basis for accreditation programs that help ensure high quality diabetes education. Today, the American Diabetes Association and the Indian Health Service both offer recognition/accreditation for programs providing high quality diabetes education. Two organizations, the American Association of Diabetes Educators and the National Certification Board of Diabetes Educators, offer certification in aspects of diabetes education and management.

DIABETES EDUCATION TODAY

Although in the course of the education process educators must provide information and help patients improve their knowledge, their role is to facilitate and support diabetes self-care. Many people with diabetes have a great deal of knowledge about their illness, yet they struggle with glycemic targets and need help and support in operationalizing that knowledge in order to improve their self-care and manage their diabetes.

Diabetes education focuses on diabetes self-care and on helping people live better with their diabetes. Fig. 1 is the Joslin Diabetes Center model for self-care domains. The triangle represents the three self-care domains of medication *(8)*, nutrition *(9)*, and physical activity *(10)*. The impact of these three domains on glucose levels is assessed by glucose monitoring *(11)*, which allows the

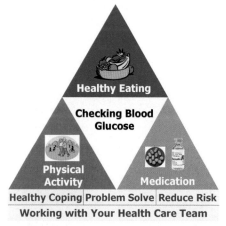

Fig. 1. Model for self-care domains.

patient to make adjustments and corrections in the three areas to obtain satisfactory glucose levels. Supporting that triangle are problem solving *(12)*, healthy coping *(13)*, and risk reduction *(14)* as well as additional self-care skills that impact living well with diabetes and that are included in the AADE7 *(15)*. Finally, the foundation for the whole triangle is a strong relationship with the health care team including diabetes educators.

MODEL OF SELF-CARE

Many factors impact how a person manages diabetes (see Fig. 2). Intra personal factors that impact self-care include knowledge and understanding of

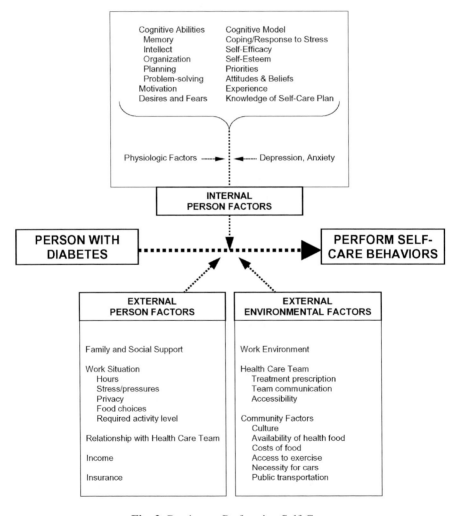

Fig. 2. Barriers to Performing Self-Care.

self-care plan and treatment prescriptions, priorities, self-esteem, self-efficacy, and innate abilities to organize and plan, to problem solve, and to cope with stress. Physiologic factors, such as insulin resistance and response to stress, also impact achievement of glycemic targets. Factors beyond the person include social support and work situation while environmental factors such as cost of food, culture, and availability of health care all influence how well one manages diabetes. During their assessments, educators must evaluate the influence of these factors to help patients realize the best strategies for success in their diabetes self-management.

PHASES OF LIVING WITH DIABETES

Because diabetes is a chronic disease, individuals' educational requirements and emotional responses shift over time as they incorporate diabetes and its treatment into their lives. Diabetes education programs must not only address the current needs of an individual based on an individualized assessment but also anticipate issues that will likely arise at different phases of living with diabetes. The emotional or psychological response of a person with diabetes influences their quality of life and their ability to follow their treatment prescription and recommendations (16,17). Psychological responses to diabetes follow a general progression though four phases beginning with the time of diagnosis until complications are so dominant that they may overshadow diabetes treatment and self-care (16–18).

DIABETES DIAGNOSIS

The diagnosis of diabetes disrupts the life of the person and the family. The person and family must accept this chronic illness, learn about what new skills and information is necessary for successfully living with diabetes, and understand the implications for his or her life. The response to the diagnosis is dependent on the person's previous experience with diabetes, how he or she copes with stress, level of family or other social support, and his or her relationship with the health care team.

For those recently diagnosed with type 1 diabetes, the diagnosis can be so overwhelming that internalizing additional information may be difficult. For these individuals, highly structured interactive instruction on survivor skills that include skills training is key. Patients must learn how to handle equipment and give themselves injections with either a syringe or a pen. Repetition of all information and of practice sessions is important, as is a contact telephone number to call for advice or information and a clearly written handout that repeats all key points. Follow-up sessions within one month are necessary in order to assess how the person is doing and to reinforce important self-care behaviors.

However, simple survivor skills are not enough for the person to successfully live with diabetes, thus newly diagnosed persons need to be enrolled in a formal group or individual education course to help facilitate the additional skills necessary for living with diabetes in the healthiest possible way.

People with type 2 diabetes are often diagnosed in adulthood. Older individuals with newly diagnosed diabetes may have subtle cognitive impairment that can impact their ability to implement a self-management plan, particularly if the diagnosis is accompanied by severe comorbidities (19). Including family members or other caretakers in setting goals and developing the self-care plan is usually helpful. Depending on the patient's age, support systems, and cognitive status, several educational sessions may be necessary to help the patient understand the care and implications of diabetes. Middle-aged individuals with type 2 diabetes without complications or comorbidities may consider the diagnosis of diabetes to be a normal part of aging, simply "taking another pill." Such individuals may not understand the importance and impact of lifestyle changes and may appear to lack the motivation to make these changes. Other health beliefs and attitudes may influence how one manages his or her diabetes and thus are important for the educator to assess.

PREVENTION PERIOD

During this phase, the person with diabetes is expected to implement lifestyle changes to stay healthy and prevent complications. However, the patient may not be experiencing distressful symptoms. This lack of symptoms may diminish motivation for lifestyle adjustments, particularly for individuals whose coping styles include procrastination and denial. Education during this phase needs to be person focused and engaging. It needs to stress healthy living and prevention of complications using interactive strategies that facilitate problem solving and engage both the person and the family. Use of threats of severe complications often scare and overwhelm patients without serving as additional motivators. However, validated behavioral interventions may be useful during this phase. For example, blood glucose awareness training helps in recognition of symptoms of low glucose levels and is useful in preventing severe hypoglycemia (20,21). Educators may find techniques based on principles of motivational interviewing useful in helping patients develop successful strategies to make needed changes in lifestyles (22,23).

As people struggle to fit diabetes into their lives, much information is forgotten or reinterpreted, different priorities emerge, and "diabetes habits" are formed. These factors influence how people manage their diabetes over time, reinforcing the importance of having regular health care visits and working relationships with their health care teams. Those patients who are successful in managing their diabetes in response to diabetes education may require reinforcement at 6 or 12 months post-education to help them stay on track *(24)*. Chapter 4 details the education process.

WORRY ABOUT COMPLICATIONS/EARLY COMPLICATIONS

Individuals who have not maintained glycemic control within their target may begin to worry about complications, particularly if they have signs of early complications. This phase often triggers patients to take action to regain control of their diabetes; this response, if unfulfilled or unstructured, may result in burnout *(6)*. Diabetes burnout is evidenced by feelings of being overwhelmed by diabetes self-care, of being controlled by diabetes, and of constantly worrying about taking care of diabetes and perhaps becoming unmotivated or unwilling to continue with diabetes self-care practices *(25)*. Patients who are overwhelmed by their recommended self-care behaviors and treatment prescriptions may require a more structured educational approach that is reminiscent of the approach used at diagnosis.

SEVERE COMPLICATIONS

When individuals with diabetes develop one or more serious complications, they may seek treatment from subspecialists who treat the complication but not the underlying diabetes. Thus, the patient is faced with several different illnesses with which to cope instead of focusing on one integrated diabetes treatment program. This phase is typically extremely stressful, and patients and families may require referral to mental health specialists experienced in care of the person with diabetes to help with coping issues.

The complexities of living with diabetes are impressive, and most educators intuitively know that diabetes education is important and helpful in supporting patients' efforts to integrate diabetes self-care into their lives. However, other health professionals and payors require scientific evidence that education is useful. Thus, we must address the question: does diabetes education work?

DOES DIABETES EDUCATION WORK?

Evaluating diabetes education is not simple. Educational strategies and outcomes are diverse and can be difficult to measure. Comparing education to a placebo arm in a randomized controlled trial is not ethically acceptable because diabetes education is considered a cornerstone of treatment *(7)*. However, meta-analyses offer a useful approach to understanding the efficacy of diabetes education. Although some still doubt whether or not diabetes education works, the research should lay the question to rest.

Diabetes education catalyzes significant improvements in many health-related variables, both physical and psychological. Many educational interventions for diabetes patients result in improved HbA1c levels and other measures of glycemic control. For example, one of the earliest meta-analyses on the subject revealed an overall mean effect size of 0.51 across many health variables showing a significantly positive effect of the interventions, particularly for knowledge gain and physical outcomes (e.g., glycosylated hemoglobin, blood glucose levels, weight loss) (26).

Similarly, another early meta-analysis revealed an initial 0.84 effect size of education on glycemic control but later found a 0.41 effect size when additional studies were included during an updated analysis (27,28). Importantly, these results likely relate to the increased knowledge (effect size of 0.49) and frequency of self-care behaviors (effect size of 0.23) after completion of a diabetes education intervention (28). The positive effect of diabetes education on psychological variables (effect size of 0.27), such as anxiety, depression, and locus of control, is also important to note (28). Thus, diabetes education is effective in improving many health variables – all of which relate to one another – that, in sum, lead to an even greater improvement in health and life with diabetes.

That being said, different kinds of diabetes education produce different effects, and more recent research shows that the incorporation of psychological principles into diabetes education is the most effective combination. For example, Whittemore (29) reviewed 72 studies focusing on lifestyle change strategies for people with diabetes. She categorized the strategies as educational, behavioral and social learning, cultural, and barrier related, and she conducted an analysis to discover the most effective strategies in terms of improvement in diabetes self-management (measured by medication adherence, diet, exercise, and frequency of blood glucose monitoring). The most effective strategies were those that focused on educating patients about self-management (and the associated necessary skills), included a behavioral component (e.g., goal setting, self-reward), and were culturally tailored to the population at hand. As the reviewed studies were published over a 14-year spectrum (1985 to 1999), Whittemore also noted that, during this time, the educational approach changed from passive to active learning, emphasizing more responsibility on the part of the person with diabetes for his or her self-care decisions and behaviors.

Specialized educational interventions aimed at improving self-care have proven to be effective for different target populations. For example, results from the Diabetes Prevention Program (30) showed that pre-diabetic participants who completed an educational lifestyle-modification program had a 58% reduced incidence of type 2 diabetes at follow-up (which averaged 2.8 years later) compared to participants in the placebo group. Notably, the lifestyle-modification program was more effective in reducing incidence of type 2 diabetes than the program that assigned taking metformin (31% reduced incidence).

Furthermore, a later meta-analysis of eight studies *(31)* of patients who were at high risk of developing type 2 diabetes revealed that those participating in lifestyle education (combined diet and exercise instruction and planned behavior changes), as opposed to more conventional education (general information about diet and/or exercise), had reduced 2-h plasma glucose levels (the glycemic response 2 hours after loading with 75 g of glucose) at 1-year follow-up. In addition, five studies revealed that, also at a 1-year follow-up, those in the lifestyle education group had a 50% reduced incidence of type 2 diabetes, thus further proving the effectiveness of lifestyle education in the prevention of type 2 diabetes.

For patients with type 2 diabetes, self-management interventions have also resulted in patients having a greater extent of diabetes knowledge, reporting healthier eating habits, and showing improved glycemic control (mostly measured by HbA1c) and self-care behaviors *(24)*. A meta-analysis of 18 studies showed the effect size of educational and behavioral interventions for reducing glycohemoglobin (including Ghb, HbA1, or HbA1c) was 0.43 *(32)*, and another review of 12 studies showed that psychological interventions further reduced glycated hemoglobin by 0.32 points *(33)*. Five of the psychological interventions were also effective in lowering psychological distress (including depression and binge eating) *(33)*.

Notably, educational strategies produced more positive effects if they included more patient involvement and collaboration within the class rather than lecture-style strategies *(24)*. In addition, patients enrolled in educational programs in which they were more frequently contacted by educational staff members were able to continue to improve or at least maintain improvement in glycemic control in the long term. Also, the educational and behavioral interventions catalyzed improvement in glycemic control regardless of whether they were conducted as a group or via individual sessions *(32)*, which is important for the interventions' cost-effectiveness.

Unfortunately, most self-management educational interventions were not able to help patients sustain improved glycemia in the long term (for more than 6 months) *(24)*. In addition, all three of the aforementioned meta-analyses *(24,32,33)* revealed that, overall, the interventions did not have any significant effect on weight loss. Furthermore, the self-management training interventions also had variable results in motivating patients to make healthy cardiovascular-related changes related to lipid levels, blood pressure, and physical activity level *(24)*. With diabetes patients being at a higher risk for cardiovascular complications, diabetes educators and researchers should work to improve the efficacy of educational strategies for motivating patients to make healthy cardiovascular-related changes.

The research on educational interventions targeted for patients with type 1 diabetes is less abundant. However, a study from the early 1980s *(34)* was one of the first to show the effectiveness of a structured diabetes education program for type 1 diabetes patients: Those patients who had participated in the program, which focused on self-management skills, had a glycosylated hemoglobin level that changed from 2.6% above normal at baseline to 1.0% above normal at 12 months post-intervention and 1.5% above normal at 22 months post-intervention. The same patients also reported significantly less hospital admissions. Randomized controlled trials have demonstrated that behavioral interventions such as Coping Skills Training have helped improve glycemia and quality of life among teenagers with type 1 diabetes (35–37).

In addition, type 1 diabetes patients who participated in an intensive insulin treatment program during the Diabetes Control and Complications Trial (DCCT) (38) had reduced A1c levels and complications at follow-up (an average of 6.5 years). The Epidemiology of Diabetes Interventions and Complications (EDIC) study continued to follow these patients, for an average (in total) of 17 years (39). During the EDIC study, the patients continued intensive insulin treatment but no longer had interaction with clinicians. Interestingly, the same patients' A1c levels increased during the EDIC study, suggesting that the educational component of the DCCT study may have partially been responsible for the original improvement in glycemic control.

CONCLUSION

Diabetes education has evolved over the years to become an essential part of diabetes care (7) as individuals with diabetes and their families struggle to integrate diabetes and its treatment into their lives. Research shows that educational interventions for patients with diabetes are most effective when the educational strategies incorporate a behavioral component, as this is likely the missing link between knowledge and action. Thus, a multidisciplinary team of physicians, nurse educators, psychologists, dieticians, exercise physiologists, and others are integral to the success of diabetes treatment and education. As a team, all health care professionals serve as educators and help their patients live better with diabetes.

ACKNOWLEDGMENTS

Work on this chapter was supported by a grant from NIH DK 60115 and in part by the Endocrinology Research Core NIHP30 DK36836.

REFERENCES

1. Barnett DM, Elliott P, Joslin MD. A Centennial Portrait. Boston: Joslin Diabetes Center; 1998.

2. Joslin EP. The Treatment of Diabetes Mellitus: With Observations Based Upon Two Thousand Cases. Philadelphia: Lea & Febiger; 1917.
3. Allen NA. The history of diabetes nursing, 1914–1936. Diabetes Educ 2003;29(6):976, 9–84, 86 passim.
4. National standards for diabetes patient education programs. From the National Diabetes Advisory Board. Diabetes Educ 1984;9(4):11–14.
5. National standards and review criteria for diabetes patient education programs: quality assurance for diabetes patient education. National Diabetes Advisory Board. Diabetes Educ 1986;12(3):286–91.
6. Funnell MM, Brown TL, Childs BP, et al. National Standards for Diabetes Self-Management Education. Diabetes Care 2007;30(6):1630–7.
7. Mensing C, Boucher J, Cypress M, et al. National standards for diabetes self-management education. Task Force to Review and Revise the National Standards for Diabetes Self-Management Education Programs. Diabetes Care 2000;23(5):682–9.
8. Odegard PS, Capoccia K. Medication taking and diabetes: a systematic review of the literature. Diabetes Educ 2007;33(6):1014–29; discussion 30–1.
9. Povey RC, Clark-Carter D. Diabetes and healthy eating: a systematic review of the literature. Diabetes Educ 2007;33(6):931–59; discussion 60–1.
10. Kavookjian J, Elswick BM, Whetsel T. Interventions for being active among individuals with diabetes: a systematic review of the literature. Diabetes Educ 2007;33(6):962–88; discussion 89–90.
11. McAndrew L, Schneider SH, Burns E, Leventhal H. Does patient blood glucose monitoring improve diabetes control? A systematic review of the literature. Diabetes Educ 2007;33(6):991–1011; discussion 2–3.
12. Hill-Briggs F, Gemmell L. Problem solving in diabetes self-management and control: a systematic review of the literature. Diabetes Educ 2007;33(6):1032–50; discussion 51–2.
13. Fisher EB, Thorpe CT, Devellis BM, Devellis RF. Healthy coping, negative emotions, and diabetes management: a systematic review and appraisal. Diabetes Educ 2007;33(6):1080–103; discussion 104–6.
14. Boren SA, Gunlock TL, Schaefer J, Albright A. Reducing risks in diabetes self-management: a systematic review of the literature. Diabetes Educ 2007;33(6):1053–77; discussion 78–9.
15. Mulcahy K, Maryniuk M, Peeples M, et al. Diabetes self-management education core outcomes measures. Diabetes Educ 2003;29(5):768–70, 73–84, 87–8 passim.
16. Jacobson AM, Weinger K. Psychosocial complications in diabetes. In: Leahy J, Clark N, Cefalu W, eds. Medical Management of Diabetes. New York: Marcel Dekker, Inc.; 2000:559–72.
17. Weinger K, McMurrich SJ. Behavioral strategies for improving self-management. In: Childs B, Cypress M, Spollett G, eds. Complete Nurse's Guide to Diabetes Care. Alexandria, VA: American Diabetes Association; 2005.
18. Hamburg BA, Inoff GE. Coping with predictable crises of diabetes. Diabetes Care 1983;6(4):409–16.
19. Sitnikov L, Weinger K. Diabetes Education in Older Adults. In: Munshi M, Lipsitz L, eds. Geriatric Diabetes. New York: Informa Healthcare; 2007:317–29.
20. Cox DJ, Gonder-Frederick L, Polonsky W, Schlundt D, Julian D, Clarke W. A multicenter evaluation of blood glucose awareness training-II. Diabetes Care 1995;18(4):523–8.
21. Cox DJ, Gonder-Frederick L, Julian D, et al. Intensive versus standard blood glucose awareness training (BGAT) with insulin-dependent diabetes: mechanisms and ancillary effects. Psychosom Med 1991;53(4):453–62.
22. Channon SJ, Huws-Thomas MV, Rollnick S, et al. A multicenter randomized controlled trial of motivational interviewing in teenagers with diabetes. Diabetes Care 2007;30(6):1390–5.

23. West DS, DiLillo V, Bursac Z, Gore SA, Greene PG. Motivational interviewing improves weight loss in women with type 2 diabetes. Diabetes Care 2007;30(5):1081–7.
24. Norris SL, Engelgau MM, Narayan KM. Effectiveness of self-management training in type 2 diabetes: a systematic review of randomized controlled trials. Diabetes Care 2001;24(3): 561–87.
25. Polonsky WH. Diabetes Burnout: What To Do When You Can't Take It Anymore. Alexandria, VA: American Diabetes Association; 1999.
26. Padgett D, Mumford E, Hynes M, Carter R. Meta-analysis of the effects of educational and psychosocial interventions on management of diabetes mellitus. J Clin Epidemiol 1988;41(10):1007–30.
27. Brown SA. Effects of educational interventions in diabetes care: a meta-analysis of findings. Nurs Res 1988;37(4):223–30.
28. Brown SA. Studies of educational interventions and outcomes in diabetic adults: a meta-analysis revisited. Patient Educ Couns 1990;16(3):189–215.
29. Whittemore R. Strategies to Facilitate Lifestyle Change Associated with Diabetes Mellitus. J Nurs Sch 2000;32(3):225–32.
30. Knowler WC, Barrett-Connor E, Fowler SE, et al. Reduction in the incidence of type 2 diabetes with lifestyle intervention or metformin. N Engl J Med 2002;346(6):393–403.
31. Yamaoka K, Tango T. Efficacy of Lifestyle Education to Prevent Type 2 Diabetes: A meta-analysis of randomized controlled trials. Diabetes Care 2005;28(11):2780–6.
32. Gary TL, Genkinger JM, Guallar E, Peyrot M, Brancati FL. Meta-Analysis of Randomized Educational and Behavioral Interventions in Type 2 Diabetes. Diabetes Educ 2003;29(3): 488–501.
33. Ismail K, Winkley K, Rabe-Hesketh S. Systematic review and meta-analysis of randomised controlled trials of psychological interventions to improve glycaemic control in patients with type 2 diabetes. Lancet 2004;363(9421):1589–97.
34. Muhlhauser I, Jorgens V, Berger M, et al. Bicentric evaluation of a teaching and treatment programme for type 1 (insulin-dependent) diabetic patients: improvement of metabolic control and other measures of diabetes care for up to 22 months. Diabetologia 1983;25(6):470–6.
35. Grey M, Boland EA, Davidson M, Li J, Tamborlane WV. Coping skills training for youth with diabetes mellitus has long-lasting effects on metabolic control and quality of life. J Pediatr 2000;137(1):107–13.
36. Grey M, Boland EA, Davidson M, Yu C, Sullivan-Bolyai S, Tamborlane WV. Short-term effects of coping skills training as adjunct to intensive therapy in adolescents. Diabetes Care 1998;21(6):902–8.
37. Grey M, Boland EA, Davidson M, Yu C, Tamborlane WV. Coping skills training for youths with diabetes on intensive therapy. Appl Nurs Res 1999;12(1):3–12.
38. The effect of intensive treatment of diabetes on the development and progression of long-term complications in insulin-dependent diabetes mellitus. The Diabetes Control and Complications Trial Research Group. N Engl J Med 1993;329(14):977–86.
39. Nathan DM, Cleary PA, Backlund JY, et al. Intensive diabetes treatment and cardiovascular disease in patients with type 1 diabetes. N Engl J Med 2005;353(25):2643–53.

2 Diabetes Mellitus Overview

Catherine Carver, MSN, APRN-BC, CDE
and Martin Abrahamson, MD

Contents

THE BURDEN: THE GROWING
    PROBLEM OF DIABETES MELLITUS
THE COST OF DIABETES MELLITUS
CLASSIFICATION AND DIAGNOSES
DIAGNOSIS
TREATMENT
DEPRESSION AND DIABETES
FEAR OF HYPOGLYCEMIA AND
    ASSOCIATED WEIGHT GAIN
LIFESTYLE CHANGES
IMPORTANCE OF SELF-MANAGEMENT
CONCLUSION
REFERENCES

Abstract

Diabetes mellitus, the most common metabolic disorder affecting the population, has many clinical and psychological implications for the patient. The provider must address these issues comprehensively. This chapter will describe the global burden and cost of diabetes mellitus, define its classifications and diagnosis criteria, detail its current treatment options, address associated complications including depression, fear of hypoglycemia, and fear of weight gain, suggest strategies for healthy lifestyle changes, and illustrate the importance of the patient's self-care and empowerment.

From: *Contemporary Diabetes: Educating Your Patient with Diabetes*
Edited by: K. Weinger and C. A. Carver, DOI 10.1007/978-1-60327-208-7_2,
© Humana Press, a part of Springer Science+Business Media, LLC 2009

Key Words: Insulin resistance, Pathophysiology, Cost, Complications, Diagnosis, Treatment, Self-care, Depression, Hypoglycemia, Self-management.

THE BURDEN: THE GROWING PROBLEM OF DIABETES MELLITUS

Diabetes mellitus is the most common metabolic disorder affecting humans and is characterized by chronic hyperglycemia. The prevalence of diabetes worldwide was recently estimated to be 171 million (2.8%) in 2000 and may rise to 366 million (4.4%) by 2030 *(1)*. There are two main types of diabetes – type 1 diabetes, which is caused by an autoimmune insulitis leading to an absolute deficiency of insulin, and type 2 diabetes, which usually includes a combination of insulin resistance and a β-cell secretory defect.

In recent years, the prevalence of type 2 diabetes, which accounts for approximately 90% of people with diabetes, has reached pandemic proportions *(1,2)*. The American Diabetes Association (ADA) estimates that 17.5 million people in the United States have been diagnosed with diabetes *(1)*. The lifetime risk of acquiring type 2 diabetes is approximately 50% in individuals with morbid obesity, an insulin resistance promoter *(3)*. Insulin resistance is a major pathophysiologic abnormality associated with type 2 diabetes that occurs initially in muscle tissue and later in the liver; it develops many years before the onset of hyperglycemia *(4)*. β cells within the pancreas initially compensate to maintain normal glucose metabolism by increasing the amount of insulin they secrete. Over time, the corporal demand for insulin exceeds the ability of the β cells to compensate, ultimately leading to pancreatic exhaustion and a major decline or halt in insulin secretion *(5)*. As insulin secretion declines there is usually a rise in postprandial glucose, which is then followed by a rise in fasting glucose. These increasing glucose concentrations further compromise insulin secretion and insulin action, a phenomenon called glucose toxicity *(4)*. Free fatty acids are also often elevated in individuals with uncontrolled type 2 diabetes; these also compromise insulin action and insulin secretion *(6)*.

More than 90% of individuals with type 1 diabetes develop this disorder as a result of autoimmune destruction of the β cells, a process which begins many years before the clinical onset of the disease. The precise mechanism precipitating the autoimmune process is not known. It is known, however, that antibodies to islet cell antigens and even insulin are present for years before overt hyperglycemia occurs *(4)*. Improvement of glucose control after presentation of the disease is often followed by a "honeymoon" phase, during which insulin requirements decrease for variable periods of time, only to be followed by further increases in insulin requirements as further β-cell destruction ensues *(7)*.

THE COST OF DIABETES MELLITUS

In 2007 the American Diabetes Association (ADA) estimated that the United States spent $174 billion in direct and indirect costs treating diabetes and its complications; this reflects an increase of 32% since only 2002. An estimated $116 billion is for medical expenditures, much resulting from treatment and hospitalization of people with diabetes-related complications. Approximately $58 billion is consumed by the indirect costs of the disease – reduced produc tivity of both those in the labor force and unpaid workers, unemployment from disease-related disability, and increased absenteeism. Approximately 1 out of every 5 healthcare dollars in the United States is spent on someone diagnosed with diabetes *(8)*.

In addition, diabetes claimed more than 284,000 lives in 2007 and remains the leading cause of blindness, end-stage renal disease, and non-traumatic lower limb amputations in the western world. Considering that an additional 6 million more people are believed to have diabetes but have not yet been diagnosed, the American Diabetes Association study estimates that the actual cost of diabetes may greatly exceed $174 billion *(8)*.

CLASSIFICATION AND DIAGNOSES

Type 1 DM

As outlined above, type 1 diabetes is characterized by β-cell destruction and leads to absolute insulin deficiency, either immune-mediated or idiopathic. It can occur at any age and presentation is usually acute. Symptoms indicative of type 1 include: polyuria, polydipsia, polyphagia, weight loss, blurred vision, recurrent vaginal or urinary tract infections, and fatigue. In older adults, type 1 may present more insidiously, similarly to type 2 diabetes, and is referred to as latent autoimmune diabetes of adults. Ninety percent of people with type 1 diabetes develop this as a result of autoimmune islet cell destruction, which is characterized by insulitis and the presence of antibodies against the β cell or insulin itself. All patients with type 1 diabetes eventually become insulin dependent *(7)*. Soon after initiation of insulin therapy in type 1 diabetes, some patients note a decline in insulin requirements.

Type 2 DM

The aging world population, increased prevalence of obesity, increased inci-dence of insulin resistance (mainly due to obesity), and a progressive decline in β-cell secretory function are the major factors that lead to hyperglycemia in patients who develop type 2 diabetes. This is a progressive disease, char-acterized by a progressive decline in insulin secretion, resulting in increasing medication requirements and ultimately insulin treatment for many patients with this disorder. At the time of diagnosis it is estimated that 50% of β-cell function has been lost in individuals with type 2 diabetes *(7)*.

The most common complications associated with diabetes are macrovascular (e.g., coronary heart disease, peripheral vascular disease, and cerebrovascular disease) and microvascular (e.g., retinopathy, nephropathy, and neuropathy). Coronary heart disease accounts for more than 55% of deaths in patients with type 1 and type 2 diabetes and is the main cause of excess mortality in individuals with diabetes *(9)*. Despite laser treatment available to halt vision loss, diabetic retinopathy is very common and often results in blindness, accounting for 11% of new cases of blindness in the United States each year *(10)*.

Diabetic nephropathy accounts for entirely one-third of all cases of dialysis-requiring end-stage renal failure in the United States *(11)*. And though diabetic neuropathy is rarely a direct cause of death, it is a major cause of morbidity and a contributor to many circumstances that impact patients' quality of life *(12)*. Symptoms of peripheral neuropathy range from numbness to severe pain in the feet. A patient with neuropathy is more likely to develop ulceration of the feet. Ulceration in someone who also has coexistent peripheral vascular disease further increases risk for the development of gangrene and/or amputation. Diabetes is the leading cause of non-traumatic lower limb amputations in the world *(12)*. While microvascular complications are not the major cause of mortality in people with diabetes, they are a source of major concern amongst patients and contribute to the morbidity associated with the disease. Early detection and aggressive treatment of these chronic microvascular complications reduce morbidity and improve quality of life for people with diabetes.

Gestational Diabetes

Gestational diabetes is defined as diabetes developing or discovered during pregnancy. The associated risks of gestational diabetes are pre-natal morbidity and mortality as well as an increased rate of cesarean delivery and chronic hypertension in the mother *(13)*. Women with gestational diabetes are more likely to give birth to babies large in weight for gestational age (macrosomia) which is the reason why more women with gestational diabetes have cesarean deliveries. These infants are also more likely to develop hypoglycemia following delivery. Women with pre-existing diabetes who become pregnant are more likely to have infants with congenital malformations if their glycemic control is suboptimal during the first trimester of pregnancy. It is thus vitally important for all women with diabetes to be counseled about the risks of hyperglycemia and pregnancy prior to conception and for women with diabetes to plan their pregnancies so as to reduce the risk for congenital malformations in their offspring

(13). Up to 50% of women with gestational diabetes go on to develop type 2 diabetes within 5 years of diagnosis with gestational diabetes *(13)*.

Other Types of Diabetes

Other types of diabetes may be caused by a variety of factors, including but not limited to genetic defects in β-cell function, genetic defects in insulin action, diseases of the exocrine pancreas (such as cystic fibrosis), and can be drug or chemical induced (such as in the treatment of AIDS or after organ transplantation) *(7)*.

DIAGNOSIS

Clinically, diabetes is defined as the following: casual plasma glucose greater than or equal to 200 mg/dl with symptoms of diabetes including polyuria, polydipsia, ketoacidosis, and unexplained weight loss *OR* fasting plasma glucose greater than or equal to 126 mg/dl *OR* a result greater than or equal to 200 mg/dl 2 h following a standard 75 g oral glucose tolerance test *(14)*. The distinction between type 1 and type 2 diabetes is usually made clinically. While either type of diabetes can occur at any age, type 1 diabetes usually affects younger people (children, adolescents, and young adults), and type 2 diabetes occurs in those over the age of 40 years. Details of diagnostic criteria for diabetes are shown in Fig. 1.

Individuals who develop type 2 diabetes are more likely to have a family history of the disease and are commonly obese or overweight. Further, the

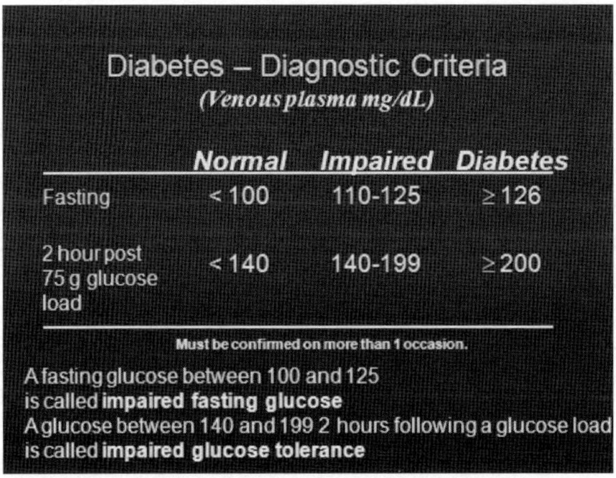

Diabetes – Diagnostic Criteria
(Venous plasma mg/dL)

	Normal	Impaired	Diabetes
Fasting	< 100	110-125	≥ 126
2 hour post 75 g glucose load	< 140	140-199	≥ 200

Must be confirmed on more than 1 occasion.

A fasting glucose between 100 and 125 is called **impaired fasting glucose**
A glucose between 140 and 199 2 hours following a glucose load is called **impaired glucose tolerance**

Fig. 1. Diabetes Diagnostic Criteria.

finding of a skin condition called acanthosis nigricans (thickening and darkening of the skin at the nape of the neck or in flexural creases) is a sign of underlying insulin resistance associated with type 2 diabetes. Measurement of the islet cell antigen antibodies and/or insulin antibodies may help distinguish type 1 from type 2 diabetes. This test is particularly useful in those individuals who have latent autoimmune diabetes of adults and who present as if they have type 2 diabetes. These individuals are usually not obese and do not have a strong family history of type 2 diabetes. Measurement of circulating insulin or C-peptide concentrations does not always help distinguish type 1 from type 2 diabetes *(14)*.

In women who are pregnant, screening for gestational diabetes is done by performing a 50-g glucose challenge test *(10)*. If the glucose is greater than or equal to 140 mg/dl 1 h after the administration of the glucose (which need not be done in the fasting state), the subject then undergoes a 3 h 100-g oral glucose tolerance test. Gestational diabetes is confirmed if there are two abnormal values out of four measured (fasting, 1-h, 2-h, and 3-h) values in this 3-h oral glucose tolerance test (abnormal values are greater than or equal to 105 mg/dl for fasting, greater than or equal to 190 mg/dl at 1 h, greater than or equal to 165 mg/dl at 2 h, and greater than or equal to 145 mg/dl at 3 h) *(15)*. Gestational diabetes usually develops toward the end of the second trimester or beginning of the third trimester and may be an indicator of predisposition for development or continuation of diabetes or the development of diabetes postpartum *(15)*. Hence, screening for this condition is usually performed between the 24th and 28th week of pregnancy, but should be done earlier in women with a previous history of gestational diabetes or those who are at greater risk for the development of this condition *(10)*.

TREATMENT

There are many pharmacologic agents available for the treatment of insulin resistance as well as the insulin deficiency in type 2 diabetes. These medications are discussed in greater detail in other chapters. In brief, the drugs used to treat insulin resistance include the biguanide metformin and the thiazolidinediones (TZDs) rosiglitazone and pioglitazone. Drugs that enhance insulin secretion include sulfonylureas, non-sulfonylurea agents that act like sulfonylureas, glucagon-like-peptide analogues, and DPP-IV inhibitors. Medications are also available that delay the absorption of glucose from the gastrointestinal tract (α-glucosidase inhibitors), and of course, insulin itself. Finally, an analogue of amylin, a peptide which is cosecreted from the β cell with insulin, is available to be used in conjunction with insulin in both type 1 and type 2 diabetes; this medication is called pramlintide (symlin) *(7)*.

Treatment of adults with hyperglycemia is detailed in an American Diabetes Association (ADA) and European Association for the Study of Diabetes (EADS) consensus statement. It details the following as primary treatment strategy: (1) intervention at diagnosis with lifestyle changes (medical nutrition therapy and exercise) and the oral agent metformin and (2) the addition of other oral agents (and, if needed, early insulin therapy) to achieve target goals. The general benchmark for gauging success of diabetes management is the hemoglobin A1c (henceforth referred to as simply "A1c" and commonly referred to as A1c or "HbA1c") test, which has a value of 6% or less in the non-diabetic population. The ADA-EASD method is to be used as the primary system to lower diabetes patients' A1c to target, which is below 7% for most patients, provided this can be achieved safely *(16)*. Achieving and maintaining glucose as close to the non-diabetic range as possible, and changing interventions at as rapid a pace as possible for safe titration, is most beneficial for patients' health in this scheme *(16)*. Treatment must be individualized with targets for glucose control based on other factors, including risk of additional complications with treatment, age of the patient, ability to comply with the treatment regimen and projected longevity of the individual, and presence or absence of chronic complications of the disease *(7)*.

The ADA-EASD algorithm took the evidence for this method of lowering A1c into account as well as its expense to the patient. Of note, this statement was developed well *before* publications and black box warnings that raised concerns about increased risk of myocardial infarction with use of rosiglitazone and congestive heart failure with both rosiglitazone and pioglitazone. Greater caution in using the thiazolidinediones may be warranted now according to individual patients' concerns. The following medications were not included in the consensus due to lack of glucose-lowering effectiveness, limited clinical data, and/or relative expense: pramlintide, exenatide, α-glucosidase inhibitors, the glinides, and DPP-IV inhibitors. Despite their exclusion in the algorithm, these are appropriate choices in individual patients to achieve glycemic and weight loss goals. Individuals presenting with weight loss and/or severe hyperglycemic symptoms require immediate initiation of insulin at time of diagnosis *(7)*.

Treatment of type 2 diabetes usually requires initiation with one or sometimes two medications together with lifestyle modification and the addition of more medications with time to achieve and maintain target goals. Because of the disease's natural history, use of insulin is ultimately required in many patients. In these patients, insulin may be initiated with just one injection of basal insulin at night, but often this is inadequate to achieve ideal glucose control; patients then require more frequent injections of insulin, ranging from twice daily to multiple daily injections (basal–prandial insulin treatment) *(7)*.

In type 1 diabetes, insulin therapy involves multiple daily insulin injections that are tailored to the individual's needs. Several studies have shown that intensive treatment with insulin in type 1 or 2 diabetes, or oral medications in type 2 diabetes, is associated with a significant reduction in risk for the development or progression of the early microvascular complications of the disease *(12,17,18)*. The United Kingdom Prospective Diabetes Study (UKPDS), a 4585-patient observational study, showed that a 1% reduction in A1c was associated with a 37% mean risk reduction for the development or progression of microvascular complications and a 14% mean reduction in risk for myocardial infarction in patients with type 2 diabetes *(12)*.

Similarly, the Kumamoto Study showed that good glycemic control achieved using insulin treatment delayed the onset and progression of diabetic retinopathy, nephropathy, and neuropathies in Japanese patients with type 2 diabetes *(18)*. A cost–effect analysis using a computer simulation to estimate lifetime benefits and costs of insulin therapy in a sample of 120,000 people with type 2 diabetes indicated great improvement in quality and longevity of life, far outweighing the disadvantages of treatment *(4)*. All studies confirm that early intensive insulin treatment in both type 1 and type 2 diabetes benefits health and quality of life for patients and is cost effective in the long term.

The benefits of intensive insulin therapy with frequent injections of insulin do come at a price, however. Insulin therapy carries the associated risk of a dangerously low level of blood glucose (hypoglycemia) in a small number of patients when the insulin dose is overmatched with the amount of food ingested. Hypoglycemia can cause dizziness and nausea and, in severe cases only, coma or death. As a result, it is the primary impediment to insulin therapy and prevents many patients from the benefits which treatment so clearly brings *(7)*.

DEPRESSION AND DIABETES

Because diabetes is a chronic disease, the burden of treatment takes a serious toll on most patients, including managing complications and the fears associated with them and dealing with weight gain and the associated social stigma. It is now common for people with any type of diabetes to be affected by major clinical depression: studies have found that up to 30% of patients with diabetes have comorbid depression *(18–20)*. If the patients' quality of life and overall health are to be a priority in diabetes treatment, this observation cannot be ignored. Studies have shown that patients with diabetes and depression have poor adherence to oral diabetes agents and other medications, have more sedentary lifestyles, and do not eat healthily when compared with non-depressed patients with diabetes *(19,21)*. Diabetes complicated by depression is also associated with higher A1c levels and obesity (defined as having a body mass index greater than $30\,\text{kg/m}^2$) when compared with people with diabetes who are not depressed *(20)*. These associations become large obstacles when insulin therapy is implemented or intensified in patients with both diabetes and depression, especially when depression is undiagnosed, which it commonly is.

Depression is thought to be associated with insulin resistance (independent of weight) and can be improved by antidepressive treatment *(22,23)*. However, because many antidepressants *cause* weight gain and diabetes, extra caution is warranted *(24)*.

FEAR OF HYPOGLYCEMIA AND ASSOCIATED WEIGHT GAIN

As mentioned previously, one common consequence of insulin treatment is the risk of hypoglycemia. However, the perceived threat of a hypoglycemic episode has been shown to greatly exceed the actual incidence of an event in patients with diabetes *(4)*. Therefore, individuals may increase caloric intake to proactively avoid such an event, which may result in weight gain. It was demonstrated in the Diabetes Control and Complications Trial (DCCT) that patients who had experienced one or more episodes of hypoglycemia gained 6.8 kg, significantly more than patients with no severe hypoglycemia (2.2 kg) *(4)*.

Two novel agents based on glucoregulatory hormones have recently become available and may be appropriate in managing weight in patients with diabetes. The amylin agonist pramlintide (Symlin®) and the incretin mimetic exenatide (Byetta®) have both demonstrated potential in improving glycemic control in patients with diabetes along with the added benefit of weight loss when compared with placebo *(25,26)*. Pramlintide is approved for use in individuals taking insulin (both type 1 and type 2 diabetes). Exenatide is approved for use in combination with metformin, sulfonylureas, and/or TZDs in subjects with type 2 diabetes.

LIFESTYLE CHANGES

The American Diabetes Association recommends that overweight patients with diabetes should lose 5%–7% of their initial weight, irrespective of its value *(27)*. For overweight people with diabetes, weight loss improves insulin sensitivity and glycemic control *(27)*, and even moderate intentional weight loss may be associated with reduced mortality *(28)*. Weight loss also improves lipid profiles and blood pressure *(29)* as well as mental health and overall quality of life *(30,31)*. These benefits, while significant, are clinically meaningful only if weight loss is sustained over time *(32)*.

Weight loss diets with low levels of carbohydrate and high levels of protein are gaining in popularity. A recent small study (n = 12) over 5 weeks compared a high-protein diet (40% carbohydrate, 30% protein, and 30% fat) to a high-carbohydrate diet (55% carbohydrate, 15% protein, and 30% fat) in patients with type 2 diabetes. Patients in both groups lost weight (-2.2 and -2.5 kg, respectively). However, mean A1c and post prandial plasma glucose decreased significantly ($p < 0.05$) only in the patients with type 2 diabetes on high-protein diet *(33)*.

Regular exercise promotes long-term weight loss, provided that the regimen is habitual and consistent *(34)*. Exercise can lower blood glucose, improve the body's ability to use glucose, and decrease the amount of insulin needed *(35)*. However, as those with type 2 diabetes generally have a lower level of fitness than non-diabetic individuals, exercise intensity should be at a comfortable level in the initial periods of training and should progress cautiously as tolerance for activity improves *(36)*.

Lifestyle changes such as those outlined above can be discussed with patients in group therapy sessions. Regular meetings with patients, possibly involving psychologists and dietitians, can help reinforce and encourage patients to continue with their diet and exercise programs *(37)*. Psychologists can help in this setting by introducing behavioral therapy aimed at improving a patient's body image and attitude to eating *(32)*.

IMPORTANCE OF SELF-MANAGEMENT

Self-management is an essential element of health in people with type 1 and type 2 diabetes. Nurses and dieticians regularly address barriers to successful self-care by identifying specific areas of self-management for improvement and setting realistic goals with the patient regarding food, medications, and insulin. A comprehensive assessment of the barriers to self-care can recognize precise areas with which the patient may need encouragement and help. Awareness of these barriers can be used to tailor the educational material received from nurses and dietitians, incorporating information and learning about these barriers can support the patient's diabetes control and care.

These ongoing, tailored self-management interventions should be integrated into routine care as they prove useful in the continuing education of the patient. The complementary nature of self-management education to diabetes clinical goals as set by the entire patient care team (including the patient, their physician, a nurse practitioner, a nurse educator, a dietitian, and, if possible, an exercise physiologist) is very constructive and can have results of surprisingly great impact; these results tend to strengthen as the relationship between the patient and the team strengthens. For example, as little as a brief self-management program aimed at helping patients to adopt low-fat eating patterns and increase physical activity levels via motivational interviews and follow-up phone contact with their patient care team has reported good success in weight maintenance *(38)*. A similar study focused on improving self-care behavior in diabetes has reported both weight loss and improvements in both healthy eating and glycemic control *(39)*.

CONCLUSION

As the incidence of diabetes grows worldwide, the importance of diabetes self-management education cannot be underestimated by any member of the patient care team. The lasting impact of the patient–team interactions is commonly reflected in the patient's commitment and success in managing their diabetes and quality of life. A sense of community and support is often the key to empowering patients to take control of their diabetes, and the patient care team must be strong enough to uphold that responsibility using good communication and quality care.

REFERENCES

1. Williamson AR, Hunt AE, Pope JF, Tolman NM. Recommendations of dietitians for overcoming barriers to dietary adherence in individuals with diabetes. *Diabetes Educ* 2002;26(2): 272–9.
2. King H, Aubert RE, Herman WH. Global burden of diabetes, 1995–2025: prevalence, numerical estimates, and projections. *Diabetes Care* 1998;9:1414–31.
3. Colditz GA, Willett WC, Rotnitzky A, Manson JE. Weight gain as a risk factor for clinical diabetes mellitus in women. *Ann Intern Med* 1995;122(7):481–6.
4. Diabetes Control and Complications Trial (DCCT). Research Group Lifetime benefits and costs of intensive therapy as practiced in the diabetes control and complications trial. *JAMA* 1996;276(17):1409–15.
5. Lipsky MS, Zimmerman BR. *Diagnosis and management of type 2 diabetes: an American family physician monograph*. 1999.
6. Joslin Diabetes Center and Joslin Clinic. Clinical Guideline for Pharmacological Management of Type 2 Diabetes. 01/12/2007.
7. Joslin Diabetes Center & Joslin Clinic. Clinical Guideline for Adults with Diabetes. 10/20/06.
8. American Diabetes Association Statement: Economic Costs of Diabetes in the US in 2007. *Diabetes Care* 2008;31(3):1–20
9. Ochi JW, Melton LJ 3rd, Palumbo PJ, Chu CP. A population-based study of diabetes mortality. *Diabetes Care* 1985;8(3):224–9.
10. Joslin Diabetes Center and Joslin Clinic. Guideline for Detection and Management of Diabetes in Pregnancy. 09/14/2005.
11. Vijan S, Stuart NS, Fitzgerald JT, Ronis DL, Hayward RA, Slater S, Hofer TP. Barriers to following dietary recommendations in Type 2 diabetes. *Diabet Med* 2005;22(1):32–8.
12. Taylor CB, Jatulis DE, Winkleby MA, Rockhill BJ, Kraemer HC. Effects of life-style on body mass index change. *Epidemiology* 1994;5(6):599–603.
13. Childs, B (ed.) et al. American Diabetes Association *Complete Nurse's Guide to Diabetes Care*. 2005
14. Brown FM, Goldfine AB. Diabetes and Pregnancy. In: *Joslin's Diabetes Mellitus*, 14th ed. Lippincott, Williams & Wilkins, 2005: 1035–1048.

15. American Diabetes Association Standards of Medical Care in Diabetes – 2008. *Diabetes Care* 2008; 31: S12–S54.
16. Abrahamson M, Aronson M (eds.) et al. *American College of Physicians Diabetes Care Guide*. 2007.
17. Gaede P, Vedel P, Larsen N, Jensen GV, Parving HH, Pedersen O. Multifactorial intervention and cardiovascular disease in patients with type 2 diabetes. *N Engl J Med* 2003; 348(5): 383–93.
18. Anderson RJ, Freedland KE, Clouse RE, Lustman PJ. The prevalence of comorbid depression in adults with diabetes: a meta-analysis. *Diabetes Care* 2001;24(6):1069–78.
19. Lin EH, Katon W, Von Korff M, Rutter C, Simon GE, Oliver M, Ciechanowski P, Ludman EJ, Bush T, Young B. Relationship of depression and diabetes self-care, medication adherence, and preventive care. *Diabetes Care* 2004;27(9):2154–60.
20. UK Prospective Diabetes Study (UKPDS) Group. UK prospective study of therapies of maturity-onset diabetes. I. Effect of diet, sulphonylurea, insulin or biguanide therapy on fasting plasma glucose and body weight over one year. *Diabetologia* 1983; 24: 404–411.
21. Engum A, Mykletun A, Midthjell K, Holen A, Dahl AA. Depression and diabetes: a large population-based study of sociodemographic, lifestyle, and clinical factors associated with depression in type 1 and type 2 diabetes. *Diabetes Care* 2005;28(8):1904–9.
22. Ross R, Janssen I, Dawson J, Kungl AM, Kuk JL, Wong SL, Nguyen-Duy TB, Lee S, Kilpatrick K, Hudson R. Exercise-induced reduction in obesity and insulin resistance in women: a randomized controlled trial. *Obes Res* 2004;12(5):789–98.
23. Katon W et al. Behavioral and clinical factors associated with depression among individuals with diabetes. *Diabetes Care* 2004; 27 (4): 914–920.
24. De Sonnaville JJ, Snoek FJ, Colly LP, Deville W, Wijkel D, Heine RJ. Well-being and symptoms in relation to insulin therapy in type 2 diabetes. *Diabetes Care* 1998;21(6): 919–24.
25. Fava M. Weight gain and antidepressants. *J Clin Psychiatry* 2000;61(suppl 11):37–41.
26. Schwartz MW. Enhanced: staying slim with insulin in mind. *Science* 2000; 289:2066–2067.
27. Buse J, Henry R, Han J et al. Effects of exenatide (exendin-4) on glycemic control over 30 weeks in sulfonylurea-treated patients with type 2 diabetes. *Diabetes Care* 2004;27: 2628–2635.
28. American Diabetes Association Position Statement: Evidence-Based Nutrition Principles and Recommendations for the Treatment and Prevention of Diabetes and Related Complications. *J Am Diet Assoc* 2002;102(1):109–18.
29. Wing RR, Marcus MD, Salata R, Epstein LH, Miaskiewicz S, Blair EH. Effects of a very-low-calorie diet on long-term glycemic control in obese type 2 diabetic subjects. *Arch Intern Med* 1991;151(7):1334–40.
30. Timonen M, et al. Insulin resistance and depression: cross-sectional study. *BMJ* 2005; 330 (7497): 965.
31. Wing RR, Koeske R, Epstein LH, Nowalk MP, Gooding W, Becker D. Long-term effects of modest weight loss in type II diabetic patients. *Arch Intern Med* 1987;147(10): 1749–53.
32. Wing RR, Epstein LH, Nowalk MP, Koeske R, Hagg S. Behavior change, weight loss, and physiological improvements in type II diabetic patients. *J Consult Clin Psychol* 1985;53(1):111–22.
33. Nuttall FQ, Gannon MC, Saeed A, Jordan K, Hoover H. The metabolic response of subjects with type 2 diabetes to a high-protein, weight-maintenance diet. *J Clin Endocrinol Metab* 2003; 88 (8): 3577–83.
34. Okamura F, et al. Insulin resistance in patients with depression and its changes in the clinical course of depression: report on three cases using the minimal model analysis. *Intern Med* 1999; 38 (3): 257–260.

35. Thomas J, Jones G, Scarinci I, Brantley P. A descriptive and comparative study of the prevalence of depressive and anxiety disorders in low-income adults with type 2 diabetes and other chronic illnesses. *Diabetes Care* 2003;26(8):2311–7.
36. Schmitz O, Brock B, Rungby J. Amylin agonists: a novel approach in the treatment of diabetes. *Diabetes* 2004;53(Suppl. 3):S233–S238.
37. Albright A, Franz M, Hornsby G, Kriska A, Marrero D, Ullrich I, Verity LS. American College of Sports Medicine position stance. Exercise and Type 2 Diabetes. *Med Sci Sports Exerc* 2000;32(7):1345–60.
38. American Diabetes Association Nutrition Recommendations and Interventions for Diabetes: A position statement. *Diabetes Care* 2007; 30: S48–S65.
39. Clark M, Hampson SE, Avery L, Simpson R. Effects of a tailored lifestyle self-management intervention in patients with type 2 diabetes. *Br J Health Psychol* 2004;9(Pt 3):365–79.
40. Jones H, Edwards L, Vallis TM, Ruggiero L, Rossi SR, Rossi JS, Greene G, Prochaska JO, Zinman B; Diabetes Stages of Change (DiSC) Study. Changes in diabetes self-care behaviors make a difference in glycemic control: the Diabetes Stages of Change (DiSC) study. *Diabetes Care* 2003;26(3):732–7.
41. Hunt LM; Valenzuela MA; Pugh JA. NIDDM patients' fears and hopes about insulin therapy. The basis of patient reluctance. *Diabetes Care* 1997; 20(3): 292–8.
42. Ohkubo Y, Kishikawa H, Araki E, Miyata T, Isami S, Motoyoshi S, Kojima Y, Furuyoshi N, Shichiri M. Intensive insulin therapy prevents the progression of diabetic microvascular complications in Japanese patients with non-insulin-dependent diabetes mellitus: a randomized prospective 6-year study. *Diabetes Res Clin Pract* 1995;28(2):103–17.
43. Stratton IM, Adler AI, Neil HA, Matthews DR, Manley SE, Cull CA, Hadden D, Turner RC, Holman RR. Association of glycaemia with macrovascular and microvascular complications of type 2 diabetes (UKPDS 35): prospective observational study. *BMJ* 2000 12;321(7258): 405–12.
44. Effect of intensive blood-glucose control with metformin on complications in overweight patients with type 2 diabetes (UKPDS 34). *Lancet* 1998;352(9131):854–65.
45. U.S. Renal Data System: *USRDS 1994 Annual Data Report*. Bethesda, Md.: National Institutes of Health, National Institute of Diabetes and Digestive and Kidney Diseases. 1994.
46. World Health Organization. Global strategy on diet, physical activity and health. http://www.who.int/dietphysical activity/publications/facts/obesity/en/. Retrieved 01/02/2005.
47. Zoorob RJ, Hagen MD. Guidelines on the care of diabetic nephropathy, retinopathy and foot disease. *Am Fam Physician* 1997;56(8):2021–8, 2033–4.
48. Sargrad K, et al. Effect of high protein vs. high carbohydrate intake on insulin sensitivity, body weight, haemoglobin A1c, and blood pressure in patients with type 2 diabetes mellitus. *J Am Diet Assoc* 2005; 105 (4): 573–80.
49. Maggio CA, Pi-Sunyer FX. The prevention and treatment of obesity. Application to type 2 diabetes. *Diabetes Care* 1997; 20 (11): 1744–1766.
50. Wild S, Roglic G, Green A, Sicree R, King H. Global prevalence of diabetes: estimates for the year 2000 and projections for 2030. *Diabetes Care* 2004;27(5):1047–53.
51. Park H, Hong Y, Lee H, Ha E, Sung Y. Individuals with type 2 diabetes and depressive symptoms exhibited lower adherence with self-care. *J Clin Epidemiol* 2004;57(9):978–84

3   Models for Diabetes Education

Linda M. Siminerio, *PhD, RN, CDE*

CONTENTS

INTRODUCTION
PATIENT–EDUCATOR INTERACTION MODELS
PRACTICE LEVEL MODELS
HEALTH SYSTEM MODELS
RECOMMENDATIONS
CONCLUSIONS
REFERENCES

ABSTRACT

Evidence-based models and frameworks have been introduced to support diabetes self-management education and support. This article presents various frameworks and models and describes their use in support of diabetes education at the patient–educator, the practice environment, and the systems/policy/environmental level. The text and tables present various models and specific recommendations and examples for educators to use at every level. Cross-cutting concepts are that models that support diabetes education at all levels include an assessment, goal setting, problem solving, and systematic follow-up; an ongoing process; and community and primary care approaches that attempt to provide outreach and sustainable programs. Tested frameworks and models serve to support the provision of diabetes education at all levels and should be used in continued implementation and evaluation.

From: *Contemporary Diabetes: Educating Your Patient with Diabetes*
Edited by: K. Weinger and C. A. Carver, DOI 10.1007/978-1-60327-208-7_3,
© Humana Press, a part of Springer Science+Business Media, LLC 2009

Key Words: Self-care, Diabetes education, Diabetes self-management education, Self-management support, Patient–educator interactions, Practice environments, Health systems.

INTRODUCTION

Diabetes is a serious disease that requires a person to make daily decisions about his or her self-care *(1)*. To promote good health, the person with diabetes needs to be proficient in key self-care behaviors that include nutrition, exercise, risk reduction, coping, monitoring, problem solving, and medication adherence *(2)*. Provision of diabetes education is critical in laying a foundation that promotes the knowledge, skills, and behavior change strategies necessary for self-care.

Diabetes education is an ever-evolving dynamic in which educators need to continually stay apprised of its changes. Acknowledged as early as 1927, "wandering nurses" calculated calories, prepared food, and gave injections while they resided with the family of a person with diabetes *(3)*. The physicians directed education and care at that time, and the patient was merely a recipient rather than a participant. Over time, themes like diabetes self-management education and self-management support approaches emerged *(4–9)*.

Self-management refers to the individual's ability to manage the symptoms, treatment, physical and psychosocial consequences, and lifestyle changes inherent in living with a chronic condition. Efficacious self-management encompasses the ability to monitor one's condition and to affect the cognitive, behavioral, and emotional responses necessary to maintain a satisfactory quality of life *(5)*.

Diabetes self-management education is defined as the ongoing process of facilitating the knowledge, skill, and ability necessary for diabetes self-care. This process incorporates the needs, goals, and life experiences of the person with diabetes and is guided by evidence-based standards *(10)*. The process of making and refining multi-level changes in the community and health-care systems to facilitate patient self-care is referred to as self-management support. Diabetes education has changed a great deal in recent years. As diabetes education has become more patient centered and theoretically based, diabetes self-management education programs are now putting a greater emphasis on providing ongoing support to sustain the self-management gains made by patients as a result of education *(4)* and incorporating self-management support into their structure *(10)*. The evidence supporting the effectiveness of diabetes self-management education and self-management support has increased dramatically over the past two decades *(9–16)*.

Because the provision of diabetes self-management education and self-management support requires that the necessary changes involve much more than direct patient education, *(11,12,17–23)* educators must consider expanding their roles and responsibilities to facilitate diabetes education at three levels. For the purpose of this chapter, the levels are categorized into direct patient–educator interactions, practice environments, and health systems. Since the importance of diabetes self-management education and self-management support has been established, reference to the provision of diabetes education will include both. The remaining sections discuss specific processes, frameworks, and models that can be used to address each of the levels with the recognition that these categories and the processes frequently overlap in implementation.

PATIENT–EDUCATOR INTERACTION MODELS

As diabetes education has evolved from a didactic to a patient-centered and now patient-directed approach, to be successful, it must be focused on the promotion of positive behavior change *(24,25)*. In years past, educators typically targeted an increase in diabetes knowledge as the critical outcome variable. Through countless studies, however, it has been demonstrated that knowledge alone does not have a potent impact on clinical outcomes such as glycemic control *(16,25,26)*. Clinical improvement is likely only when knowledge prompts a positive change in self-care behavior. Without doubt, behavior change is the major mediating variable linking diabetes self-management training and positive clinical outcomes *(27)*. Although the idea of behavior change seems straightforward, frameworks and models serve to ultimately support the facilitation of behavior so that common conceptual mistakes are avoided. The teaching–learning process, theoretical frameworks, and the 5As model serve to remind educators of the key elements in suppporting a comprehensive, step-wise approach for a positive patient interation to promote self-care.

The Teaching–Learning Process

The teaching–learning process was one of the earliest models used as a framework to support the process of changing the behavior patterns of people. Teaching is defined as a system of actions that include the provision of experiences and guidance to facilitate learning. Learning is a change in behavior that involves a process of transforming new knowledge, insights, skills, and values into new behavior *(28–31)*. Learning is goal directed. It comes as no surprise that the terms are familiar. The elements described in the teaching–learning process have sustained the test of time and remain a guide for educators. The critical components of the process are assessment, planning, implementation, and evaluation, which are discussed in more detail in other chapters.

Theoretical Models and Diabetes Education

Diabetes educators should also be familiar with educational theories, philosophies, and conceptual models that are often used to explain or predict an individual's learning and behavior. Diabetes educators are encouraged to use a variety of theoretical constructs because they serve as a framework for a comprehensive plan of care, provide guidelines for teaching, and facilitate clinical practice and research (32). Although there are many theoretical models, four models frequently used and tested in diabetes education include (but are not limited to) the *health belief model*, the *empowerment model, self-efficacy* and the *social cognitive theory*, and the *transtheoretical model (33–37)*.

The *health belief model* helps educators understand a patient's health-related choices (33). This model hypothesizes that adherence to medical advice depends on holding a particular set of beliefs. These beliefs include the following:

- a motive to comply
- recognition that one has the disease and is susceptible to serious sequelae
- that adherence would be beneficial in reducing problems
- that one has the ability to follow health recommendations
- the benefits of care outweigh the cost

The *health belief model* in relation to diabetes suggests that the person's willingness to adhere to the management plan largely depends on accepting the seriousness of the condition and believing that the benefits of the health action outweigh the costs.

The *empowerment model*, based on the frameworks of self-determination and autonomy support (38), has served as the philosophical basis for diabetes self-management education for more than 15 years (4). The patient empowerment approach to diabetes education is intended to enable patients to make informed decisions about their own diabetes care and to be fully responsible members of the health-care team (34). People are empowered when they have sufficient knowledge to make rational decisions, sufficient control and resources to implement those decisions, and sufficient experience to evaluate effectiveness. Facilitating patient empowerment requires a specific set of skills and attitudes on the part of diabetes educators and has been demonstrated to be an effective model for facilitating self-management (35).

The concept of self-efficacy is based on *social cognitive theory*, which describes the interaction between behavioral, personal, and environmental factors in health and chronic disease, has also been proposed as a basis for identifying strategies to enhance diabetes self-management (36). The more confident and capable the person feels about performing a set of behaviors, the more likely it is that the person will actually perform those behaviors. The theory of self-efficacy can be used to learn more about a patient's convictions and beliefs regarding his or her ability to carry out recommendations for care. As the effectiveness of diabetes management depends on self-care, the adoption of the self-efficacy theory for diabetes care appears logical.

The *transtheoretical model* is a model that focuses on stages of behavior change. The central hypothesis of this model is that not all individuals are prepared to take action to change their behavior at any given time. Stages included in this readiness model include precontemplation, contemplation, preparation, action, and maintenance. This model offers an approach in helping diabetes educators to identify where a patient is in the learning process and to develop complimentary interventions *(37)*.

The 5A's Model

In a report on implementing practical interventions to self-management, Glasgow et al. *(39)* suggested the use of the *5A's model*. The *5A's* has been recommended as a practical and efficient evidence-based approach for clinicians (educators) to ask, advise, agree on goals, assist, and arrange follow-up *(39,40)*. Consistent with the traditional *teaching/learning process*, a well-designed patient interaction system begins with an assessment of the patient's knowledge, psychosocial needs, beliefs, and behaviors. The educator then advises the patient by providing specific information about diabetes and its risks for complications and health benefits in implementing specific interventions. Patient data

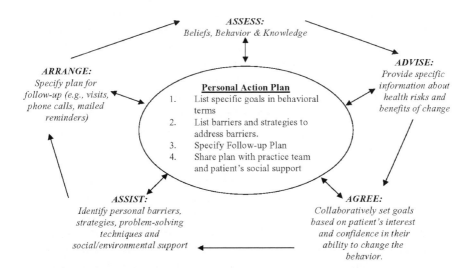

Fig. 1. Five A's Model of Self-Management Support Adapted from Glasgow et al. *(4)*.

that includes a history, laboratory values, and physical exam findings are used together with the patient information as a framework in developing an educational plan. Within the plan, goals are discussed and agreed upon. Patients are then assisted to develop goals and work on problem solving. Finally, a follow-up plan is arranged. The 5A's framework presented in Fig. 1 is a useful tool in implementing effective diabetes education.

PRACTICE LEVEL MODELS

Beyond the patient–educator interaction, the provision of diabetes education requires attention at the practice level so that adequate services are provided to support diabetes self-management education (17–23,39). Unfortunately, because the numbers of patients who currently receive diabetes self-management education are disappointingly small (41–43), with reported estimates that < 50% (probably closer to 35–40%) of all patients with diabetes ever attend a diabetes education/behavioral intervention program (43), it is critically important that educators use systematic approaches to address barriers to education services (44). Educators familiar with self-management processes rooted at the individual level (e.g., assessment, goal setting, problem solving) should consider and apply these processes in developing practice changes in an effort to provide diabetes self-management education to the growing number of people with diabetes.

It has been reported that access to education may be a potential barrier to the provision of diabetes self-management education (44). Another potential problem may be the traditional way in which education is prescribed and delivered. Most health-care practices are based on the traditional model of acute, episodic care (45,46). In many areas, physicians are encouraged by their affiliated institutions to refer patients with diabetes to a centralized hospital-based diabetes self-management education program to a one-time series of education classes. Because diabetes self-management education and self-management support are also rarely integrated into the medical care provided to the patient (8,47), exploring new strategies to redesign practices need to be considered (44,47,48).

An ecological approach, parallel to the 5A's model used to assist patients, has been introduced by Fisher et al. to identify key elements for the support of diabetes self-management practices (19,49). The resources and supports for self-management model extended the framework of the 5A's as a structure for planning and implementing ongoing services to support patients' self-management at multiple levels (19,49,50). The resources and supports for self-management model elements include an individualized assessment, collaborative goal setting, skills enhancement, follow-up and support, access to resources, and continuity of quality clinical care. Although these elements are quite similar to those outlined in the 5A's framework, the difference is one of emphasis. In contrast to self-management that emphasizes the individual, an ecological approach to self-management explores the services and support the individuals need and receive from (1) their environment, including family, friends, worksites, organizations, and cultures and (2) the physical and policy environments of neighborhoods, communities, and governments (19,49). Table 1 illustrates the comparative features of the 5A's Model outlined by Glasgow et al. to the resources and supports for self-management model presented by Fisher et al.

Both the 5A's and the resources and supports for self-management approaches emphasize identification of goals, problem solving, and facilitation and reinforcement of the use of those skills. The resources and supports for self-management framework may be especially helpful in understanding and organizing different tactical approaches for practice change (19). The first step is to assess the practice to determine if and to what extent that diabetes self-management education and self-management support are being provided.

Table 1
Correspondence of Core Concepts of Self-management with the "5A's"
and Resources and Supports for Self-Management

Core Concepts of Self-Management	"5A's"	Resources and Supports for Self-Management
Identification	Assess Advise	Individualized Assessment
	Agree	Collaborative goal setting
Skills	Assist	Skills for-problem solving, "temptation" management stress/emotion management healthy diet, physical activity managing specific diseases
Facilitation, incentives, support for maintaining behavior	Arrange	Ongoing follow-up and support Access to resources in daily life
Link to Clinical care	Implicit in assumption that in most cases, 4A's are implemented within clinical settings	Continuity of quality clinical care

Note. For "5A's," see Whitlock et al.[149]
From Fisher et al. (19)

For example, are patients referred to diabetes self-management education programs, are there follow-up resources to assure communication with the educator on a plan?

Advice, the second step, involves obtaining recommendations for practice change based on the assessment information. This advice is customized to fit the given practice or program. The advice should be based on the findings from the assessment process. For example, the educator may advise the practice to facilitate evening follow-up group visits based on a need's assessment survey that indicated most of the patients could not accommodate time off during the work day.

The third step is for the practice team to agree upon a philosophy and common vision to support diabetes self-management education and self-management support because many professionals have been trained within an acute care model of delivery and are more comfortable with directive approaches *(39,51–54)*. Integrating the principles of diabetes self-management education and behavioral change into all aspects of diabetes care for all practitioners in the program or practice, not just for behavioral and educational specialists, is critical for success.

The fourth step is to assist the practice by identifying barriers and implementing problem-solving strategies to support diabetes self-management education and self-management support. Finally, practice teams need to arrange follow-up and evaluate progress and results. For example, the "Arrange" of the 5A's can easily be re-focused to address the need for a diabetes team to "arrange" program resources for follow-up supports through telephone calls or case management *(39)*.

Practices, like patients, need ongoing training and support to sustain behavior changes. Glasgow et al. also stress that it is important that teams experiment and feel able to try practice changes and recommend that teams conduct rapid cycle improvements through a model for improvement called the plan–do–study act (PDSA) cycle. PDSA affords practice teams the opportunity to rapidly test and create new plans as needed *(55–57)*. Strategies used for patients, like making small changes first and re-evaluating, also work for practice change. These strategies can help teams to sustain new practice patterns.

HEALTH SYSTEM MODELS

The delivery of diabetes education resides within programs and practices that are often part of a larger health system environment where educators find themselves as advocates for system changes. A recent Institute of Medicine on chronic illness care reports *(58)* that programs based on the chronic care model

(59) are helping health-care systems provide more clinically effective and cost-efficient care *(60–63)*. Several health-care organizations and state governmental organizations are currently organizing care around the model.

The chronic care model provides a paradigm shift from our current model of health-care delivery that is designed to handle acute problems, to a system that is prevention based, and focused on avoiding long-term problems, including diabetes complications *(59,60)*. Due to its multi-faceted nature, quality diabetes care requires an integration of the patient into a health system that promotes long-term management *(62)*, rather than one where care is provided episodically. Unlike acute illnesses, diabetes encompasses behavioral, psychosocial, psychological, environmental, and clinical factors, all of which require team-based support from a variety of health-care disciplines *(13,17,64,65)*. The premise of the model is that quality diabetes care is not delivered in isolation, but with community resources, delivery system design, decision support and clinical information systems working in tandem leading to productive interactions between a proactive practice team and prepared activated patient *(60,64)*. Elements of the model are presented in Fig. 2.

An integral facet of the chronic care model is the importance of self-management support. Because it emphasizes self-management, it provides an ideal framework for a systematic approach and supports the inclusion of all members of the diabetes health-care team in contrast to traditional methods. The model has already been shown to be an effective means of implementing and sustaining diabetes self-management education programs *(44,47)*.

Educators can refer to the following elements of the model to address and assure diabetes self-management education and self-management support at the system level:

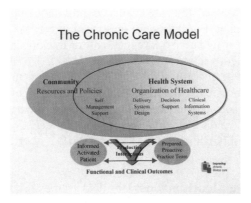

Fig. 2. The Chronic Care Model Adapted from Wagner.

1. Health care organization provides the structural foundation (philosophically and literally) upon which the remaining four components of the model rely. Understanding the mission, goals, and values of the provider organization and its relationship with purchasers, insurers, and health-care providers are key to successful implementation of programs. It is doubtful that meaningful improvement in chronic disease care can be achieved without committed leadership and resources *(47,60)*. Educators who are able to gain their health system and organization's support are more likely to facilitate and sustain their programs *(47,60)*.
2. Community resources and policies provide individuals with diabetes, their caregivers, clinicians, and educators with a variety of ancillary services that provide support for self-management support. Within a community policies define relationships between various agencies (e.g., networks, how services are accessed and provided, etc). Working with communities to facilitate diabetes self-management education and self-management support and to establish policies are critical for follow up, reimbursement, and sustainability.
3. Decision support uses specialist expertise to establish evidence-based clinical practice guidelines, standards, and protocols. Use of the evidence-based tools, like the National Standards for Diabetes Self-Management Education *(10)*, provides a framework for educators to assure quality and consistency.
4. Self-management engages the patient in the active self-management of their illness. When informed patients take an active role in managing their disease, and providers are prepared, proactive, and supported with time and resources, their interaction is likely to be productive *(51)*. It is the responsibility of the diabetes educator to customize care and services to the needs and circumstances of each individual and community.
5. Clinical information systems are necessary for collecting and housing timely, useful data about individual patients and populations of patients, using tools such as patient registries and databases. The information system allows quality measures to be assessed and care evaluated, providing ongoing feedback to the provider and patient. Educators not only need to rely on information systems for patient monitoring but to a larger extent for tracking and reporting data for practice and system's reports and feedback *(41,47)*.
6. Delivery system design affords opportunities to restructure medical practices to facilitate team care, define team roles, and delegates tasks. In an effort to expand diabetes self-management education and self-management support services, educators could explore reconfiguring the delivery of care in primary care and community clinic settings *(11,54,59–65)*.

The Chronic Care Model provides an ideal framework to support diabetes self-management education as a template for diabetes educators to explore collaboration with (heretofore) unlikely partners in their local health-care systems and communities. Potential partners include organization administrators, financial officers, information systems, insurers, employers, and policy makers. This leads to search for opportunities outside of traditional educator roles, such as the development of business models for sustainability, strategic planning, and integrating technological approaches and data management. The model also challenges diabetes educators to (1) develop partnerships with community facilities such as wellness and senior centers, (2) seek opportunities to collect and share data, (3) overlap responsibilities with other team members, and (4) form consortia and/or organize system-wide quality initiatives. Developing systems that promote accessible, sustainable diabetes self-management education programs that impact metabolic outcomes have large-scale public health implications.

RECOMMENDATIONS

Frameworks and models can also serve as useful templates for educators at all levels for continued exploration and evaluation in expanding the pool of evidence in support of diabetes education. The RE-AIM (reach, effectiveness, adoption, adoption, implementation, and maintenance) framework has been developed to evaluate and translate initiatives into an even larger public health realm *(66–68)*. In building the evidence for widespread dissemination of diabetes education, educators should consider using the RE-AIM model.

In using RE-AIM, it has been recommended that initiatives be evaluated by examining all five of the following RE-AIM dimensions at both the patient and the setting level. Reach and efficacy are individual levels of impact, whereas adoption and implementation are organizational levels of impact. Maintenance can be both at an individual and organizational levels of impact.

For example, educators can determine reach into the target population by performing a needs assessment to determine patient demographics and characteristics, and the numbers of patients reached with services. Educators assure the efficacy/effectiveness of the diabetes self-management education intervention by measuring their patient's behavioral, clinical, and psychosocial outcomes, while they consider the adoption of the education interventions on a larger scale at their institutions, in their community, and by their colleagues.

Diabetes educators need to assess implementation at the patient and practice levels. At the patient level, implementation refers to patients' use and adherence of various intervention strategies, while at the practice level, evaluating the team's intervention efforts and their adherence to the various elements of the program is equally as important.

Within the RE-AIM framework, maintenance also applies to the individual and practice level. At the individual level, maintenance has been defined as the effects of a program on outcomes after 6 or more months. The extent to which a program or policy becomes institutionalized or part of the routine organizational practices and policies is a measure of maintenance at the practice level.

CONCLUSIONS

As the incidence of diabetes continues to increase at rapid pace, systematic approaches need to be established so that DSME may be accessible to the ever-increasing pool of people with diabetes. Leveraging an increased interest in evidence-based processes, frameworks and models (to further foster diabetes education in the current health care environment) may help diabetes educators to provide new avenues of support for appropriate reimbursement and dissemination.

REFERENCES

1. Glasgow RE, Anderson RM. In diabetes care, moving from compliance to adherence is not enough: something entirely different is needed. *Diabetes Care* 22:2090–2097, 1999.
2. Mulcahy K, Maryniuk M, Peeples M, et al: Diabetes Self-Management Education Core Outcome Measures. *Diabetes Educ* 29:768–803, 2003.
3. Barnett DM: Elliot P. Joslin, MD: A centennial portrait. Joslin Diabetes Center, 1998.
4. Funnell MM, Tang TS, Anderson RM: From DSME to DSMS: Developing empowerment-based diabetes self-management support. *Diabetes Spectr* 20:221–226, 2007.
5. Barlow JH, Wright C, Sheasby J, et al: Self-management approaches for people with chronic conditions: A review. *Patient Educ Couns* 48:177–187, 2002.
6. Glasgow RE, Funnell MM, Bonomi AE, et al: Self-management aspects of the improving chronic illness care Breakthrough Series: Implementation with diabetes and heart failure teams. *Ann Behav Med* 24:80–87, 2002.
7. Clark NM, Becker MH, Lorig K, et al: Self-management of chronic disease by older adults: A review and questions for research. *J Aging Health* 3:3–27, 1991.
8. Funnell MM, Anderson RM: Changing office practice and health care systems to facilitate diabetes self-management. *Curr Diabetes Rep* 3(2):127–133, 2003.
9. Norris SL, Engelgau MM, Narayan KM: Effectiveness of self-management training in type 2 diabetes: Systematic review of randomized controlled trials. *Diabetes Care* 24:561–587, 2001.
10. Funnell, M, Brown T, Childs B, Haas L, Hosey G, Jensen B, Maryniuk M, Peyrot M, Piette J, Reader D, Siminerio L, Weinger K, Weiss M. National standards for diabetes self-management education". *Diabetes Care* 30(6):1630–1637, 2007.
11. Lorig KR, Sobel DS, Stewart AL, et al: Evidence suggesting that a chronic disease self-management program can improve health status while reducing hospitalization. *Med Care* 37:5–14, 1999.
12. The Diabetes Prevention Program Research Group: Reduction in the incidence of type 2 diabetes with lifestyle intervention or metformin. *N Eng J Med* 346:393–403, 2002.
13. Wagner EH, Austin BT, Davis C, et al: Improving chronic illness care: Translating evidence into action. *Health Aff* 20:64–78, 2001.
14. Norris SL, Lau J, Smith SJ, Schmid CH, Engelgau MM: Self-management education for adults with type 2 diabetes. *Diabetes Care* 25(7):1159–1171, 2002.

15. Bodenheimer TS, Lorig K, Holman H, et al: Patient self-management of chronic disease in primary care. *JAMA* 288:2469–2475, 2002.
16. Brown SA: Effects of educational interventions and outcomes in diabetic adults: A Meta-analysis revisited. *Patient Educ Couns* 16:189–215, 1990.
17. Skovlund SE, Peyrot M: DAWN International Advisory Panel: Lifestyle and behavior: The Diabetes Attitudes, Wishes and Needs (DAWN) program: A new approach to improving outcomes of diabetes care. *Diabetes Spectr* 18:136–142, 2005.
18. Rubin R, Peyrot M, Siminerio L. Health care and patient-reported outcomes: Results of the cross-national diabetes attitudes, wishes and needs (DAWN) study. *Diabetes Care* 29(6):1249–1255, 2006.
19. Fisher EB, Brownson CA, O'Toole ML, Shetty G, Anwuri VV, Glasgow RE: Ecological approaches to self-management: The case of diabetes. *Am J Public Health* 95(9): 1523–1535, 2005.
20. Fiore MC, Bailey WC, Cohen SJ, et al. *Treating tobacco use and dependence: Clinical practice guideline*. June. 2000. Rockville, MD, U.S. Department of Health and Human Services, Public Health Service.
21. Whitlock EP, Orleans CT, Pender N, et al: Evaluating primary care behavioral counseling interventions: An evidence-based approach. *Am J Prev Med* 22:267–284, 2002.
22. Goldstein MR, DePue J: Models for provider-patient interaction: Applications to health behavior change, in Shumaker S, Schron EB, McBee WL (Eds): *The handbook of health behavior change*. New York, Springer, 1998, pp. 85–113.
23. Siminerio L, Piatt G, Emerson S, Ruppert K, Saul M, Solano F, Stewart A, Zgibor J: Deploying the chronic care model to implement and sustain diabetes self-management training programs. *Diabetes Educ* 32(2):1–8, 2006.
24. Peeples M, Tomky D, Mulcahy K, Peyrot M, Siminerio L: Evolution of the American Association of Diabetes Educators' diabetes education outcomes project. *Diabetes Educ* 33(5):794–817, 2007.
25. Piette JD, Glasgow R: Strategies for improving behavioral health outcomes among patients with diabetes: self-management education. *Evidence-Based Diabetes Care*. Gerstein HC, Haynes RB, Eds. Ontario, Canada: BC Decker Publishers, 207–251, 2001.
26. Padgett D, Mumford E, Hynes M, Carter R: Meta-analysis of the effects of educational and psychosocial interventions on management of diabetes mellitus. *J Clin Epidemiol* 41: 1007–30, 1992.
27. Peyrot M: Behavior change in diabetes education. *Diabetes Educ* 25(6):62–73, 1999.
28. Cecco J, Crawford W: The psychology of learning and instruction. New Jersey: Prentice-Hall, Inc., 1974.
29. Rollnick S, Mason P, Butler C: *Health behavior change: A guide for clinicians*. New York, Churchill Livingstone, 1999.
30. Lorenz R: Training health professionals to improve the effectiveness of patient education programs. *Diabetes Educ* 12:204–209, 1986.
31. McLeod B: Diabetes program development education. Ontario, Canada: Canadian Diabetes Association, 1988.
32. Siminerio L (Ed.) McLaughlin S and Polonsky W (Contributing Ed.) Diabetes Education Goals 3rd Edition. American Diabetes Association. Alexandria, VA, 2002.
33. Becker MH, Janz N: The health belief model applied to understanding diabetes regimen compliance. *Diabetes Educ* 11:41–47, 1985.
34. Anderson RM, Funnell MM, Butler PM, Arnold MS, Fitzgerald JT, Feste CC: Patient empowerment: Results of a randomized control trial. *Diabetes Care* 18:943–949, 1995.
35. Anderson R, Funnell M: The art of empowerment. Stories and Strategies for Diabetes Educators 2nd ed. American Diabetes Association, 2005.

36. Bandura A: Social foundations of thought and action: A social cognitive theory. Englewood Cliffs, NJ, Prentice Hall, 1986.
37. Ruggerio L, Prochaska JO (Eds): Readiness for change: application of the transtheoretical model to diabetes. *Diabetes Spectr* 6:22–60, 1993.
38. Williams, GC. "Improving patients' health through supporting the autonomy of patients and providers." *Handbook of Self-Determination Research.* Ed. EL Deci and RM Ryan, Rochester, NY; University of Rochester Press, 233–54, 2002.
39. Glasgow RE, Davis FL, Funnell MM, Beck A: Implementing practical interventions to support chronic illness self-management. *Jt Comm J Qual Saf* 29(11):563–574, 2003.
40. Whitlock EP, Orleans CT, Pender N, et al: Evaluating primary care behavioral counseling interventions: An evidence-based approach. *Am J Prev Med* 22:267–284, 2002.
41. Pearson J, Mensing C, Anderson R. Medicare reimbursement and diabetes self-management training: national survey results. *Diabetes Educ* (30):914–927, 2004.
42. Coonrod BA, Betschart J, Harris MI. Frequency and determinants of diabetes patient education among adults in the U.S. population. *Diabetes Care* (17): 852–858, 1994.
43. Polonsky WH, Anderson BJ, Lohrer PA, Welch G, Jacobson AM, Schwartz C: Assessment of diabetes-specific distress. *Diabetes Care* 18:754–760, 1995.
44. Siminerio L, Piatt G, Zgibor J: Implementing the chronic care model in a rural practice. *Diabetes Educ* 31(2):225–234, 2005.
45. Hiss RG: Barriers to care in non-insulin-dependent diabetes mellitus, The Michigan experience. *Ann Intern Med* 124(1):146–148, 1996.
46. Glasgow RE, Hiss RG, Anderson RM, et al: Report of Health Care Delivery Work Group: Behavioral research related to the establishment of a chronic disease model for diabetes care. *Diabetes Care* 24:124–130, 2001.
47. Siminerio L, Piatt G, Emerson S, Ruppert K, Saul M, Solano F, Stewart A, Zgibor J. "Deploying the chronic care model to implement and sustain diabetes self-management training programs". *Diabetes Educ* 32(2):1–8, 2006.
48. Wagner EH, Grothaus LC, Sandhu N, et al: Chronic care clinics for diabetes in primary care: A system-wide randomized trial. *Diabetes Care* 24:695–700, 2001.
49. The Robert Wood Johnson Foundation and Center for the Advancement of Health. Essential elements of self-management interventions. December 2001. Available at: http://www.cfah.org/pdfs/EssentialElementsReport.pdf.
50. Glasgow RE, Goldstein M, Ockene J, Pronk JP: Translating what we have learned into practice: principles and hypotheses for addressing multiple behaviors in primary care. *Am J Prev Med* 27:88–101, 2004.
51. Anderson RM: Patient empowerment and the traditional medical model. *Diabetes Care* 18:412–415, 1995.
52. Funnell MM, Anderson RM: The problem with compliance in diabetes. *JAMA* 284:1709, 2000.
53. Funnell MM, Anderson RM: The problem with compliance in diabetes. *JAMA* 284:1709, 2000.
54. Anderson RM, Fitzgerald JT, Gorenflo DW, Oh MS: A comparison of the diabetes-related attitudes of health care professionals and patients. *Patient Educ Couns* 21:41–50, 1993.
55. Wagner EH, Glasgow RE, Davis C, et al: Quality improvement in chronic illness care: A collaborative approach. *J Jt Comm Health Care Qual* 27:63–80, 2001.
56. Von Korff M, Gruman J, Schaefer J, et al: Collaborative management of chronic illness. *Ann Intern Med* 19:1097–1102, 1997.
57. Langley GJ, Nolan KM, Nolan TW, et al: *The improvement guide: A practical approach to enhancing organizational performance.* San Francisco, Jossey-Bass, 1996.
58. Institute of Medicine: Chapter 1: A New Health System for the 21st Century. Crossing the Quality Chasm. Ed. R Briere, National Academy Press, Washington, D.C. 2001.

59. Wagner EH, Austin BT, Von Korfs M: Improving outcomes in chronic illness. *Manag Care Q* 4(2):12–25, 1996.
60. Siminerio L, Zgibor J, Solano FX: Implementing the chronic care model for improvements in diabetes practice and outcomes in primary care: The University of Pittsburgh Medical Center experience. *Clin Diabetes* 22(2):54–58, 2004.
61. Piatt GA, Orchard TJ, Emerson S, Simmons D, Songer TJ, Brooks MM, Korytkowski M, Siminerio LM, Ahmad U, Zgibor JC. Translating the chronic care model into the community: Results from a randomized controlled trial of a multi-faceted diabetes care intervention. *Diabetes Care* 29(4): 811–817, 2006.
62. Wagner EH, Austin BT, VonKorfs M: Improving outcomes in chronic illness. *Milbank Q* 4(2):12–25, 1996.
63. Wagner, EH, Davis C, Schaefer J, Von Korff M, Austin B: A survey of leading chronic disease management programs: are they consistent with the literature? *Manag Care Q*: 56–66, 1999.
64. Wagner EH: The role of patient care teams in chronic disease management. *Br Med J* 320: 569–572, 2000.
65. Siminerio L, Funnell M, Peyrot M, Rubin R. US nurses' perceptions of their role in diabetes care: Results of the cross-national diabetes, attitudes, wishes and needs (DAWN) study. *Diabetes Educ* 33(1):152–162, 2007.
66. Glasgow RE, Nelson CC, Strycker LA, King DK: Using RE-AIM metrics to evaluate diabetes self-management support interventions. *Am J Prev Med* 30(1):67–73, 2006.
67. Glasgow RE: Evaluation of theory-based interventions: the RE-AIM model. In: Glanz K, Lewis FM, Rimer BK, eds. Health behavior and health education. 3rd ed. San Francisco: John Wiley & Sons: 531–544, 2002.
68. Glasgow RE, McKay HG, Pietter JD, Reynolds KD: The RE-AIM framework for evaluating interventions: what can it tell us about approaches to chronic illness management? *Patient Educ Couns* 44:119–127, 2001.

4 Diabetes Education Process

Amy P. Campbell, MS, RD, CDE
and Elaine D. Sullivan, MS, RN, CDE

CONTENTS

INTRODUCTION
ASSESSMENT: THE FIRST STEP
SAMPLE OPEN-ENDED ASSESSMENT QUESTIONS
EDUCATION PLAN
PLANNING: A STANDARD OF PROFESSIONAL
    PERFORMANCE FOR DIABETES EDUCATORS
GOAL SETTING
IMPLEMENTING THE EDUCATION PLAN
THE NEXT STEP: EDUCATION FOLLOW UP
DOCUMENTATION AND INFORMATICS
CONCLUSION
REFERENCES

ABSTRACT

Diabetes self-management is well recognized as the cornerstone of a person's diabetes care. A person with diabetes must have the knowledge and skills to successfully manage his diabetes. The healthcare team is an integral part of a person's diabetes treatment plan. The team typically consists of a physician, a nurse educator, and a dietitian, although other healthcare providers may be part of the team, such as an exercise physiologist, a pharmacist, and a mental health counselor. The diabetes educator is primarily responsible for developing the patient's education plan with input from the patient, and support and reinforcement from the rest of the team. Individualized goal setting is a key component of the education plan and is

From: *Contemporary Diabetes: Educating Your Patient with Diabetes*
Edited by: K. Weinger and C. A. Carver, DOI 10.1007/978-1-60327-208-7_4,
© Humana Press, a part of Springer Science+Business Media, LLC 2009

essential to help the person with diabetes change behaviors to improve health and quality of life. The education plan is not static; it must be continually adjusted and updated to reflect the patient's changes in priorities and goals, the progression of diabetes, and life circumstances. Finally, the education plan must be appropriately documented in the patient's medical record to help monitor progress and to meet quality and accreditation standards.

Key Words: Assessment, Education plan, Goal setting, Readiness to learn, Documentation.

INTRODUCTION

Diabetes self-management education is well recognized as the cornerstone of a person's diabetes care. Considering that the majority of diabetes care is up to the person with diabetes, and not the healthcare team, it's critical that the person with diabetes have the knowledge and behavioral skill set to appropriately and successfully manage diabetes. The educator facilitates learning and behavior change. Hopefully, the result of healthy behavior change is improved outcomes and quality of life, despite a chronic illness.

Day-to-day diabetes management involves meal planning, taking medication, monitoring, and preventing or treating acute complications, such as hypoglycemia. However, the person with diabetes must also take measures to prevent or limit the occurrence of long-term complications, such as retinopathy, neuropathy, nephropathy, and cardiovascular disease. Risk reduction, therefore, is an integral part of the diabetes care and education process. Many people who have diabetes report that managing it is a full-time job. Also, lack of financial and educational resources, plus inadequate psychosocial support, are major obstacles that often stand in the way of optimal diabetes management.

The healthcare team is an integral and critical part of a person's diabetes treatment plan. The team typically consists of physicians (primary care, endocrinologist), a nurse educator, and a dietitian, but may also include a nurse practitioner, an exercise physiologist, a pharmacist, a gynecologist/obstetrician, a podiatrist, an ophthalmologist, and a mental health counselor. The job of the healthcare team is to help the person develop the self-care, problem-solving, and coping skills and behaviors necessary for optimal diabetes management.

ASSESSMENT: THE FIRST STEP

The first step in developing a person's education plan is to complete a thorough assessment. The initial assessment establishes the relationship between the educator and the person with diabetes. It also determines priorities and the most effective process for education. If the educator establishes priorities based on "academic" diabetes (his or her own expertise), content may be "covered" to meet reimbursement expectations, but the patient may not benefit. Personalized diabetes education can happen only if the educator knows the patient and has established rapport with that patient.

Assessment Components

Assessment can be done in a face-to-face interview, a group discussion, by phone, via Internet, and/or using a self-assessment tool. The Diabetes Initiative of the Robert Wood Johnson Foundation has published a wide range of assessment tools on their website at http://diabetesnpo.im.wustl.edu/resources/topics/IndAssessment.html. Assessment must be ongoing in the education process, and, in fact, should happen at the beginning and end of each education session. A careful assessment addresses medical, psychosocial, and behavioral issues and lays out the patient's priorities. Additional assessments of cultural influences, literacy, language, and learning style need to be considered in developing an educational plan *(1)*.

The medical assessment includes current diagnoses, diabetes complications, past medical history, recent lab results, and current medications. The referring provider should provide much of this if the request-for-service form is well designed. Educators should verify the patient's understanding of information from the healthcare provider. Some of the medical data can be gathered on the first appointment, including blood pressure, weight, height, waist circumference, and BMI. If recent laboratory results including A1C, lipids, and microalbumin are not included on the request for service, encourage the patient to follow up with the healthcare provider to obtain these results before the next appointment. Educators should ask the patient to bring a list of current medications.

The psychosocial assessment can be done using a variety of tools. The Problem Areas in Diabetes Tool (PAID) is a simple, well-validated questionnaire to determine psychosocial distress with diabetes *(2)*. Two simple questions can screen for depression, a common risk for people with diabetes:

- During the past month have you been bothered by feeling down, depressed, or hopeless?
- During the past month have you been bothered by little interest or pleasure in doing things? *(3)*

Social questions include information about both the financial barriers to successful diabetes management and the people who provide support or interfere with self-management. Use the psychosocial assessment to determine if mental health services are needed to improve the patient's chances of successful diabetes management.

The behavioral assessment focuses on what the patient is currently doing and is willing to do to improve diabetes control. Knowledge does not always translate into action. Including behavioral questions like "How often do you check your blood glucose?" or "How often do you follow a meal plan?" can give baseline measurements that can be compared in follow-up assessments. When doing a nutrition assessment, explore the patient's typical eating patterns and food preferences. If the patient says, "I know I shouldn't drink regular soda, but I hate the taste of diet soda," ask about other non-caloric beverages the patient likes or would consider trying. Seven self-care behaviors are important to diabetes management: being active, healthy eating, taking medication, monitoring blood glucose, problem solving, reducing risks, and healthy coping (4). Joslin Diabetes Center adds working with the healthcare team to that list. Asking the patient to complete a behavioral questionnaire pre- and post-education can prioritize and focus discussion.

Additional components of the assessment include cultural issues, language, learning style, and health literacy. In assessing cultural issues, avoid making assumptions that any culture is homogenous. Use an open-ended question like "Is there anything you want me to understand about how your culture and religion influence your choices in managing your diabetes?" For patients who do not speak, understand, and/or read English, a professional interpreter is the best solution. Do not assume that a patient who does not read English will be able to read material written in his or her own language. For the hearing-impaired patient, provide assistive devices or an interpreter as required by law.

Educators should assess the patient's preferred learning style – demonstration, discussion, written material, or audio/video material. Further, educators should determine if the patient has any learning impairments – hearing, vision, dexterity, or cognitive dysfunction (5). It is imperative to accommodate for all these issues.

Health literacy is a stronger predictor of health status than is socioeconomic status, age, or ethnicity (6). The Test of Functional Health Literacy in Adults (TOFHLA) is currently the gold standard for health literacy but it is time consuming and therefore not practical for clinical practice (7). A tool called the Newest Vital Sign uses a nutrition label with six questions to assess health literacy (8). Numeracy, or quantitative literacy, is the ability to perform calculations using numbers found in printed materials (9). Counting carbohydrates and making insulin adjustments require quantitative literacy. Roughly half the adult population in the United States functions at an inadequate literacy level. Consider the patient's literacy level when providing written instructions or asking him or her to complete paperwork.

Group Assessment

Group assessment can be done by asking open-ended questions and then circling around the group to give everyone a chance to respond. This method gives the group a chance to know each other and to find others with common issues. Use a white board to record responses or have patients put their answers on a table tent. The advantage of the white board is that you can cross off patient topics as they are addressed. The table tent has the advantage of helping the educator refer back to the patient responses later in the session. Another strategy to help the educator remember participants' specific issues is to draw a seating chart of the room and put participants' specific information on the chart for later feedback and documentation.

SAMPLE OPEN-ENDED ASSESSMENT QUESTIONS

1. What is one thing you want to be sure we talk about today?
2. What is the most difficult thing about living with diabetes?
3. What parts of your diabetes management are you doing well?
4. What makes you afraid when you think about your diabetes?
5. How do you think a diabetes educator can help you?

Educators should ask the patient explicitly about his or her goals for the education session. Validate conclusions from the assessment by reflecting back your understanding of the patient's priorities for learning. A comment like "What I hear you saying is that you are afraid of going blind and you want to know what to do to prevent that" is an example. After confirming the patient's fear, educators should ask if anyone else in the group has that fear. Also, reassure the group that by the end of the session they will have several strategies to prevent blindness.

Readiness to Learn

Finally, the diabetes educator must determine the level of the patient's readiness to learn. Many newly diagnosed people with diabetes are understandably overwhelmed and may not be able to assimilate all the knowledge and skills that educators feel they need. The focus, initially, may need to be on survival skills. On the other hand, a newly diagnosed person may be very eager to embrace behavior change to avoid complications. The person with long-standing diabetes and complications may be discouraged and difficult to engage in the change process. In addition, common co-morbid conditions such as depression or obesity can present more challenges to the diabetes team. The Transtheoretical Model *(10)* provides a basis for evaluation and interventions to support behavior change utilizing diverse psychotherapeutic approaches. This approach starts with identification of the patient's stage of change related to the specific behavior: pre-contemplation, contemplation, preparation, action, and maintenance *(11)*. If the educator wants to focus on smoking cessation, but the patient says "I can't think about that right now" help the patient select another behavior. Continue to ask about readiness to stop smoking on subsequent visits. Asking the question may help move the patient to action in the future.

Educators need to be expert interviewers to complete a comprehensive assessment efficiently. The assessment is the foundation of the education plan. Without it, education is impersonal, may result in knowledge acquisition, but probably will not result in successful self-care by the patient. Educators must recognize that the person with diabetes is the expert in his or her disease. The educator facilitates learning and behavior change with a goal of improved outcomes and quality of life *(12)*.

EDUCATION PLAN

Once the assessment is complete, the next step is to develop a diabetes education plan. The education plan is much like a road map. It serves to lead the team and the patient through a process of education, negotiation, skill demonstration, application, and goal setting *(1)*. The plan will change over the course of time, depending on circumstances such as the patient's goals, rate of learning and understanding, functional health literacy, health status, and life events.

For the patient with long-standing diabetes, inquiring about what has worked in the past, what has not, and the reasons why is important. For example, it is common, when talking to patients about meal planning, to hear that they have seen dietitians before and that the diets "just didn't work." Careful probing of a statement such as this can reveal that perhaps dietitians did not tailor the person's meal plan to his or her lifestyle or that may be the meal plan was too low in calories. Maybe the patient did not understand the concept of exchanges or carbohydrate counting or was dealing with other life events and could not take the necessary time for meal planning. It is understandable that some patients may be reluctant to work with a dietitian, nurse educator, or exercise physiologist again, unless they feel reassured that the education plan will be developed based on the individualized assessment.

Motivational interviewing *(13)* is a patient-centered education and counseling method that involves exploring and resolving ambivalence. This is an effective approach when working with people who have a chronic disease, such as diabetes *(14)*. This approach encourages the educator to ask questions, has patients rate the importance of change, and explores readiness to change. The focus is to help a person find his inner motivation in order to elicit behavior change, rather than the educator telling the patient what he or she must do to take care of his or her diabetes *(15)*. While motivational interviewing encourages the person with diabetes to work on those areas that are important to them, an educator must also balance a person's motivation with a person's safety. For example, someone who takes insulin is at an increased risk of having hypoglycemia. This person must learn about the signs and symptoms of hypoglycemia, be able to monitor his or her blood glucose levels, appropriately treat the hypoglycemia, and possibly involve a friend or family member in learning how to use glucagon. If the educator relies solely on what the patient wants to learn about at every visit, the patient's safety could be compromised if the patient is unwilling or resistant to discussing other topics. Therefore, the healthcare team must be upfront about what skills and behaviors need to be acquired for the patient to manage his diabetes, ensuring that safety issues are addressed early on.

PLANNING: A STANDARD OF PROFESSIONAL PERFORMANCE FOR DIABETES EDUCATORS

Planning is a Standard of Professional Performance for Diabetes Educators *(16)*. The diabetes educator is responsible for developing the education plan with input from the patient; the patient, the healthcare team, the patient's referring provider, and the patient's support system then work to support the plan to achieve the expected outcomes. This team approach, which stems from a concept called collaborative management, is a way to help patients with diabetes (and other chronic diseases) to better handle self-management tasks *(17)*.

What comprises a patient's diabetes education plan? According to this performance standard *(16)*, an education plan should include or address:

- Specific outcomes
- Specific instructional strategies that will be used
- The individual's cultural, lifestyle, and health beliefs
- Measurable, behaviorally focused objectives
- Evaluation of the plan's effectiveness

In addition, the diabetes educator and the team must remember that the plan may need to change, based on the patient's diabetes, abilities, and possible lifestyle changes, as well as new diabetes technologies and research.

GOAL SETTING

The education plan is based on collaborative management, an approach that focuses on self-care by the chronically ill in partnership with effective medical, preventative and health maintenance strategies *(17)*. Collaborative management is enhanced by goal setting, which is essential to help the person with diabetes change behaviors to improve health. It is clear that behavior change does not happen overnight. Some goals may be more difficult to achieve than others. For example, a person may have no difficulty monitoring his blood glucose level three times daily. However, that same person may struggle with fitting a 30-minute walk into his schedule three times per week. Goal setting is a technique that helps to focus the patient on a particular behavior *(18)*.

Both the educator and the patient should mutually agree on the problem areas that need to be addressed. This is a step-wise process:

- Identify the problem area
- Select action steps for addressing the problem
- Put the plan into action
- Evaluate the results

Part of the diabetes self-management education process involves the patient acquiring the necessary knowledge needed to sufficiently manage his or her diabetes. However, much of the process involves developing and practicing specific skills needed for diabetes management, as well. For example, a patient can read the manual that comes with his blood glucose meter or be able to list foods that contain carbohydrates. However, knowledge does not necessarily translate into action. This same patient must be able to perform a blood glucose check using a meter and accurately determine the amount of carbohydrate he or she plans to eat at a meal in order to gauge how much insulin to take. This is where goal setting comes in: the educator and the patient agree upon a specific set of behavior change goals that will ideally result in behaviors that improve the patient's health and quality of life.

Many patients, especially those who are newly diagnosed with diabetes, are unfamiliar with setting behavioral goals and frequently will state a poorly defined, vague goal, such as "I will exercise more." Here's where the concept of SMART goals comes in. A SMART goal is Specific, Measurable, Achievable, Realistic, and Time bound. Let us take another look at this goal:

"I will exercise more."

What is missing here is a description of how that patient will do more exercise, what he or she will do for exericse, and over how much time. A more focused and SMART way of reworking this goal is as follows:

"I will walk for 20 minutes during my lunch break Monday through Friday for the next four weeks."

This goal requires the patient to take a specific action for a defined period of time, with the end result, hopefully, being more physically active. Goals, then, must be clearly written as being measurable and observable, allowing both the patient and the educator to determine if those goals have been achieved *(19)*.

The healthcare team's job is to assess how well the patient is meeting his or her goals at each visit. The responsibility of goal reinforcement and adjustment may lie primarily between the educator and the patient, but the chances of successful behavior change can be improved if the entire healthcare team is involved in the diabetes self-management education process *(20)*. In many cases, behavioral goals or objectives will need to be revised, based on the patient's circumstances and abilities. Documenting the defined behavioral goals and progress toward those goals at every visit is crucial. If the only goal the patient ever sets is to walk during lunch, but ends up working during her lunch break, the long-term goal of being more physically active may not happen, and the person may struggle with diabetes control.

IMPLEMENTING THE EDUCATION PLAN

The process of delivering diabetes self-management education has evolved over the years. Many diabetes educators are familiar with the days of limitless individual education sessions. However, changes to the payor system and regulations put forth by Medicare have shifted the focus away from individual or one-on-one sessions to group-counseling sessions. Evidence shows group counseling to be both effective and efficient from an educational standpoint and a cost perspective *(21–23)*.

The process of group education has evolved, as well. While many educators still teach using a didactic approach whereby the educator "lectures" and the patients passively participate, research tells us that engaging the patient in the education process is more effective in implementing behavior change *(24)*. A format that uses group discussion, questions and answers, or one of the newest approaches, using Conversation Maps (www.healthyi.com) allows the educator to take the role of "facilitator" rather than "teacher" and also helps ensure that the session better meets the needs and interests of the participants. The participants also will benefit from sharing experiences and tips with each other.

Many educators who are unaccustomed to leading groups are concerned about performing an assessment and setting behavioral goals with participants, especially if the group is large. While this concern is understandable, it requires the educator to make a paradigm shift: put the onus on the patient to complete the assessment and goal-setting process. Patients can complete a brief, focused self-assessment that is then reviewed by the healthcare team. Patients can also easily determine their own behavioral objectives by either stating them or using a simple checklist tool. The educator must be attuned to patients who may have psychosocial or learning issues that would impede them from successfully participating in a group setting. While group education is recognized as being effective, it is not appropriate for all people with diabetes. Some patients simply learn better in individual sessions. The educator must also pay attention to patients who may have particular acute or chronic complications that require more immediate intervention.

The assessment skills of the educator can help determine how a particular patient best learns. A person who has learning difficulties or who does not speak English may not be suited to a group class; instead, this person would benefit from an individual session that incorporates lower literacy education tools. On the other hand, a busy executive who frequently travels may not have time to attend a series of diabetes classes. That person may do better with Internet-based learning modules or DVDs, for example *(5)*. The point, then, is not necessarily the education setting but, rather, the process and interventions that help the patient to implement behavior change.

In summary, an education plan is a crucial component of the diabetes self-management education process. Each person with diabetes should have his or her own individualized education plan, as no two people with diabetes are alike nor are their self-management goals alike. Furthermore, the education plan is not static; rather, it is a living document in that it must continually be adjusted and updated to reflect a patient's lifestyle circumstances. The entire healthcare team (including the patient) should "buy-in" and support the plan in order for it to be successful. Finally, the education plan must be documented in every patient's medical record to help monitor progress and to meet quality and accreditation standards. *(5)*

THE NEXT STEP: EDUCATION FOLLOW UP

Educators understand the value of follow up to treat this challenging chronic disease, but patients may see diabetes education as a single or short-term experience. Try to convey the message that treatment strategies change as a result of new research, individual circumstances, and changes in physiology. Additional education can help the person with diabetes respond to these changes.

Follow up consists of:

- Monitoring of status and self-management
- Encouragement and facilitation of regular clinical care
- Encouragement and motivation of self-management
- Facilitating skills for coping with changes in circumstances or emergent problems *(25)*

There is no set follow-up pattern. Some patients will require frequent educator contact, others may do fine with primary care provider follow up, and still others may benefit most from community support. Since the goal is to self-manage diabetes, follow up should be scheduled to help the patient reach that overarching goal.

The follow-up process includes assessment, evaluation of goals, and setting new goals. One way to measure goal attainment is to ask "What percent of the time do you. . .?"

This allows for quantitative measurement for goal tracking. It also helps to ask the questions: "How important is this goal for you?" and "How confident do you feel about attaining this goal?" *(26)*. Compare the answers to the previous education session and share and discuss the changes with the patient. This is an easy way to generate discussion about goal achievement and the need to change the plan. Ask patients if they found the plan helpful. If not, reassure them that the plan is designed to be changed to best meet their needs *(27)*.

Follow up does not have to be in a formal education session. Individualize the follow up by offering individual or group interactions, including phone, email, or regular mail as follow-up methods. Use caution in offering phone and email support, both non-reimbursable efforts that can become extremely time consuming. Most of an educator's time should be spent face-to-face educating patients to assure the financial viability of the program. Share with patients the community resources that can be helpful including: diabetes support groups, Weight Watchers, Overeaters Anonymous, walking clubs, exercise facilities, community pharmacists, and mental health providers.

An essential component of follow up is referral back to the primary care provider. Stress to the patient the importance of regular visits to the healthcare provider and timely laboratory testing. Knowledge of key diabetes numbers including A1C, blood pressure, lipid levels, and microalbumin results, along with frequency of eye and foot exams, is the most important way to evaluate the effectiveness of the education plan as well as to identify and prevent complications. Clarify when the patient needs to contact the healthcare provider for urgent evaluation: sick days, unexplained hyper or hypoglycemia, medication side effects, new symptoms of complications, unexplained weight gain or loss, problems taking prescribed medications, and any time he/she does not feel well.

Educators have a responsibility to develop a supportive community by working with community leaders and public health officials and link patients to that ongoing support. One great resource for ongoing support is the program developed by the Centers for Disease Control and Prevention and the National Institutes of Health titled *New Beginnings: A Discussion Guide for Living Well with Diabetes*. This notebook is designed to guide lay or professionally run support groups *(28)*.

Use caution in trying to take ownership of your patient's diabetes. There are not enough trained diabetes educators to see everyone with diabetes forever. The goal of diabetes education is self-management. Educators support the patient in the behavior change process, but it is up to the patient to do the work. If patients resist your efforts to help, reassure them that the door is always open when they are ready for more assistance in managing diabetes and try to link them to community support.

DOCUMENTATION AND INFORMATICS

Documentation is an essential component of the diabetes education process. In fact, Standard 7 of the National Standards for Diabetes Self-Management Education states:

An individual assessment and education plan will be developed collaboratively by the participant and instructor(s) to direct the selection of appropriate educational interventions and self-management support strategies. This assessment and education plan and the intervention and outcomes will be documented in the education record. (29)

Purpose of Documentation

Documentation of the education plan and the patient's outcomes may seem obvious to the healthcare provider. The documentation of each patient visit serves as a communication tool for the healthcare team, can help to prevent duplication of services (thus saving time and resources), and provides a picture of the patient's adherence to the diabetes care and education plan. In addition, documentation is required in order for a program to be accredited and to receive payment for services. *(5)*

Consumers of Documentation

The patient's medical record is generally the primary documentation tool. The medical record might be a paper chart, although more and more diabetes centers are using electronic medical records. When documentation of the diabetes care process is done properly, including an assessment, goals and objectives, and educational interventions and outcomes, the patient's progress (or lack of progress) is clearly defined and can help determine the next step in both the medical and the educational process. For example, a patient may refuse to start on insulin and instead persuade the healthcare team to allow that patient more time to focus on meal planning and physical activity. However, after several months of consistent high blood glucose readings and an elevated A1C, the team may be able to convince the patient to begin insulin. Without documentation of the patient's efforts and the team's interventions, appropriate diabetes treatment could be delayed. Therefore, the consumers of documentation are the patient, the diabetes educator, the physician, and any of the other team members involved in the patient's care.

Components of Documentation

What is truly needed when one documents the outcomes of a patient encounter? In order to help answer this question, it is helpful to remember the purpose of documentation. As Funnell and Mensing state in the *Complete Nurse's Guide to Diabetes Care*, "The documentation should provide enough information so that others can follow up and reinforce content as needed and assess goal attainment *(5)*." Because visits to diabetes educators are often limited based on Medicare and insurance regulations, it is critical to optimize each visit and encounter. Having to search for information from a previous visit or working with incomplete or poorly documented medical records wastes time and impedes the education and diabetes treatment process. Documentation becomes especially crucial if a diabetes educator works in private practice or has little contact with the patient's physician and other healthcare team members.

Given that the patient's medical record is the venue for determining progress and adherence, it helps to view the documentation process according to the steps of diabetes self-management: assessment, outcomes identification, planning, implementation, and evaluation *(30,31)*. Think of documentation of diabetes education as an on-going process that supports all the above steps of diabetes self-management education *(32)*. No matter in which stage of DSME the patient is engaged, documentation of that visit should include the following:

- Date and time of visit and of any assessments and interventions
- Patient's readiness and willingness to make changes, along with his or her values and perceptions
- Treatment and behavioral goals and any identified barriers to achievement
- Identified clinical and behavioral outcomes, as determined by the assessment
- Descriptions of specific interventions, including educational materials and tools
- Patient's receptivity and understanding of those interventions
- Progress toward identified goals and objectives
- Clinical and behavioral outcomes
- Plans for follow-up or for discontinuation of care
- Referrals to other providers or programs
- Any communication with the referring provider *(31)*

Obviously, there is a lot of information to organize and document. Unless there is a central and convenient area in the medical records in which to document this information, being able to identify progress, track outcomes, or readily make changes to the treatment plan can be difficult. Using forms and checklists is one way to help organize and document pertinent information. In addition, using these tools may help the busy educator document the "right amount" of information – neither too much nor too little. Time is usually of the essence for a busy educator, and the use of documentation forms can ensure that documentation is done in an efficient manner.

One example of a form that can help to track patient progress is the AADE 7 Self-Care Behaviors™ Goal Sheet *(4)*. This particular form serves a dual purpose: it can ensure that the educator covers the seven critical self-care behaviors with the patient, and it allows the diabetes team (including the patient) to view and track goals and progress in a systematic way. The Goal Sheet is helpful in that it allows progress toward these self-care behaviors to be documented at the initial visit (baseline), and then at 1-, 3-, 6-, and 12-month intervals. Use of this form, or a similar form, will also help in the aggregate documentation process, which is necessary for education program recognition, reimbursement, and continuous quality improvement.

To further help the educator focus on what is most essential for documentation, it is beneficial to remember that the diabetes self-management education process focuses primarily on outcomes: measuring outcomes, monitoring outcomes and finally, managing outcomes in order to evaluate an individual's progress and the diabetes education program, as a whole *(33)*.

Medical Records: Paper vs. Electronic

More and more diabetes programs are using electronic medical records, or EMRs. Strides in technology have helped to improve the ease of use and overall functioning of EMRs, although changing over to an EMR is often difficult and rife with growing pains. Of course, many diabetes programs and provider offices do not have the funds necessary to implement an EMR in their setting; thus, paper charts remain the mainstay for many. Some educator and providers are hesitant or even fearful about switching over to an EMR. This reluctance may stem from a fear of technology or mistrust that the system might fail and data could be lost. With a little instruction, time, practice, and patience, along with a competent data back-up system, these fears can be dispelled.

If implementation of an EMR is not feasible, another alternative is to use a diabetes registry. A registry helps the provider or practice keep track of its diabetes patients, target high-risk patients, send reminders to patients regarding appointments (e.g., for classes or lab work), and monitor the outcomes *(34)*. Use of diabetes registries has been shown to be cost-effective. One recent report showed that diabetes registries save $14.5 billion over 10 years *(35)*.

CONCLUSION

In conclusion, unlike many other chronic diseases, diabetes is truly a condition of self-management. It is the responsibility of the person with diabetes to acquire the knowledge and behaviors that he or she needs to effectively manage his or her diabetes, maintain overall health, and improve or maintain quality of life. The educator, in turn, has a responsibility to ensure that each person with diabetes receives quality education and has the behavioral skill set needed to live healthfully with a chronic disease. The diabetes education process, as discussed in this chapter, is a means of ensuring that the person with diabetes, the educator, and the entire healthcare team can work together to implement a successful diabetes education and treatment plan.

REFERENCES

1. Blair, E. Patient education. In: Beaser, RS and the Staff of Joslin Diabetes Center. Joslin's Diabetes Deskbook: A Guide for Primary Care Providers, 2nd ed. Boston: Joslin Diabetes Center, 2007:385–402.
2. Polonsky, WH, Anderson BJ, Lohrer, PA, Welch, G, Jacobson, AM, Aponte, JE, Schwartz, CE. Assessment of diabetes-related distress. Diabetes Care 1995;18:754–760.
3. Whooley, MA, Avins AL, Miranda J et al. Case-finding instruments for depression. Two questions are as good as many. J Gen Intern Med 1997; 12:439–45.
4. Mulcahy K, Maryniuk M, Peeples M, Peyrot M, Tomky D, Weaver T, Yarborough P. Diabetes self-management education core outcomes measures. Diabetes Educ 2003;29:768–70, 773–84, 787–8.
5. Funnell, MH, Mensing, CR. Diabetes education in the management of diabetes. In: Childs BP, Cypress M, Spollett G. Complete Nurse's Guide to Diabetes Care. Alexandria: American Diabetes Association 2005:188–198.
6. Williams, MV, Baker DW, Parker RM et al. Relationship of functional health literacy to patients' knowledge of their chronic disease: A study of patients with hypertension and diabetes. Arch Intern Med 1998; 158:166–72.
7. Osborn CY, Weiss, BD, Davis TC et al. Measuring adult literacy in health care: performance of the newest vital sign. Am J Health Behav 2007; 31 (Suppl 3):S36–46.
8. Weiss, BD, Mays MZ, Martz W et al. Quick assessment of literacy in primary care: the newest vital sign. Ann Fam Med 2005;3:514–22.
9. Committee on Performance Levels for Adult Literacy. Measuring literacy: performance levels for adults. Washington, DC: National Academies Press; 2005. http://newton.nap.edu/catalog/11267.html#description.
10. Prochaska, JO, DiClemente, CC. Stages and processes of self-change of smoking: Toward an integrative model of change. J Consult Clin Psychol 1983;51:390–395.
11. Highstein, GR, O'Toole, ML, Shetty, G, Brownson, CA, Fisher, EB. Use of the Transtheoretical Model to enhance resources and supports for diabetes self-management. Diabetes Educ 2007;33(Suppl 6):193S–200S.
12. Swenson, K, Brackenridge, B. The Art of Diabetes Education: Discover Your Path to Excellence 2006; Diabetes Management & Training Center, 30–43.
13. Rollnick S, Miller WR. What is motivational interviewing? Behav Cogn Psychother 1995;23:325–334.
14. Welch G, Rose G, Ernst D. Motivational interviewing and diabetes: What is it, how is it used and does it work? Diabetes Spectr 2006;19:5–11.
15. Bundy C. Changing behavior: using motivational interviewing techniques. J R Soc Med 2004;97(Suppl 44):43–47.
16. Martin C, Daly A, McWorter LS, Shwide-Slavin C, Kushion W. The scope of practice, standards of practice, and standards of professional performance for diabetes educators. Diabetes Educ 2005;31:487–512.

17. Von Korff M, Gruman J, Schaefer J, Curry S, Wagner E. Collaborative management of chronic illness. Ann Intern Med 1997;127:1097–102.
18. Langford, AT, Sawyer DR, Gioimo S, Brownson CA, O'Toole ML. Patient-centered goal setting as a tool to improve diabetes self-management. Diabetes Educ 2007;33(Suppl 6): 139S–144S.
19. Hill JVC. Writing behavioral objectives: tips from an educator and auditor. On the Cutting Edge 2005;23:682–9.
20. Glasgow RE, Funnell MM, Bonomi AE et al. Self-management aspects of the Improving Chronic Illness Care Breakthrough series: design and implementation with diabetes and heart failure teams. Ann Behav Med 2002;24:80–87.
21. Rickheim PL, Weaver TW, Flader JL, Kendall DM. Assessment of group versus individual diabetes education: a randomized study. Diabetes Care 2002;25:269–74.
22. Heller SR, Clarke P, Daly H, et al. Group education for obese patients with type 2 diabetes: greater success at less cost. Diabetes Med 1988;5:552–6.
23. Campbell EM, Redman S, Moffitt PS, Sanson-Fisher RW. The relative effectiveness of educational and behavioral instruction programs for patients with NIDDM: a randomized trial. Diabetes Educ 1996;22:379–86.
24. Barlow J, Wright C, Sheasby J et al. Self-management approaches for people with chronic conditions: A review. Patient Educ Couns 2002;48:177–187.
25. Fisher, EB, Brownson, CA, O'Toole, ML, Anwuri, VV. Ongoing follow-up and support for chronic disease management in the Robert Wood Johnson Foundation Diabetes Initiative. Diabetes Educ 2007;3(Suppl 6):201S–207S.
26. Zweben A, Zuckoff A. Motivational interviewing and treatment adherence. In: Motivational Interviewing: Preparing People for Change. Miller WR, Rollnick S, eds. New York: Guilford Press, 2002:299–319.
27. Weigner, K, Murrich, SJ. Behavioral strategies for improving self-management. In: Complete Nurse's Guide to Diabetes Care. Childs BP, Cypress M, Spollett G. Alexandria: American Diabetes Association, 2005:199–206.
28. Centers for Disease Control and Prevention and the National Institutes of Health New Beginnings: A Discussion Guide for Living Well with Diabetes, 2005, www.ndep.nih.gov.
29. Funnell MM, Brown TL, Childs BP et al. National standards for diabetes self-management education. Diabetes Care 2007;30:1630–37.
30. Report of the Task Force on the Delivery of Diabetes Self-Management Education and Medical Nutrition Therapy. Diabetes Spectr 1999;12:44–7.
31. American Association of Diabetes Educators. The scope of practice, standards of practice, and standards of professional performance for diabetes educators. Diabetes Educ 2005;31: 487–513.
32. Lacey K, Pritchett E. Nutrition care process and model: ADA adopts road map to quality care and outcomes management. J Am Diet Assoc 2003;103:1061–72.
33. American Association of Diabetes Educators. Standards for outcomes measurement of diabetes self-management education. Diabetes Educ 2003;29:804–16.
34. Gabbay RA, Khan L, Peterson KL. Critical features for a successful implementation of a diabetes registry. Diabetes Technol Ther 2005;7:958–67.
35. Bu D, Pan E, Johnston D et al. The value of information technology-enabled diabetes management. 2007. Available on the Internet at: www.citl.org/research/ITDM.htm.

5 Making the Most of the Outpatient Visit

Carolè Mensing, RN, MA, CDE and
Deborah Hinnen, ARNP, BC-ADM, CDE, FAAN

Contents

Introduction
Role of the Team
Healthy Eating
Monitoring
Ketone Testing
Height and Weight Monitoring
Being Active
Taking Diabetes Medications
Medication Review by Type and Action
Commonly Asked Questions
Summary
References

Abstract

Primary care providers deliver more outpatient diabetes management than any other group of health care professionals. However, primary care providers are faced with several challenges in providing diabetes education. Time restraints, high patient volumes, and other medical issues that must be addressed are just some of the many factors that may impede effective diabetes education. Solutions to these issues include involving the entire outpatient office staff in the diabetes management of the patient; focusing on issues of most concern to the patient; providing basic,

From: *Contemporary Diabetes: Educating Your Patient with Diabetes*
Edited by: K. Weinger and C. A. Carver, DOI 10.1007/978-1-60327-208-7_5,
© Humana Press, a part of Springer Science+Business Media, LLC 2009

"survival" skill education; and referring, when appropriate, to other specialists, including endocrinologists and diabetes educators.

Key Words: Outpatient Diabetes, Patient Education, Diabetes Self-Management Education, Outpatient Interdisciplinary Team Care.

INTRODUCTION

Managing diabetes in the outpatient practice setting is critical to the successful outcomes of improved metabolic control, reduced risk for complications, improved health, and overall quality of life for people with diabetes. Enhancing self-care skills and behaviors is key to helping people with diabetes achieve successful outcomes. Providers working in the outpatient setting are charged with providing effective educational information that in turn will help patients learn self-care skills and behaviors to better manage their diabetes.

It is widely accepted that primary care providers deliver more outpatient diabetes management than any other group of health care professionals. The standards of care *(1)* suggest that it is incumbent on the providers to assure that comprehensive education is available for people with diabetes. With the ever-growing complexity of insulin delivery devices, diabetes medications, and blood glucose monitoring tools it is more challenging than ever to tailor treatment protocols to the patient.

Primary care providers seldom have more than a few minutes to spend with each patient, and therefore may be able to only teach basic diabetes skills and provide "survival" education. Therefore, prioritizing and implementing initial treatment protocols, delivering basic education, and making appropriate referrals to diabetes educators and other specialists is probably the most realistic expectations for today's outpatient practitioner.

The clinicians and educators in the outpatient setting often must integrate diabetes education into a visit when diabetes itself may not be the primary reason for the visit, as evidence shows that comprehensive care and education are essential for the person with a chronic disease, such as diabetes *(2)*. Medical office staff, including medical assistants, licensed practical nurses, and even office managers, are important members of the outpatient care team to help ensure that diabetes patients are given the time and information that they need to effectively manage their diabetes.

ROLE OF THE TEAM

The "diabetes team" in the outpatient setting may extend well beyond the clinical staff in the provider's office. The provider and office staff work to coordinate care and education. Their role is to provide treatment recommendations and basic diabetes education; begin the process of teaching problem solving and coping skills; and provide additional resources and referrals for more comprehensive education. Too many patients continue to receive little or no diabetes education in the community (3).

One concern of office staff is choosing the appropriate diabetes-related topic to address first. This challenge is easily addressed by asking the patient what he or she would like to discuss. Letting the patient guide the educational session will help ensure that the most relevant information to the patient during the visit is provided. For patients who are newly diagnosed with diabetes and unsure of what they need to know, providing a list of various topics or a simple education brochure can help guide the discussion. In addition, the provider should be prepared to help the patient set one or two realistic and achievable goals to work on between visits. These initial diabetes education goals are identified in Table 1.

Because time is limited and patient volume is high, the outpatient team needs to quickly establish a "connection" with their patients. A simple yet direct approach recommended by Pichert and Schlundt (5) is to create an environment that encourages people to be comfortable discussing goals, feelings, and problems; use a variety of assessment and interviewing skills and a variety of strategies to elicit what the patient wants and needs from the visit; and develop an understanding of the patient's specific problems and motivations. Anderson and Patrias (6) recommend having the patient complete a short assessment prior to his or her visit. This assessment allows an opportunity to write down issues the patient would like to discuss with the provider and asks the patient to indicate areas of difficulty in terms of self-management.

At the conclusion of the visit, it is helpful if the provider writes down a plan of action in collaboration with the patient and those in attendance (see Table 2). A written plan of action serves to clarify specific behaviors and goals to be carried out between visits, gives the patient an opportunity to ask questions or voice concerns, and helps ensure that the patient feels engaged in their care planning.

Table 1
Survival Skills

Survival skill education (4):

(a)   Initiate healthy eating guidelines, including consistent carbohydrate intake
(b)   Teach the patient how to safely take medication
(c)   Initiate self-monitoring blood glucose (SMBG) to evaluate treatment
(d)   Instruct on hypoglycemia treatment and prevention if on hypoglycemic-inducing medications
(e)   Provide information on how and when to call the provider
(f)   Refer for comprehensive diabetes education including medical nutrition therapy
(g)   Involve family and care partners as directed by patient

Table 2
Diabetes Action Plan

Diabetes Action Plan

1. Medication:
     Time/dose_____
     Special instructions_____

2. Meal plan: _____

3. Blood glucose/urine ketone monitoring:

   Your target blood glucose goal is _____mg/dl before meals
                                      _____mg/dl before bedtime
                                      _____mg/dl 2 h after a meal

   Check blood glucose_____times a day/week:

       ☐ before breakfast   ☐ _____hour after breakfast
       ☐ before lunch   ☐ _____hour after lunch
       ☐ before dinner   ☐ _____hour after dinner
       ☐ at bedtime   ☐ Other _____

   Call your physician or diabetes educator if your blood glucose is higher
   than_____mg/dl for more than _____readings/day in a row.

       If you have type 1 diabetes or you are using insulin, and blood glucose levels are above
   250 mg/dl, check your urine for ketones.

       If the ketones are moderate or large (deep purple on the color chart), call your physician
   immediately.

4. Activity/Exercise Plan
     Type _____Frequency _____Duration _____
     If you are not already exercising, discuss a safe exercise plan with your
     physician first.
     Special Instructions _____

5. Important Information:
     Your primary physician is _____Phone #_____Next appointment is_____
     Your diabetes physician is _____Phone #_____Next appointment is_____
     Your diabetes educator is _____Phone #_____Next appointment is _____
     Your dietitian is _____Phone #_____Next appointment is _____
     Other appointments: _____
   Telephone number to call for questions or problems: _____

6. Self-management behaviors/goals are
       1. Meal plan _____
       2. Activity _____
       3. Monitoring _____
       4. Medication _____
       5. Other Risk Reduction, Tobacco/Alcohol use _____
       Follow-up: Call:_____
            Visit: _____

Future office visit timelines, topics, and informational planning guidelines are shown in Table 3.

The following section offers brief, topic-specific information and considerations for clinical staff and their patients when providing diabetes management and education in the outpatient setting.

Table 3
Office Flow for the Person with Diabetes

At time of symptoms or annual physical	*Staff*
Initial	
1. Confirm diagnosis of T2DM:	Provider (Physician,
a. FBS $\geq$ 126 mg/Random > 200 mg	nurse practitioner)
2. Write Rx for glucose monitor	
a. Request tests fasting and 2 h after meals 3 days per week	Provider
3. Determine medication need	
a. Diabetes	Provider
b. Lipids	
c. Hypertension	
4. Advise on healthy eating	
5. Refer for diabetes education/dietitian appt	Nurse
2 weeks/1 month follow-up	
1. Review blood glucose log	Provider
a. If fastings elevated (above 110 mg), increase metformin	
b. If post-meal glucose elevated, consider sitagliptin, secretagogue, TZD, exenatide, or basal insulin	
2. Begin standards of care monitoring	
a. Foot exam with monofilament	
b. Blood pressure	
c. Weight/waist circumference	
d. Continue diabetes education/MNT or verify referral	
3-month follow-up visits	
1. Review blood glucose log/down load glucose meter	Provider
2. Repeat A1C	
3. Repeat lipid panel, if appropriate	

(Continued)

Table 3 *(Continued)*

At time of symptoms or annual physical	*Staff*
4. Titrate meds as needed	
5. If glucose stable refer for dilated eye exam	
6. Continue education reinforcement	
7. Recheck BP/Wt/waist circumference	
Annual visit	
1. Repeat A1C	Provider
2. Repeat lipid panel	
3. Check microalbumin	
4. Check BP/Wt/waist circumference	
5. Complete foot exam with monofilament	
6. Provide flu and pneumonia vaccines, as indicated	
7. Refer for annual dilated eye exam	
8. Refer for dental exam	
9. Continue diabetes education reinforcement/referral	
10. Titrate meds as needed	
11. Renew prescriptions	
a. Glucose testing strips/lancets/control solution	
b. Meds: Diabetes/Lipids/HTN	
Documentation every visit	All Staff
1. Flow sheet	
2. Plan of case	

HEALTHY EATING

People with diabetes can and should eat the same as people without diabetes. Eating a variety of foods is necessary for overall health. Many people with type 2 diabetes are overweight and may have other complications in addition to their diabetes, such as hypertension or heart disease. Teaching these patients to eat smaller portions and reduce their intake of fat and sodium is important *(1)*. For others, emphasizing consistency in terms of meal and snack times can help minimize fluctuations in blood glucose levels. All patients with diabetes will benefit from learning which foods contain carbohydrate and how to read a food label. Outpatient providers can be instrumental in providing basic meal planning guidelines to the patient until he or she meets with a registered dietitian for an individualized meal plan.

Considerations

1. Help people get started with healthy eating. Begin by using the term "meal plan" rather than "diet." Easy patient instruction examples are to

   a. Reduce portion sizes, eat all foods in moderation, and eat from all the food groups.

   b. Aim to eat about the same amount of carbohydrate foods at meals and snacks every day. Foods that contain carbohydrate include bread, pasta, rice, fruit, milk, and desserts.

   c. Eat fiber-rich foods including whole grain breads and cereals, and fruits and vegetables.

   d. Choose beverages with little or no carbohydrates such as water, seltzer, and sugar-free soft drinks.

   e. Demonstrate the use of the plate method: fill half of the plate with vegetables, a quarter with a carbohydrate food, such as brown rice, and the other quarter with a lean protein, such as chicken, fish, or lean meat. Add a serving of fruit or non-fat or low-fat milk or yogurt.

2. Encourage patients to keep a food record for at least several days during the week. Providers, in turn, must take the time to review and briefly discuss food records at each visit; failing to do so devalues the importance of record keeping.

3. Schedule an appointment with a registered dietitian for medical nutrition therapy (1). While all clinicians can provide general meal planning advice and guidance, the team member with the most expertise and demonstrated effectiveness for medical nutrition therapy is a registered dietitian, and only dietitians can bill for medical nutrition therapy.

4. Help correlate blood glucose values with food intake and activity. Suggest that patients occasionally check glucose levels after meals to learn how a particular food or meal affects their blood glucose. If glucose levels are high after a meal, discuss ways that the patient might prevent this, such as eating smaller portions or going for a walk after a meal.

Each of the above actions helps to increase the patient's awareness about food intake in relation to glucose levels (4) and begins the process of establishing healthy eating habits. Patients may also be more likely to learn more about meal planning and achieving and maintaining a healthy weight.

MONITORING

The concept and process of self-monitoring of blood glucose can be overwhelming for both the person with diabetes and the provider. One of the first hurdles to overcome is the fear of sticking oneself with a lancet in order to obtain a blood sample. Some patients may require more time and patience in learning this skill than others. Patients must then learn when and how often to monitor and what to do with the information. The key is to start with only the basic information that patients need to complete an accurate blood glucose check.

There are a variety of meters to choose from, but essentially the procedure for obtaining a blood sample and performing a glucose check is the same from meter to meter. Meter choice is determined by several factors, including insurance coverage, lifestyle, manual dexterity, and visual acuity. Medical assistants and licensed practical nurses can be trained on the technical aspects of teaching patients the process of blood glucose monitoring, as well as when and how often to check, with guidance from the provider. However, the provider should reinforce the importance of bringing in the meter and logbook and review blood glucose data with the patient at every visit. Most meters also allow results to be easily downloaded with appropriate software available from the manufacturer.

Continuous glucose monitoring is now available. This technology allows one to check interstitial glucose values every 5 min. An internal sensor is worn, much like an insulin pump infusion set, and glucose data is transmitted to a receiver. However, one must continue to monitor blood glucose levels with a meter; the use of continuous glucose monitoring does not replace fingersticks.

Considerations

1. Help the patient select an appropriate meter, based on such factors as insurance, visual ability, and manual dexterity. People with vision impairment and the elderly often have specific monitoring issues that can be addressed by referring to a diabetes education program for individualization and appropriate adaptive equipment.
2. Encourage the patient to monitor at specific times, such as before and after meals and at bedtime; that will help to determine if the diabetes treatment plan is working.
3. Instruct the patient to record glucose results in a logbook, and always review and discuss the results at every visit.

KETONE TESTING

Urine (or blood) ketone testing provides information about the metabolic status of the patient. Patients with type 1 diabetes are prone to ketosis in the absence of insulin; the presence of ketones can signify impending diabetic ketoacidosis, a serious and life-threatening condition if not treated promptly. Patients with type 2 diabetes are less prone to ketosis, but those requiring insulin are often advised to check for ketones in certain circumstances, such as illness. Also, women with gestational diabetes are taught to check for ketones in the morning urine; the presence of ketones can indicate overnight starvation, which is remedied by increasing food intake in the evening. Additional monitoring guidelines can be found in the American Diabetes Association's Standards of Medical Care in Diabetes (1).

HEIGHT AND WEIGHT MONITORING

It is common practice for outpatient staff to routinely check weight at each clinic visit. Weight changes have significant implications for chronic disease care and can be a first indicator of poorly controlled diabetes. Weight gain or loss may also indicate fluid retention, eating disorders, and depression, for example; therefore, weight accuracy and consistency is important. It is also important to routinely measure the patient's height, especially in older women if osteoporosis is a concern. Body mass index, a common weight status measure, cannot be accurately calculated without an accurate height measurement.

In addition to height and weight, the measurement of a patient's waist circumference is an important indicator of obesity and heart disease risk. Instructions are available elsewhere for obtaining an accurate measurement using a measuring tape. A waist circumference of greater than 40 inches for men and greater than 35 inches for women is indicative of increased risk for heart disease *(7)*.

Considerations

1. Accuracy in measurements is essential.
2. Accuracy in Documentation is important.

BEING ACTIVE

Encouraging people to be physically active is challenging. For most people, getting started is the hardest part. Many people think they need to enroll in a gym and purchase special equipment, when, in fact, a simple walking program or even routine housework are effective ways to become more physically fit. Encouraging patients to increase their daily activities of living, such as taking the stairs one or two flights or parking the care further away, is another way to ease patients into becoming more active. The important short-term goals surrounding physical activity are to make some modest lifestyle changes *(8,9)*.

Considerations

1. Get moving. Start an activity or increase current activity by 5 min each day. Choose an activity that is enjoyable, such as walking, dancing, or bicycling.
2. Plan to do 30 min of activity most days of the week. Breaking activity into shorter, 10-min segments is allowable.
3. Advance to 150 min of activity a week.
4. Consider wearing a pedometer to measure steps. The long-term goal for most people is to aim for 10,000 steps per day.

Some patients will need a medical evaluation, including a stress test, before increasing their level of activity. Patients with diabetic complications, such as retinopathy or neuropathy, may have certain limitations; refer these patients to a qualified exercise physiologist or physical therapist.

To prevent hypoglycemia, encourage patients who take insulin or certain diabetes medications that can lead to hypoglycemia to monitor their blood glucose before and after activity. Patients should also be instructed to carry treatment for hypoglycemia, such as glucose tablets or glucose gel, carry identification, wear appropriate footwear, and to stop activity immediately and seek medical attention if pain or shortness of breath occurs.

TAKING DIABETES MEDICATIONS

Medication management is based on the metabolic defects of diabetes. In type 1 diabetes mellitus, an autoimmune-triggered destruction of the beta cells, insulin is required. Type 2 diabetes mellitus has multiple defects *(10)*. Insulin resistance is the distinguishing feature of type 2 diabetes.

A variety of medications are available as treatment options. Most pharmacologic therapies reduce A1C 1–2% *(11,12)*. These are summarized in Tables 4 and 5. This section reviews type of medicines commonly prescribed, how it works in the body, instructions or cautions, and coaching tips for staff.

Considerations

1. Initiate medication therapy that is safe and effective.
2. Teach patients how medication works, when to take it, and what side effects to watch for.

MEDICATION REVIEW BY TYPE AND ACTION

Metformin

Metformin reduces hepatic glucose release by two mechanisms: reducing gluconeogenesis and glycogenolysis. To a lesser degree it also improves peripheral glucose utilization much like the thiazolidinediones.

Metformin is the most commonly prescribed oral agent for type 2 diabetes. In fact, the treatment protocol developed by the American Diabetes Association and the European Association for the Study of Diabetes recommends metformin as initial therapy *(11)*.

CONSIDERATIONS

1. Creatinine should be less than 1.5 mg/dl in men and less than 1.4 mg/dl in women before starting metformin.
2. Gastrointestinal problems, such as flatulence and diarrhea, can be minimized if taken with food or immediately after the meal.

Table 4
Oral Agents

Generic name	Trade Name	When to take	Doses	Side Effects
Secretagogues (Hypoglycemia Agents) – Stimulates the pancreas to produce more insulin				
Sulfonylureas				
Glyburide	Diabeta or Micronase	30 min before meals	1.25, 2.5, 5 mg (Max: 20 mg)	
Glyburide-press tab	Glynase	30 min before meals	1.5, 3, 6 mg (Max: 12 mg)	Low blood glucose-Hypoglycemia
Glipizide	Glucotrol	30 min before meals	5, 10 mg (Max: 40 mg)	Weight gain
Glipizide	Glucotrol XL	before or with meals	5, 10 mg (Max: 20 mg)	
Glimepiride	Amaryl	before or with meals	1, 2, 4 mg (Max: 8 mg)	
Meglitinides				
Repaglinide blood glucose;	Prandin	5-30 min before meals	0.5, 1, 2, mg (Max: 16 mg)	Low
				Headaches
Nateglinide	Starlix	5-30 min before meals	120 mg, 60 mg	
Biguanides – Decrease hepatic glucose production				
Metformin (Glucophage, Riomet-liquid)		Take with meals	500, 850, 1000 mg	Nausea; Diarrhea;
Metformin Extended Release				Metallic Taste;
(Glucophage XR; Glumetza, Fortamet)			500&1000 mg (Max: 2550 mg)	Lactic Acidosis; Hypoglycemia
COMBINATION PILLS				Lactic Acidosis
Glyburide/Metformin	Glucovance	Take with meals	25/250; 2.5/500; 5/500 mg	(also hypoglycemia)
Metformin/Glipizide	Metaglip	Take with meals	2.5/250; 5/500; 5/500 mg	
Rosiglitizone/Metformin	Avandamet	Take with meals	1mg/500 mg, 2/500, 4/500	
Pioglitazone/Metformin	Acto*plus*met	Take with meals	15mg/500mg; 15/850	
Rosiglitazone/Glimepiride	Avandaryl	Take same time of day	4mg/1mg; 4/2; 4/4	
Pioglitazone/Glimepiride	Duetact	Take with meals	30 mg/2 mg; 30/4 mg	Low Blood Glucose; Weight Gain; Fluid Retention
Sitagliptin/Metformin	JanuMet	Twice daily with meals	50 mg/500 mg; 50/1000 mg	Runny nose; Fever; Nausea; Diarrhea
Note: Stop if having kidney dye study; Check creatinine & liver function; need good oxygenation in body.				
Alpha- glucosidase Inhibitors -- Slow down carbohydrate absorption in intestines				
Acarbose	Precose	Take with first bite	25, 50, 100 mg (Max: 300 mg)	Nausea, Diarrhea Flatulence
Miglitol	Glyset	Take with first bite	25, 50, 100 mg (Max: 300 mg)	
Note: For low blood glucose treatment, use honey or glucose gel/tablets; do not use table or brown sugar				
Thiazolidinediones (Insulin Sensitizer) – Improve peripheral insulin sensitivity				
Pioglitazone	Actos	With or without meals	15, 30 mg (Max: 45 mg)	Possible liver dysfunction
Rosiglitazone	Avandia	With or without meals	2, 4, 6 mg (Max: 8 mg max)	Possible anemia, edema

Note: May take 6 weeks to work best; need liver function studies before starting and periodically thereafter; do not use in patients with heart failure; may decrease effectiveness of birth control.

INCRETINS- - Gliptins: for patients with type 2 diabetes on secretagogue, metformin, or TZDs:

1. Byetta (exenatide injection) 5-10mcg 2x/d. Stimulates insulin release when blood glucose is increasing; regulates food release~stomach, slows liver glucose release, increases satiety. Side effect: weight loss & nausea.

2. Januvia (oral agent) 100mg 1x/d. Increases GLP1 (gut hormone) by stopping breakdown of internal GLP1. Increases insulin release and slows hepatic release of glucose.

---

3. Starting metformin with the evening meal for several days, then adding the breakfast dose will further minimize gastrointestinal side effects. Extended release formulations may also reduce gastrointestinal disturbances.

4. Titrate up by 500 mg (or 850 mg) once a week, until the clinical therapeutic dose of 1000 mg, 2000-2450 (1700 mg) twice daily, is reached.

5. Women of childbearing age should be advised that metformin may increase ovulation; therefore, birth control measures should be implemented to avoid pregnancy.

Another major metabolic defect of type 2 diabetes is the loss of pancreatic beta-cell function. As beta-cell failure occurs, post-prandial glucose elevations become evident *(10)*. To attain the target A1C level, post-prandial glucose control must be maintained *(13–16)*.

Incretins

Newer medications, called incretins, are available that can minimize post-prandial glucose excursions. Incretins mimic the action of certain gut hormones that help facilitate first-phase insulin release and post-prandial glucagon suppression, both of which are defective in type 2 diabetes *(10)*. Exenatide (Byetta), an injectable medication for patients with type 2 diabetes not taking insulin, stimulates the beta cells to release insulin after eating. While nausea is a common side effect, exenatide also helps suppress the appetite and can aid with weight loss. Exenatide can be used in combination with metformin, thiazolidinediones, and sulfonylureas. It is not yet approved as monotherapy.

Dipeptidyl peptidase IV (DPP-IV) inhibitors are a new class of diabetes medications taken in pill form. These medications are weight neutral *(12)* and work to lower post-prandial blood glucose levels, along with suppressing glucose release from the liver.

CONSIDERATIONS

1. Demonstrate a Byetta injection with a "demo" pen to reduce fears about injections.
2. Ask patients to take their first Byetta injection 15 min before the evening meal. Ask them to eat slowly and stop eating when they feel full to help reduce nausea. If no problems occur, they may begin injections twice daily, before breakfast and the evening meal the next day.
3. If the patient is on a secretagogue, the dose is usually reduced by 50% before starting Byetta to prevent hypoglycemia.
4. Sitagliptin (Januvia), a DPP-IV inhibitor, may work best early in the onset of type 2 diabetes. Clinical experience suggests that it does not work as well in the later stages.

Secretagogues

Secretagogues work by increasing endogenous insulin secretion and should be taken up to 30 min before meals. Hypoglycemia is the primary side effect if meals are missed or delayed. Secretagogue doses must be titrated and re-evaluated until the A1C goal is reached (typically less than 7% for most people with diabetes) *(1,15)*.

CONSIDERATIONS

1. Glimepiride- or glipizide-extended release are 24-h medications and will increase the likeliness of medication compliance since patients only have to remember to take it once a day.
2. If glipizide or glyburide is started once a day, but 2-h post-prandial glucose levels are above target, consider twice-daily dosing.
3. Meglitinides and D-phenylalanine derivatives must be given with each meal.
4. Advise patients to carry treatment for hypoglycemia, such as glucose tablets.

Thiazolidinediones

Thiazolidinediones, commonly called "TZDs," include pioglitazone (Actos) and rosiglitazone (Avandia). These primarily treat the insulin resistance of type 2 diabetes. They take up to 6–8 weeks to achieve maximum benefit. Liver function tests must be checked prior to initiating and then periodically during the use of these medications. Recent concerns *(17,18)* have arisen linking rosiglitazone with cardiovascular issues and rosiglitazone. Patients taking rosiglitazone should discuss its continued use with their providers. Patient with congestive heart failure should not take thiazolidinediones.

CONSIDERATIONS

1. Patients should watch for edema and weight gain when taking thiazolidine-diones.
2. Women of childbearing age should be advised that these medications may increase ovulation, and therefore birth control measures should be implemented if pregnancy is not desired.

Alpha-glucosidase Inhibitors

Alpha-glucosidase inhibitors slow the absorption of the glucose in the intestine by inhibiting the enzyme that breaks down carbohydrate. This class of medication specifically targets post-prandial glucose levels. The main side effects of alpha-glucosidase inhibitors are flatulence and diarrhea.

CONSIDERATIONS

1. Start these medications at a low dose and titrate up slowly to minimize side effects.
2. These medications must be taken right before a meal.

Insulin

Insulin is needed when endogenous (internal) insulin reserves are depleted or if the glucose toxicity at diagnosis is such that the patient is not able to respond to oral agents. Table 5 summarizes insulin types, brand, and duration. Selecting an insulin regimen that best mimics non-diabetic endogenous insulin patterns requires basal/bolus therapy or physiologic insulin therapy *(19–22)*. If extenuating circumstances are present, such as lack of insurance coverage to

Table 5
Insulin

Type/Name	Manufacturer	Source	Onset	Peak	Duration
RAPID-ACTING (Bolus/Meal Insulins)					
Lispro (Humalog)	Lilly	Human rDNA	5 - 10 min	0.5-3 hrs	3-5 hrs
Aspart (Novolog)	Novo Nordisk	Human rDNA	5 - 10 min	0.5-3 hrs	3-5 hrs
Glulisine (Apidra)	Aventis	Human rDNA	5 + min	0.5-3 hrs	3-5 hrs
REGULAR					
Humulin R	Lilly	Human rDNA	30 min	2 - 3 hrs	6 -8 hrs
Novolin R	Novo Nordisk	Human rDNA	30 min	2 - 4 hrs	6 - 8 hrs
INTERMEDIATE-ACTING (Basal/Background Insulins)					
NPH					
Humulin N	Lilly	Human rDNA	2 hrs	6 - 8 hrs	10 -12 hrs
Novolin N	Novo Nordisk	Human rDNA	2 hrs	6 - 8 hrs	10 -12 hrs
LONG-ACTING (Basal/Background)					
Glargine (Lantus	Aventis	Human rDNA	1-2 hrs	nearly flat	up to 24 hrs
Detemir (Levemir)	Novo Nordisk	Human rDNA	1-2 hrs	nearly flat	up to 24 hrs
MIXTURES					
Pre-MIXED		all are rDNA Human			
Humalog75/25Mix Lilly		75% NPL /25% lispro			
Novolog Mix 70/30 NovoNordisk		70% N/30% aspart			
Humulin 70/30	Lilly	70% NPH/30% regular			
Novolin 70/30	Novo Nordisk	70% NPH/30% regular			
Humulin 50/50	Lilly	50% NPH/50% regular			
Humalog Mix 50/50 Lilly		50% NPL/50% lispro			

INSULIN CARTRIDGES: For insulin pens (Novo Pen 3, Innovo) R, N, 70/30, Novolog; Humalog 3ml for Memoir and Luxura HD, Lantus for OptiClick

INSULIN PREFILLED PENS – Humalog, NPH and 75/25 (Lilly); InnoLet 70/30, R and NPH (Novo); Novolog, Novolog Mix 70/30; SoloStar (Lantus), KwikPen (Humalog & mixes)

For patients on Insulin:

Pramlintide (Symlin) (amylin hormone) injection. Type 1 diabetes: 15-30 mcg 2-4x/d; type 2 diabetes: 60-120mcg - 2-4x/d. To start: Pramlintide with the first bite of food, insulin with the last bite.

cover the cost of insulin or patient resistance, preclude use of insulin analogs for multiple daily injections (MDI); premixed insulins can be prescribed to provide similar outcomes.

Many insulins and insulin protocols are available *(19–22)*, and the provider must work with the patient to determine what will work best. Insulin initiation can be difficult for clinicians who do not have much experience with insulin therapy. Clinical inertia, a delay in starting insulin or not changing therapy when it is needed, is seen in academic settings as well as in primary care *(23–25)*. A referral to a diabetes educator is prudent rather than a delay in therapy change.

CONSIDERATIONS

1. Type 2 diabetes is a progressive disease. People will gradually lose nearly all beta-cell function *(26)*. It does not mean they have done anything wrong, but it does mean that insulin is necessary.
2. Avoid using words like oral agent *"failure."* Patients think "they" have failed, when in fact their beta-cell destruction was likely inevitable.
3. Basal insulin or one injection of mixed insulin at supper can improve the fasting glucose level.
4. Post-prandial monitoring can determine if mealtime insulin is warranted.
5. Fear of insulin injections (another form of "insulin resistance") can be minimized by having the patient do a "practice" injection using saline. This can be done in a busy office in a matter of minutes *(23–25)*.
6. If there are no extenuating circumstances (i.e., immunosuppression), it is acceptable to inject through clothing. This makes injecting easier and more convenient *(27)*.
7. If insurance coverage is adequate, insulin pens make multiple daily injections easier and safer.
8. Refer patients to comprehensive diabetes self-management education programs for more information on insulin adjustments and treatment of hyper- and hypoglycemia.

COMMONLY ASKED QUESTIONS

Providers and office staff are often faced with questions from patients that require quick, accurate responses. The following are common questions and answers to help keep messages consistent and accurate. All staff may benefit from reviewing:

Q. What do I eat?

A: Until patients meet with a registered dietitian, help patients with the following meal planning concepts:

1. Eat healthy foods in smaller portions.
2. Drink water, diet soda, and tea/coffee with non-nutritive sweeteners instead of sugared soft drinks and fruit juices.

3. Eat about the same amount of carbohydrate at meals/snacks. Do not eliminate all carbohydrate from the eating plan.
4. Eat about the same amount of food at the same time every day.

Q. Will this go away if I lose weight?

A: No. But diabetes can be controlled with a healthy eating plan and regular physical activity, and sometimes medication. Losing just 5–10% of body weight can help the body's insulin work better, thus reducing the insulin resistance.

Q. Will I go blind?

A: Research *(26,28–30)* shows that diabetes complications such as blindness and kidney disease are linked to poorly controlled diabetes. Keeping the A1C level under 7% helps reduce the risk of complications.

Q. Is "sugar-free" candy okay to eat?

A: "Sugar-free" usually means a food is sweetened with sugar alcohols, such as sorbitol and mannitol. Sugar-free candies and other products may still contain carbohydrate, which can affect blood glucose levels. Always read the Nutrition Facts label to learn how much carbohydrate is in a product.

Q. Did I get diabetes because I ate too much sugar?

A: Diabetes is not caused by eating too much sugar. Type 2 diabetes, which is genetic, is triggered by extra weight that leads to insulin resistance. When the pancreas cannot make enough insulin to overcome insulin resistance, or when the body cannot use its own insulin effectively, diabetes results. Type 1 diabetes is an autoimmune disease likely triggered by a virus or other environmental factors.

Q. Should I see a diabetes doctor?

A: If you are working in close partnership with your primary care provider, maintaining your target A1C, blood pressure, and cholesterol levels, and have received sufficient diabetes self-management education, you may not need to see a diabetes doctor.

Q. Can I still have children?

A: Many women with diabetes who adequately control their diabetes can have healthy babies. Pregnancy is a time when working with a diabetes specialist is advised. Tighter glucose levels, frequent insulin adjustments, and careful meal planning are often needed during pregnancy. Pre-pregnancy education and tight glucose control are recommended.

Q. I am having blurry vision since I was diagnosed. Am I going blind?

A: No. This is not the permanent blindness that can result from years of poorly controlled diabetes. Blurry vision can result from high blood glucose levels that cause a change in the shape of the eyeball. As blood glucose levels improve, normal vision will be restored. If glasses are needed, it is advised to wait several weeks until diabetes control has improved and the shape of the eyeball and lens has returned to normal.

Q. My provider said I do not have to check my blood sugar since I am not on insulin. Is that true?

A: Self-monitoring of blood glucose is the only way to tell on a daily basis whether diabetes is in control. Most people do not have any symptoms of hyperglycemia until glucose levels are near 300. Research suggests that damage to the nerves, blood vessels, eyes, and kidneys can occur when glucose levels are consistently above 140–150 mg *(26,28–30)*. Glucose monitoring provides important information as to how the diabetes treatment plan is working. However, there is no consensus on how often to monitor. Providers may suggest several times a day at different times. This pattern of monitoring allows the provider to determine if the meal plan, medication, and level of physical activity are all in balance.

Q. Why will not my insurance cover diabetes education?

A: Many insurance companies reimburse for diabetes education if the program has attained American Diabetes Association (or Indian Health Services) national recognition. Ten hours of diabetes education are covered if the program has received American Diabetes Association education program recognition. Two hours of additional education is covered every year (12 months) thereafter. Contact your health plan, state insurance commissioner, or the American Diabetes Association for more information.

Q. Will I always have diabetes?

A: Yes, diabetes does not go away, but it can be controlled with a healthy eating plan, regular physical activity, medication if needed, and regular self-monitoring of blood glucose.

Q. I have no time to go to a gym and I cannot afford it anyway. What can I do?

A: Activity helps the insulin (internal from the pancreas or external from injections) work better. Any type of activity that moves large muscle groups will help to lower blood glucose levels. Walking is a great, low-cost activity that can be done just about anywhere, at any time. The goal is to work up to a minimum of 30 min, most days of the week *(31)*.

Q. Does starting on insulin mean that my diabetes is getting worse?

A: No. Type 2 diabetes is progressive, meaning that it changes over time. Eventually, the insulin-producing beta cells of the pancreas die, and insulin injections are needed. It does not mean you have done anything wrong if you need insulin shots *(32)*.

SUMMARY

Diabetes management is complex, requiring a combination of lifestyle and medication management along with problem solving and coping skills. The person with diabetes must live with the disease and balance the nuances of meal planning, glucose monitoring, activity, and stress management on a daily basis.

Table 6
Diabetes Resources

1. Comprehensive diabetes self-management education:
   Find an American Diabetes Association-recognized education program at
   www.diabetes.org/recognition
2. Diabetes Educator:
   Find a diabetes educator at American Association of Diabetes Educators at
   www.aadenet.org or www.diabeteseducator.org or 1-800-TEAM UP4
3. Medical Nutrition Therapy:
   Find a registered dietitian at American Dietetic Association at www.eatright.org
4. Nutrition resources:
   Find resources at www.mypyramid.gov or www.platemethod.com

Acquiring the skills necessary to maintain good control is an ongoing process for the person with diabetes and must be facilitated by the provider and health care team. Perseverance with these challenges will have a positive impact on improving patient outcomes. Referrals and use of community resources assist the provider in obtaining support for their patients. Common diabetes resources are listed in Table 6.

Improving patients' knowledge about diabetes is not enough. Patients need ongoing education and support to effectively manage their diabetes. Because time and resources in the outpatient setting are limited, the challenge becomes making the most of the visit. The entire office staff can be instrumental in helping to educate and support the patient with diabetes. Providers are advised to spend time in the areas of enhancing skills for self-care and creative problem solving which, in turn, can affect and improve patient outcomes *(33)*.

REFERENCES

1. American Diabetes Association. Standards of medical care in diabetes. Diabetes Care 2008; 31:S12–S54.
2. Brown S. Effects of educational intervention in diabetes care: a meta-analysis. Nursing Res 1988; 4:223–230.
3. Center for Disease Control and Prevention. Preventative care practices among persons with diabetes. JAMA 2002; 288:2814–2815.
4. Leontos C, Geil PB. Individualized Approaches to Diabetes Nutrition Therapy: Case Studies. Alexandria: American Diabetes Association 2002:657.
5. Pichert JW, Schlundt DG. Assessment: Gathering information and facilitating engagement. In: Mensing, C. The Art and Science of Diabetes Self-Management Education: A Desk Reference for Healthcare Professionals. Chicago: American Association of Diabetes Educators 2006:578–595.
6. Anderson R, Patrius R. Getting out ahead: The diabetes concerns assessment form. Clin Diabetes 2007; 25:141–144.

7. National Heart Lung and Blood Institute. Clinical guidelines on the identification, evaluation and treatment of overweight and obesity in adults: The evidence report; Obes Res 1998; 6:51S–209S.

8. Camp KK. Being active. In: Mensing, C. The Art and Science of Diabetes Self-Management Education: A Desk Reference for Healthcare Professionals. Chicago: American Association of Diabetes Educators 2006:670–688.

9. Bardsley JK, Ratner RE. Pathophysiology of the metabolic disorder. In: Mensing, C. The Art and Science of Diabetes Self-Management Education: A Desk Reference for Healthcare Professionals. Chicago: American Association of Diabetes Educators 2006:143–161.

10. Hinnen D, Nielsen L, Waninger A, Kushner P. Incretin Mimetics and DPP-IV Inhibitors: New Paradigms for the Treatment of Type 2 Diabetes. J Am Board Fam Med. 2006; 19: 612–620.

11. Monnier L, Lapinski H, Colette C. Contributions of fasting and postprandial plasma glucose increments to the overall diurnal hyperglycemia of type 2 diabetic patients: Variations with increasing levels of HbA(1c). Diabetes Care. 2003; 26:881–885.

12. Gerich JE. Clinical significance, pathogenesis, and management of postprandial hyperglycemia. Arch Intern Med. 2003; 163:1306–1316.

13. American Association of Clinical Endocrinologists/American College of Endocrinology Diabetes Recommendations Implementation Writing Committee. ACE/AACE Consensus conference on the implementation of outpatient management of diabetes mellitus: Consensus conference recommendations. Endocr Pract. 2006; 12:(Suppl 1): 6–12.

14. American Association of Clinical Endocrinologists. Medical guidelines for clinical practice for the diagnosis and treatment of dyslipidemia and prevention of atherogenesis. Endocr Pract. 2000; 6:162–213.

15. Ohkubo Y, Kishikawa H, Araki E, et al. Intensive insulin therapy prevents the progression of diabetic microvascular complications in Japanese patients with non-insulin-dependent diabetes mellitus: A randomized prospective 6-year study. Diabetes Res Clin Pract. 1995; 28:103–117.

16. UKPDS Group. Intensive blood glucose control with sulphonylureas or insulin compared with conventional treatment and risk of complications in patients with type 2 diabetes (UKPDS 33). Lancet. 1998; 352:837–853.

17. DCCT/EDIC Group. Retinopathy and nephropathy in patients with type 1 diabetes four years after a trial of intensive therapy. N Engl J Med. 2000; 342:381–389.

18. DCCT/EDIC Group. Intensive diabetes treatment and cardiovascular disease in patients with type 1 diabetes. N Engl J Med. 2005; 353:2643–2653.

19. Nathan DM, Buse JB, Davidson MB, et al. Management of hyperglycemia in type 2 diabetes: A consensus algorithm for the initiation and adjustment of therapy. Diabetes Care. 2006; 29:1963–1972.

20. Nathan DM. Finding new treatments for diabetes—How many, how fast. . .how good. N Engl J Med. 2007; 365:437–440.

21. Skyler JS. Insulin treatment. In: Lebovitz HE, ed. Therapy for Diabetes Mellitus and Related Disorders. Alexandria: American Diabetes Association 2004:207–223.

22. Hirsch IB, Bergenstal RM, Parkin CG, et al. A real-world approach to insulin therapy in primary care practice. Clin Diabetes. 2005; 23:78–86.

23. Riddle MC, Rosenstock J, Gerich J. The Treat-to-Target Trial: Randomized addition of glargine or human NPH insulin to oral therapy of type 2 diabetic patients. Diabetes Care. 2003; 26:3080–3086.

24. Gavin JR. Practical approaches to insulin therapy. Diabetes Educ. 2007; 33:66S–73S.

25. Mullooly CA. Physical Activity. In: Mensing, C. The Art and Science of Diabetes Self-Management Education: A Desk Reference for Healthcare Professionals. Chicago: American Association of Diabetes Educators 2006:297–319.

26. Polonsky WH, Fisher L, Guzman S, et al. Psychological insulin resistance in patients with type 2 diabetes. Diabetes Care. 2005; 28:2543–2545.

27. Pergallo-Dittko V. Removing barriers to insulin therapy. Diabetes Educ. 2007; 33:60S–65S.
28. Peyrot M, Rubin RR, Lauritzen T, et al. Resistance to insulin therapy among patients and providers. Diabetes Care. 2005; 28:2673–2679.
29. Fleming, D, Jacober SJ, Vandenberg MA et al. The safety of injecting insulin through clothing. Diabetes Care. 1997; 20: 244.
30. Singh S, Yoon K. Loke YK, Furberg CD. Long-term risk of cardiovascular events with rosiglitazone: A meta-analysis. JAMA. 2007; 298:1189–1195.
31. Nissen, SE, Wolski K. Effect of rosiglitazone on the risk of myocardial infarction and death from cardiovascular causes. N Engl J Med. 2007; 356: 2457–2471.
32. American Diabetes Association. A Resource Guide. Diabetes Forecast January, 2008: RG11–RG14.
33. Zgibor J, Peyrot M, Ruppert K. Using the AADE outcomes system to identify patient behavior change goals and diabetes educator responses. Diabetes Educ 2007; 33:840–41.

6

Meeting the Challenge of Inpatient Diabetes Education: An Interdisciplinary Approach

Jane Seley, GNP, MPH, MSN, CDE
and Marisa Wallace, MS, FNP

CONTENTS

INTRODUCTION
INPATIENT DIABETES
    SELF-MANAGEMENT EDUCATION PROCESS
CONCLUSION
REFERENCES

ABSTRACT

Teaching diabetes self-management to the growing number of hospitalized patients with diabetes and hyperglycemia is a challenging task. Inpatients are acutely ill and in an environment that is fraught with frequent interruptions and other concerns related to the admitting diagnosis. Because of these competing priorities, limited time, and an ill-conducive learning environment, the primary focus for diabetes self-management education should be on those skills that are essential for the patient to be able to return home safely. This chapter explores the inpatient diabetes self-management education process including assessment, identifying barriers and advantages, goal setting, key topics of content, delivery, communication among providers, and discharge. Practical tips are offered to help integrate diabetes self-management education into current clinical practice in the inpatient setting.

From: *Contemporary Diabetes: Educating Your Patient with Diabetes*
Edited by: K. Weinger and C. A. Carver, DOI 10.1007/978-1-60327-208-7_6,
© Humana Press, a part of Springer Science+Business Media, LLC 2009

Key Words: Inpatient Education, Diabetes Education, Diabetes Self-Management, Patient Education, Hospitalized Education, Nursing.

INTRODUCTION

The diabetes epidemic has created both challenge and opportunity for our health-care system to provide comprehensive services for people with diabetes across all settings. Just as the number of Americans diagnosed with diabetes has grown from 5.6 to 15.8 million people in the past 25 years, the number of hospital discharges carrying a diagnosis of diabetes has escalated from 2.2 million in 1980 to 5.1 million in 2003 *(1)*. Although these figures are staggering, the true number of inpatients with diabetes is probably much higher. The majority of patients with diabetes are hospitalized not strictly for diabetes, but rather with a co-morbidity. Because the focus of attention is on the admitting diagnosis, glycemic control is often overlooked or placed on the back burner *(2)*.

Until recently, a common belief was that it was safer for blood glucose to remain somewhat elevated in the acute care setting because of the potential risk of overtreating and causing hypoglycemia. There is now a growing body of knowledge that suggests that ignoring short-term hyperglycemia in an acutely ill patient has serious consequences *(3)*. Many times, it is the diabetes educator who is the voice of reason in advocating for strict glycemic management of the hospitalized patient.

The benefits of glycemic control and diabetes self-management education in the outpatient setting are well established. Recently, many studies have validated the need for attention to the importance of inpatient glycemic control as critical to successful outcomes in the acute care setting. Pivotal studies have demonstrated that hyperglycemia management decreases the risk of mortality and morbidity post-myocardial infarction, and coronary artery bypass surgery; in the critically ill, it reduces infections and promotes wound healing, as well as shortening length of stay and reducing readmissions *(3,4)*. The heightened awareness regarding optimal diabetes management in the acute care setting presents a unique opportunity for improvements in both glycemic control and self-management education. Because diabetes is often not the primary reason for admission, educational opportunities may be missed. Just as glycemic control is overlooked in the acute care setting, so too is diabetes self-management education.

INPATIENT DIABETES SELF-MANAGEMENT
EDUCATION PROCESS

Evidence supports that educational interventions increase patient knowledge and are an essential component of health care for the chronically ill *(5)*. Inpatient diabetes education is associated with earlier discharge and improved outcomes post-discharge *(3)*. Inpatient diabetes self-management education is a process that includes assessment, identifying barriers, goal setting, key topics of content, delivery, communication among providers, and discharge.

Assessment

In order to facilitate diabetes self-management education, a patient with diabetes should be assessed for current self-care practices, barriers to self-management, and outpatient support. Just as in the outpatient arena, it is ineffective for a clinician to enter a hospital room and begin educating the patient about diabetes without assessing the patient and developing an education plan. This step is frequently overlooked in the fast-paced acute care environment. Staff nurses are in a unique position to take on the role of diabetes educator because much of diabetes self-management education can be built into current nursing practice.

The initial assessment will help identify which "survival skills" are necessary and even possible for the patient to learn. Adaptations may be needed depending on each patient's cognitive and physical abilities during and after acute illness and family support. It is vital to convey to the patient that achieving glycemic control will improve outcomes following discharge. To determine glycemic control and self-care practices prior to admission, it is important to obtain a diabetes history including type and duration of diabetes, previously established dietary and exercise plans, medications for hyperglycemia management, assessment of blood glucose control (including self-monitoring of blood glucose, frequency, and results), acute symptoms of hypoglycemia and hyperglycemia, substance abuse, and other barriers to self-care.

The American Diabetes Association 2004 technical review on the management of diabetes and hyperglycemia in hospitals lists the following components to the educational assessment as critical before initiating education:

- Knowledge, psychomotor skills, and affective domains
- Current level of self-care
- Preferred learning styles
- Psychological status
- Stress factors that impair learning
- Social/cultural/religious beliefs
- Literacy skills
- Readiness to learn
- Assessment of abilities – age, mobility, visual acuity, hearing loss, and dexterity *(3)*

Because many patients have shortened lengths of stay and education should begin as soon as possible, this assessment is best accomplished at admission whenever possible.

Identifying Potential Barriers and Advantages

Teaching diabetes self-management to hospitalized patients is a challenging task. Patients are hospitalized because they are acutely ill, under increased stress, and in an environment that is not conducive to learning *(3)*. Frequent interruptions, distractions, and noise (such as alarms) are common in hospital rooms. Patients may have other concerns related to their hospitalization and are often being seen by multiple providers and are not yet focused on discharge planning and learning diabetes self-management skills. It is often up to health-care professionals such as nurses and dietitians to seek opportunities to educate the patient and build on prior diabetes self-management skills and knowledge.

The inpatient setting does offer a few advantages over outpatient diabetes education. Family members are more easily accessible to include in the educational process because they are often visiting the patient. In addition, education can be offered in small segments over several days with the learner able to build on new knowledge over time. When defining what is essential for the patient to learn for a safe discharge home, the clinician must work with the patient and family to set individualized and appropriate goals for learning diabetes self-management skills. In an acutely ill patient, sessions should be shorter and more frequent in relation to the patient's condition, ability to concentrate, level of pain, expected length of stay, and complexity of the discharge plan *(3)*.

Goal Setting

Trying to teach all aspects of diabetes care is overwhelming to inpatients, especially if diabetes is not the primary reason for admission and other self-care skills need to be learned. Because of these competing priorities, limited time and a less than ideal learning environment, the primary focus for diabetes self-management education should be on those skills that are essential for the patient to go home safely *(6)*. Many clinicians refer to this as diabetes "survival skills" education.

Determining each patient's "survival skills" depends on medical necessity and the discharge plan e.g. own home versus short-term rehabilitation *(3)*. Inquiries to help determine educational goals and special considerations following discharge should include:

- Does the patient require further immediate outpatient diabetes self-management education?
- Does the patient need help with meal preparation?
- Can the patient take his or her diabetes medications or insulin independently?
- Can the patient monitor his or her blood glucose and take appropriate action?

- Is there a family member who can assist at least temporarily with any of these tasks that the patient cannot perform at the time of discharge?
- Is a visiting nurse needed to facilitate safe transition to the home? *(7)*

Hospitalized patients who have deficits in learning or self-care abilities will need "survival skills" goals tailored to fit their individual needs. Most hospitalized diabetes patients would benefit most from a simple plan which can be expanded upon as an outpatient. Simplified goals for patients should include

- Correct timing and dosing of diabetes medications in relation to meals, sometimes using fixed doses initially until the patient can learn to adjust medications to match blood glucose levels over time
- Planning and spacing consistent carbohydrate meals
- Need for home glucose monitoring to evaluate treatment efficacy
- Individualized glycemic targets over time and knowledge of when to seek help
- Identification of symptoms and appropriate treatment for hypoglycemia *(7)*

Key Topics of Content

Once the learning needs assessment is accomplished and goals are set, the education can begin. The education plan is now focused on new learning needs and the review and reinforcement of any former skills. It is important to review former knowledge and skills since many patients have received minimal or no education in the past *(4)*. In addition, time may have passed and the information the patient received may be outdated. For example, it is not uncommon for patients to receive blood glucose meters from pharmacies or by mail order without instruction and attempt to self-learn.

For patients who have a new diagnosis or have had little previous education, Nettles suggests a brief explanation of the following topics:

- The role of glucose and insulin in the disease process
- The relationship between glycemic control and diabetes complications
- Nutritional counseling by a registered dietitian and/or certified diabetes educator
- Medication management including insulin self-administration, with special emphasis on any changes made to a prior regimen
- How to self monitor blood glucose and individualized glycemic targets
- How to recognize and treat high and low blood glucose
- The importance of follow-up care, including when to contact a health-care provider or go to the emergency department *(7)*

During hospitalization is a great time to look at whether or not the patient is properly using the lancing device, coding the meter if applicable, and applying the blood sample correctly onto the test strip. Many patients are discouraged from checking their blood glucose at home because they have never been shown how to use the equipment and ways to make the procedure more comfortable. Survival skills education focuses on meal planning, taking diabetes medication safely, and blood glucose monitoring to facilitate self-care after discharge. Additional diabetes education should take place in an outpatient setting.

MEAL PLANNING

Dietitians are generally more available in acute care than in outpatient settings to instruct patients in consistent carbohydrate counting. Simple handouts should capture basic principles such as spacing meals, identifying which foods have carbohydrates, appropriate portion sizes, and reading nutrition facts labels. Bedside nurses should become familiar with the carbohydrate counting handout used by the dietitians so that they can reinforce the information with patients. One strategy may be for the bedside nurse to sit in on a few sessions with the dietitian as an observer. We have adopted the trainer approach where certified diabetes educators and the nurse educators have taught staff nurses how to use a one page handout on carbohydrate counting to reinforce the dietitian's instruction. For patients that are newly diagnosed or have never learned carbohydrate counting, identifying which foods have carbohydrates and portion sizes of foods they commonly eat may be all that can be accomplished during a brief hospitalization. Meal-planning lessons are best scheduled when family members are present, especially those that shop and prepare meals in the home.

There are many opportunities to reinforce nutritional counseling in the hospital setting. Menus and meal trays can become learning tools. Ask patients to identify the carbohydrates and portion sizes on the meal tray and compare their answers with the actual menu. Nutrition facts labels from food brought in by visitors can be read and discussed. The nutritional counseling received during hospitalization may be the patient's only exposure to formal instruction in carbohydrate counting.

MEDICATIONS

Oral agents are often held during hospitalization and then reinstated at discharge. This is partially because acute illness often requires insulin therapy, as well as the potential danger of using oral agents during hospital procedures (5). Because many patients will be returning to oral medications at home or perhaps started on new ones, a discussion about the disease process and how each oral agent the patient will be taking works is essential. A simple handout that lists oral agents according to category and defect is useful for nurses and other clinicians to review with patients. Copies of handouts written in languages other than English, particularly Spanish should be readily available in clinical care areas.

Patients often require insulin during hospitalization. It is not always easy to determine whether or not a patient taking insulin in the hospital will continue insulin therapy at home. One can make an educated guess based on levels of glycemia, insulin dosage requirements, and whether steroids are going to be continued or tapered. Common sense dictates that it is better to teach a patient insulin self-administration whenever insulin is administered then to wait for confirmation of the need just prior to discharge. In reality, nurses often reserve insulin instruction until the last moment when it is a mandate and an emergency. This is unfortunate because this approach unnecessarily denies the patient ample time to learn and practice a new skill and can delay discharge.

Teaching insulin self-administration needs to be a key component of the nursing care of the patient with diabetes. Patients would benefit from knowing that they can safely and correctly administer insulin, should the need present itself at a later time. It can be taught as soon as the patient can perform at least some of the steps, including while in intensive care (4). With shortened lengths of stay, patients are sometimes discharged from or soon after being in intensive care.

Teaching a patient how to self-administer insulin is a great example of how diabetes education can be integrated into routine nursing practice. Every time a patient receives subcutaneous insulin, the nurse should be preparing the dose in front of the patient and family and coaching the patient through self-injection. If the patient is not ready to learn how to prepare the dose, the nurse can show the patient the steps while performing them. The most important step to include the patient and family in is the injection itself. Patients will be relieved to practice in front of the trained eyes of the nurse rather than at home unsupervised. Once the patient masters self-injection, much of the anxiety of insulin therapy will be alleviated.

Just as in the outpatient setting, insulin self-administration should include when and how much to take, the importance of matching mealtimes to insulin action, storage of insulin, disposal of syringes or pen needles, and hypoglycemia identification and treatment.

Teaching insulin self-administration to the hospitalized patient can be challenging at best. Patients are often anxious, in pain, and may have poor concentration which limits ability to learn (3). In addition, patients may have physical barriers that brought them into the hospital such as surgery and fractures which may limit manual dexterity. Creativity in choosing regimens and delivery methods that match each patient's abilities is important. This may mean that family members need to be enlisted to perform a portion of the survival skills, at least initially. For example, a patient with a recent shoulder fracture may not be able to master drawing up the dose at this time but can safely administer it. A family member may be willing to take on a shared responsibility until the patient can master it independently.

It is difficult to practice insulin delivery with the patient if the device that the patient will go home with is not available in the hospital. However, the hospital setting can be an effective place for nurses to teach patients, for example, use insulin pens for rapid acting insulin and using basal insulin with a vial and syringe. This gives the patient an opportunity to see both methods and make an informed choice for discharge.

BLOOD GLUCOSE MONITORING

Monitoring blood glucose in the hospital is a great learning tool. Patients can participate in the procedure by assisting in getting an adequate blood sample and correctly applying it to the test strip. Even though home-monitoring equipment is different, these basic skills are transferable. The next important step in teaching patients about blood glucose monitoring using hospital equipment is to explain the differences between pre and post-prandial checks and the value of each. Patients should know that the frequency of monitoring in the hospital may differ from at home and why. Every time a blood glucose check is performed, the nurse should engage the patient in interpreting the value. Glycemic targets should be discussed and ways to achieve these goals. Patients should be encouraged to keep blood glucose logs during hospitalization and to review their values daily with the health-care team. This is a great way to show patients the value of glucose monitoring and how the results are utilized to make treatment changes.

Some hospitals have programs with meter companies or home care suppliers to distribute home meters to patients prior to discharge. This is a great way to ensure that the patient is properly trained in how and when to use the monitor at home. It is best to train patients early in the hospitalization so that they can practice the skill. Diabetes educators can train nurse educators, clinical nurse specialists, and staff nurses in how to use home meters. It is important that the approved hospital meter is used for all treatment and charting, not the patient meter. The patient can use their own equipment to obtain the blood sample and apply it to both the hospital meter (for treatment) and the home meter (for teaching purposes only). This is a great way for patients to practice blood glucose monitoring and get comfortable with the skill.

ADDITIONAL EDUCATION

Whether or not a hospitalized patient is able to learn beyond survival skills is a judgment call. If the patient has not yet mastered meal planning, monitoring, and medication, new topics such as foot care should be introduced in the outpatient setting. Well-meaning clinicians may overload the patient with too much information, leading to confusion and a greater potential for error. Ideally, an inpatient can learn survival skills on an ongoing basis by being an active participant in their diabetes care during the hospital stay.

Educational Delivery

CHOOSING PATIENT EDUCATION MATERIALS FOR INPATIENTS

Educational materials in the hospital setting may not necessarily be the same materials that are useful in outpatient centers. Because the focus of inpatient education is survival skills, the handouts should be restricted to key information to support survival skill education, facilitate a safe discharge, and prevent readmission. Diabetes educators, nurse educators, and clinical nurse specialists are excellent resources for choosing handouts that meet these criteria. For example, at New York Presbyterian Hospital, a team of clinicians, educators, and content experts (certified diabetes educators) assembled to develop a series of simple, one page handouts that addressed basic topics such as carbohydrate counting (See Fig. 1), insulin self administration, and hypoglycemia treatment. These handouts are available on the hospital infonet in English and Spanish. Specialty areas such as pediatrics and antepartum may want to develop or acquire customized material to serve the special needs of their populations. In addition, the patient education channel is an excellent way to provide general diabetes information such as disease process and meal planning to patients and family members. Program guides can be placed at the bedside to remind patients to view topics of interest.

MAKING HOSPITALS DIABETES FRIENDLY

Patients who have mastered diabetes self-management skills in the outpatient setting are often frustrated when they become inpatients. The timing of glucose checks, insulin administration, and meal tray delivery may lack coordination in the hospital and result in unnecessary hypo and hyperglycemia *(8)*. Patients will complain that they can do a better job of taking care of their diabetes at home. A further concern is that patients will model their own diabetes care behaviors after what they observe in the hospital such as poor timing of glucose testing, insulin delivery, and meals as well as ignoring hyperglycemia *(9)*.

Similar problems exist in the United Kingdom, where patients reported inappropriate timing of diabetes medications and meals, staff's lack of knowledge about diabetes, and nurse discomfort with patients participating in self-care management in the hospital setting *(10)*. In an effort to rectify this and promote self-management, the use of unit-based "link" nurses and inpatient diabetes specialty nurses has been tried. Link nurses receive additional education in inpatient diabetes management and work closely with the inpatient diabetes specialist nurse. Similar to an inpatient-certified diabetes educator role in the United States, the diabetes specialist nurse assists in clinical decision making and patient and staff education. Although the diabetes specialist nurse role has

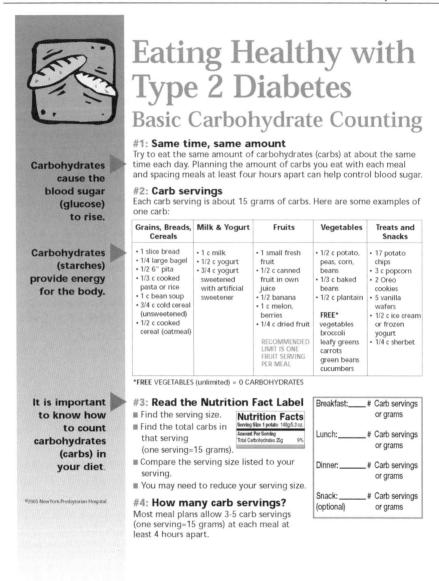

Eating Healthy with Type 2 Diabetes
Basic Carbohydrate Counting

Carbohydrates cause the blood sugar (glucose) to rise.

Carbohydrates (starches) provide energy for the body.

#1: Same time, same amount
Try to eat the same amount of carbohydrates (carbs) at about the same time each day. Planning the amount of carbs you eat with each meal and spacing meals at least four hours apart can help control blood sugar.

#2: Carb servings
Each carb serving is about 15 grams of carbs. Here are some examples of one carb:

Grains, Breads, Cereals	Milk & Yogurt	Fruits	Vegetables	Treats and Snacks
• 1 slice bread • 1/4 large bagel • 1/2 6" pita • 1/3 c cooked pasta or rice • 1 c bean soup • 3/4 c cold cereal (unsweetened) • 1/2 c cooked cereal (oatmeal)	• 1 c milk • 1/2 c yogurt • 3/4 c yogurt sweetened with artificial sweetener	• 1 small fresh fruit • 1/2 c canned fruit in own juice • 1/2 banana • 1 c melon, berries • 1/4 c dried fruit RECOMMENDED LIMIT IS ONE FRUIT SERVING PER MEAL	• 1/2 c potato, peas, corn, beans • 1/3 c baked beans • 1/2 c plantain **FREE*** vegetables broccoli leafy greens carrots green beans cucumbers	• 17 potato chips • 3 c popcorn • 2 Oreo cookies • 5 vanilla wafers • 1/2 c ice cream or frozen yogurt • 1/4 c sherbet

*FREE VEGETABLES (unlimited) = 0 CARBOHYDRATES

It is important to know how to count carbohydrates (carbs) in your diet.

©2005 New York-Presbyterian Hospital

#3: Read the Nutrition Fact Label
- Find the serving size.
- Find the total carbs in that serving (one serving=15 grams).
- Compare the serving size listed to your serving.
- You may need to reduce your serving size.

Nutrition Facts
Serving Size 1 potato 148g/5.3 oz.
Amount Per Serving
Total Carbohydrates 25g   9%

#4: How many carb servings?
Most meal plans allow 3-5 carb servings (one serving=15 grams) at each meal at least 4 hours apart.

Breakfast:_____ # Carb servings or grams

Lunch:_____ # Carb servings or grams

Dinner:_____ # Carb servings or grams

Snack:_____ # Carb servings (optional) or grams

Fig. 1. Carbohydrate Counting Handout Example.

proven to be effective in reducing length of stay and increasing patient satisfaction, the effectiveness of the link nurse has been somewhat limited. This was attributed to staff turnover and lack of sufficient knowledge of diabetes management to assume a unit-based resource role. Ideally a unit-based resource nurse could be cultivated over time by the certified diabetes educator to help create a climate on their unit where diabetes self-management education is part of routine nursing care.

DOCUMENTATION

Each institution has a way of documenting patient education in the medical record. Whether it is a checklist or free text, paper, or electronic, it is important to know where and who actually documents patient teaching and more importantly, who reads it. The status of patient teaching and the level of need for reinforcement should be in a prominent place in the medical record that is viewed by most providers. The status of diabetes self-management education is important to know in discharge planning. The mechanism for requesting diabetes self-management education should be pre-determined, easy, and well known. Although diabetes education does not require an order, it often places it at the head of the list of things to do. Diabetes education can be included in electronic orders and order sets. This helps remind providers of the need to start teaching sooner rather than later. Teaching checklists can be developed to streamline documentation.

The priority for documenting diabetes education is not to meet Joint Commission requirements, but rather to communicate the status of goals from clinician to clinician so each of us knows how to proceed to meet those goals. Documentation should highlight barriers and any helpful adaptations made along the way. For example, a patient is having difficulty obtaining an adequate blood sample and is frustrated having to stick himself multiple times. A nurse helps the patient achieve success by washing the hands with warm water and soap first and massaging the finger in a dependent position. Each subsequent nurse should know this and remind the patient to perform these steps. Documentation should be brief and focus on whether or not the patient is able to perform each skill independently or needs review. If the patient is unable to learn or will need assistance, an alternative plan should be formulated as soon as possible. Family members may need to be called in to meet with staff to brainstorm a safe discharge plan.

Communication Among Providers

In order to facilitate appropriate inpatient diabetes self-management education and improve outcomes post-discharge, it is best to have an interdisciplinary team. This may include physicians and other providers, nurses, dietitians, diabetes educators, pharmacists, social workers, case managers, home care coordinators, and physical therapists. To assist with this coordination of care, communication across disciplines is crucial. Appropriate documentation of the learning needs assessment and goals are not only useful for communication purposes but are a requirement of the Joint Commission in order to demonstrate that proper plans for patients' discharge are being met.

THE ROLE OF THE CERTIFIED DIABETES EDUCATOR

When a certified diabetes educator is available, there is often confusion about the role of the staff nurse in diabetes self-management education versus the role of the certified diabetes educator. Roles vary from institution to institution and are somewhat related to the number of beds and the number of certified diabetes educators on site. With the number of inpatients with hyperglycemia constantly rising, it is virtually impossible for certified diabetes educators to meet with and educate all diabetes patients. In addition to the role of educator, certified diabetes educators often spend their time addressing hyperglycemia and facilitating prompt and effective treatment. This takes away from time available to educate and practice skills. Additionally, it is not necessarily the best use of an expert's time to instruct a patient in a survival skill that any bedside nurse could be trained to do. It is better to utilize the certified diabetes educator to fine tune and individualize the education, discussing topics such as how to adjust insulin, food, and activity based on blood glucose levels.

EDUCATING THE STAFF TO BE DIABETES EDUCATORS

Some staff nurses will have more of an interest in diabetes care than others. Those nurses should be cultivated. We offer continuing education in a variety of ways including a monthly Diabetes Resource Nurse committee, day-long courses, and unit-based inservices that cover a variety of topics including teaching glucose meters, insulin delivery devices, and meal planning. The idea is to empower the nurse to feel comfortable with diabetes self-management education and to help brainstorm ways to incorporate it into usual nursing care. The goal is to have at least one diabetes resource nurse on each shift in all clinical areas. Use of diabetes handouts can help guide a nurse when educating patients and ensure that information is uniform and not contradictory from nurse to nurse. Staff should be encouraged to go to diabetes seminars such as certified diabetes educator review courses where they can expand their knowledge and comfort level in a short period of time.

QUALITY IMPROVEMENT PROJECTS

The effectiveness of diabetes resource nurses is one of many possible diabetes quality improvement projects to consider. Many of our nursing practice changes were results of such projects. We implemented a policy that fasting blood glucose could not be checked more than 1 h before breakfast to correct a common practice on the night shift of checking glucoses between 5 and 6 AM. Monitoring point of care testing data helped identify units that were not following the new policy so that they could be counseled. Prandial insulin was often skipped if the patient had started eating the meal prior to administration. Since rapid acting insulin remains effective when given up to 20 minutes after the start of the meal, a new policy allowed insulin to be given within 20 minutes of the start of the meal.

The last piece of the puzzle was to coordinate the meal to match the new and more appropriate timing of monitoring and medication. Our solution was to deliver the meal trays to patients with diabetes first, thus making the meal tray delivery time more predictable. In the end, patients could now be in a more diabetes friendly environment and follow this schedule at home. Quality improvement projects can also be applied to improving the provision of diabetes self-management education to patients in need.

Discharge

For effective discharge planning, collaboration among health-care professionals is essential to transition the patient back to the outpatient setting *(3)*. Safe and effective discharge planning must include follow-up care, which should be clearly defined, discussed, and documented. Referrals to community resources will provide additional support for the patient and family.

SMOOTHING THE TRANSITION FROM INPATIENT TO OUTPATIENT

By the time of discharge, the patient should be able to state when to monitor blood glucose, take diabetes medications, and eat meals. Writing out a tentative schedule with the patient is helpful. The patient or family member should know how many carbohydrate servings are recommended per meal and how to calculate portion sizes. The patient should have a working blood glucose meter and know how to use it and keep records. Prescriptions should be given for test strips and lancets. Oral medications should be reviewed so that the patient knows the dose, time taken, and mechanism of action. It is important to review oral agents taken prior to admission and make sure that the patient does not resume prior medications that are no longer needed. Errors have occurred where, for example, a patient was given a prescription for metformin at discharge and went home taking metformin and resumed taking a prior prescription for Glucophage.

If going home on insulin for the first time, the patient should be able to differentiate between basal and bolus insulin and know the names of each insulin, differences in action in relation to meals, and when and how much to take. This is also important if the patient was taking insulin before and the regimen has now been intensified. Prescriptions for insulin pen needles and syringes should be based on individualized needs in respect to needle length and type of syringe or needle. For example, a 3/10 cc insulin syringe with a short needle will be easier to dose accurately if the dose is less than 30 units and also will be less intimidating to the patient. Other information to review at the time of discharge includes where to store the insulin and meter supplies, disposal of sharps, hypoglycemia detection and treatment, when and who to call for help, and follow-up

Diabetes Discharge Checklist

Name_____DOB_____MR#_____Date_____

CONSISTENT CARBOHYDRATE COUNTING: # SERVINGS/MEAL

Breakfast:_____ Lunch:_____Dinner:_____Who will prepare meals?_____

Received diet instruction ☐ Received handout ☐ Needs Review ☐ Independent ☐

PILLS FOR DIABETES: NEED RXS

Name of Drug	Dose	When to take	Special Instructions

GLUCOSE MONITORING

<u>Need Rx's</u> Glucose meter? ☐ Test strips? ☐ Lancets? ☐
Test Times:_____Who will check BG?_____

Demonstration ☐   Return Demonstration ☐   Needs Review ☐   Independent ☐

INSULIN

FAST ACTING ☐ Name of Insulin:_____Instructions:
Units/Times_____

Demonstration ☐   Return Demonstration ☐   Needs Review ☐   Independent ☐

LONG ACTING ☐ *or* PRE MIX ☐ Instructions: Take_____at_____
Name of Insulin_____Who will draw up & inject_____

Demonstration ☐   Return Demonstration ☐   Needs Review ☐   Independent ☐

<u>Need Rx's</u> For each insulin: Insulin vial & syringes OR Insulin Pens & Pen Needles
_____

Follow up appointment for diabetes management:
_____

Comments:
_____
_____
_____
_____

Signature/Title_____ Date:_____

© 2007 NewYork-Presbyterian Hospital

Fig. 2. Diabetes Discharge Checklist Example.

appointments. Taking the extra time to review this information just prior to discharge can identify any learning deficits or misunderstandings and allow the opportunity to provide further instruction. We have started a program where staff nurses call patients after discharge to find out how they are doing. This presents a great opportunity to review the complex treatment plan and the blood glucose log. This model should become a standard of care for patients going home with a new diagnosis of diabetes or a more intensive regimen.

Constructing a discharge plan that is in keeping with the patient's resources is important. Insurance reimbursement may dictate which blood glucose meter or insulin delivery device the patient may use. Co-pays can be expensive when a patient is asked to take multiple medications for a long list of co-morbidities. Use of a diabetes-specific communication tool can be helpful in making sure the patient has all the necessary skills, knowledge, and equipment for a safe discharge. Fig. 2 is an example of a Diabetes Discharge Checklist used at the Weill Cornell Medical Center to facilitate communication between clinicians and social workers, case managers, and home care coordinators. Staff were trained in the importance of considering all the items listed in the tool so that important components of self care were not overlooked. Patients are more likely to receive instruction in survival skills and necessary equipment and prescriptions when the tool is utilized. This served as a reminder, making it less likely that the patient will go home with an insulin pen, for example, without a prescription for pen needles.

Many patients can benefit from a home health agency referral for at least a safety visit or for continued support and education at home if insurance reimbursement permits. Candidates for home care include those patients who are newly diagnosed and/or taking insulin for the first time, the elderly, those with co-morbidities that require additional care, and a history of an inability to follow treatment recommendations leading to adverse outcomes *(3)*.

CONCLUSION

The numbers of patients with diabetes and hyperglycemia will most likely continue to grow. This presents a dilemma for already overburdened clinicians in inpatient and outpatient settings. Diabetes education is an ongoing process. It is time for nurses and other health-care professionals in close proximity to inpatients with diabetes to take action so that patients do not go home unable to self-manage their disease. Too many patients continue to receive little or no diabetes education in the community *(11)*. The hospitalization may be the only opportunity for the patient to receive individualized instruction in diabetes self-management. Hospitals should continue to look at routines that are not diabetes friendly and work toward change. And most importantly, the certified diabetes educator, as change agent, is often the captain of this journey and needs to remain steady on the course however difficult it may be.

REFERENCES

1. Centers for Disease Control and Prevention. National Diabetes Fact Sheet, General Information and National Estimates on Diabetes in the United States, 2005. Atlanta, Ga: U.S. Department of Health and Human Services, Centers for Disease Control and Prevention; (2005). Available from http://apps.nccd.cdc.gov/DDTSTRS/template/ndfs_2005.pdf Accessed September 26, 2007.
2. Pollom, R., Pollom, D. (2004) Utilization of a Multidisciplinary Team for Inpatient Diabetes *Care Critical Care Quarterly* **2**, 185–188.
3. Clement, S., Braithwaite, S., Magee, M., Ahmann, A., Smith, E., Schafer, R., Hirsch, I. (2004) American Diabetes Association Diabetes in Hospitals Writing Committee: Management of Diabetes and Hyperglycemia in Hospitals *Diabetes Care* **27** 553–591.
4. English, S., Young, S. Diabetes Care in the Hospital in Childs, B., Cypress, M., Spollett, G. (2005) Complete Nurse's Guide to Diabetes Care pp 342–360. Alexandria, VA: American Diabetes Association.
5. Brown, S. (1988) Effects of Educational Interventions in Diabetes Care: A Meta-analysis of Findings *Nursing Research* **4**, 223–230.
6. American Diabetes Association. Clinical Practice Recommendations (2007) *Diabetes Care* **31** (suppl 1):S41.
7. Nettles, A. (2005) Patient Education in the Hospital *Diabetes Spectrum* **18** 44–48.
8. ACE/ADA Task Force on Inpatient Diabetes (2006) American College of Endocrinology and American Diabetes Association Consensus Statement on Inpatient Diabetes and Glycemic Control *Diabetes Care* **29** 1955–1962.
9. Cohen, L., Sedhom, L., Salifu, M, Friedman, E. (2007). Inpatient Diabetes Management: Examining Morning Practice in an Acute Care Setting *The Diabetes Educator* **33** 483–492.
10. Pledger, J. (2005) The effect on inpatient care of a dedicated diabetes specialist nurse *Journal of Diabetes Nursing* **9.7** 252–256.
11. Centers for Disease Control and Prevention (2002). Preventative care practices among persons with diabetes – United States, 1995 and 2001. *JAMA* **288** 2814–2815.

7   Optimizing Self-Care
with Diabetes Complications
and Comorbidities

Belinda P. Childs, MN, ARNP, BC, CDE
and Jolene Grothe, BSN, RN, CDE

CONTENTS

INTRODUCTION
IMPACT OF DIABETES COMPLICATIONS
    AND COMORBIDITIES ON SELF-CARE
POLYPHARMACY WITH DIABETES
    COMPLICATIONS AND COMORBIDITIES
EDUCATION CONSIDERATION FOR
    MACROVASCULAR COMPLICATIONS
CEREBROVASCULAR DISEASE
PERIPHERAL ARTERIAL DISEASE
DIABETIC EYE DISEASE
NEPHROPATHY
DIABETIC NEUROPATHIES
COMORBIDITIES
RESOURCES
ADAPTING GROUP EDUCATION
SUMMARY
REFERENCES

ABSTRACT

Diabetes complications and comorbidities present challenges and opportunities for the diabetes educator when assisting the individual with diabetes to set

From: *Contemporary Diabetes: Educating Your Patient with Diabetes*
Edited by: K. Weinger and C. A. Carver, DOI 10.1007/978-1-60327-208-7_7,
© Humana Press, a part of Springer Science+Business Media, LLC 2009

realistic self-care goals. This chapter utilizes self-care behaviors as a framework for educational considerations, taking into account many of the common diabetes complications including myocardial infarction, heart failure, visual impairment, diabetic kidney disease, and peripheral neuropathy. Optimizing self-care can be overwhelming for the individual with diabetes complications and comorbidities. Assisting the individual to identify barriers, prioritize needs, and develop strategies to overcome those barriers move them closer to the goal of optimum self-care.

Key Words: Diabetes complications, Comorbidities, Resources, Microvascular disease, Macrovascular disease.

INTRODUCTION

Optimizing self-care can be challenged by the presence of diabetes complications and comorbidities. The role of the diabetes educator is to assist the individual in identifying barriers to self-care, prioritizing needs, and developing strategies to overcome the identified barriers. For the individual who has complications and/or comorbidities, the educator should assist the individual to identify risk factors that may be modified to prevent the progression of the complication or development of new complications.

According to the 2005 Center for Disease Control Fact Sheet, heart disease and stroke account for 65% of the deaths associated with diabetes (1). Diabetic retinopathy was responsible for 12,000–24,000 new cases of blindness. Between 60 and 70% of patients with diabetes had some neuropathy, and in one year, nearly 82,000 amputations were performed. The report also indicates that 153,730 individuals had end-stage renal disease resulting in the need for kidney transplantation or dialysis. These numbers quantify the impact that microvascular and macrovascular diseases can have on the individual with diabetes. The statistics do not begin to reflect the personal impact on the individual with diabetes or their family.

Most adults with diabetes also have one comorbid condition and up to 40% reported three comorbid conditions (2). These conditions may be associated with diabetes such as thyroid disease and macular degeneration or may include cancer, arthritis, and other diseases associated with aging.

IMPACT OF DIABETES COMPLICATIONS AND COMORBIDITIES ON SELF-CARE

Complications and comorbidities can have a significant impact on the patient's ability to manage their self-care. Krien and colleagues evaluated the effect of pain on one's ability to carry out self-care. Sixty percent of the patients with diabetes reported pain and those with chronic pain reported more difficulty in following the recommended exercise and dietary plans. When patients with severe or very severe pain were compared with those that had moderate to mild pain, those with severe pain have more difficulty taking medications and exercising (3). Aljasem and colleagues reported in a study of type 2 patients that those with complications tended to skip medications. However, in this study complications did not affect other self-care behaviors such as exercising, eating, or testing of blood glucose levels (4).

Safford and colleagues found that individuals with diabetes spend an average of 48 min a day on self-care. In addition, they found that those with severe neuropathy were more than twice as likely to spend time caring for their feet as those without neuropathy, yet one in four reported spending no time on foot care (5). Even when comorbid chronic diseases do not directly limit one's ability to self-manage their diabetes, these comorbidities represent competing demands (6).

There is little research on the effect of comorbidities on the ability to perform self-care. But clinically, one can expect that cancer and chemotherapy treatments can lead to alteration in one's ability to consume adequate consistent calories. The impact of steroid use on blood glucose levels is well known whether the steroids are given orally for a number of autoimmune diseases like rheumatoid arthritis, as premedication for chemotherapy, to manage chronic obstructive pulmonary disease (COPD) or as an intra-articular treatment for osteoarthritis (7). The impact of psychosocial issues such as depression and anxiety is addressed in another chapter.

During the assessment phase, the educator will need to assist the individual to determine what barriers to self-care, if any, are present as a result of any diabetes complications or comorbidities. Once the barriers have been identified, it will be important for the educator to assist the patient in prioritizing the needs and goals. When there are multiple complications and comorbidities, patients often struggle with managing these complex problems and complicated regimens. Petite and Kerr note that clinicians and patients often must set priorities and focus on specific health goals (8). It may not be possible to achieve every goal when there are multiple problems present. Commonly, multiple health specialists care for patients with complications. This may complicate the messages that patients receive regarding which self-care behaviors are a priority. The individual may be overwhelmed by the multiple goals set by multiple health care providers. The diabetes educator can facilitate the communication between the patient and the health care specialists and assist in setting realistic goals.

Educators help the patient identify strategies, including the use of available resources, to overcome the barriers to carry out self-care. Once the barriers have been identified, the educator can assist by providing information, developing strategies with the patient to overcome these barriers, and identifying potential resources to overcome the identified barriers.

Each patient is unique in duration of diabetes; presence of complications and/or comorbidities; and physical, cognitive, psychological, social, and economic status. The AADE 7^{TM} Self-Care Behaviors of healthy eating, being active, taking medication, monitoring, problem solving, healthy coping, and risk reduction provide a framework for evaluating the potential barriers and strategies that may be associated with each of the complications and should be considered for the impact of individual comorbidities (9).

POLYPHARMACY WITH DIABETES COMPLICATIONS AND COMORBIDITIES

Polypharmacy is a natural consequence of practicing evidence-based care with individuals with diabetes with or without complications (10). There is conflicting information regarding whether polypharmacy reduces the patients adherence to the treatment of a chronic condition. Studies with patients who have hypertension or hyperlipidemia suggest that patient adherence to medication regimens is poor. A large study conducted in Italy with 16,000 patients with hypertension found that 64.9% were not adherent to their medication regimen over a 1-year period (11). A British study of patients with diabetes who were on simvastatin demonstrated a clinically significant rate of nonadherence to the medication regimen (12). A study evaluating the records of 653 patients with diabetes and dyslipidemia prescribed statin therapy in a managed diabetes care program found a correlation between adherence to the statin therapy as reflected by computing a 9-month medication possession ratio (MPR). This study found that LDL goal achievement appeared to increase when the MPR is greater than 80% (13).

Similar issues have been cited in patients with diabetes using oral hypoglycemic agents (14). A study of patients with diabetes with prescription coverage found medication adherence rates between 31 and 60%. Furthermore, financial issues were not the primary cause for poor adherence. A study of patients with diabetic nephropathy and hypertension also showed that reduced medication adherence was an important issue in their management (15).

In contrast, a recent study in patients with diabetes claimed that treatment regimens with multiple medications did not reduce the adherence of patients with diabetes (16). However, its findings were based on subjective patient reports during telephone interviews. These findings were in contrast to many previous studies as cited above, as well as an earlier study, which addressed the same question but measured actual pills that, arguably, had a stronger methodology (17).

Supplements and complementary treatments, as well as over-the-counter medications, also must be accounted for when obtaining a medication history.

Najm and colleagues found that 48% of the elderly surveyed in their study used complementary and alternative medicine during the past year, and 62% of the elderly who used these did not tell their health care providers about their use of these therapies *(18)*.

Medication Strategies

Medications play such a critical role in the management of the complications and comorbidities associated with diabetes. When assessing medication behaviors, the educator should

- Make sure the medication list is accurate by asking the patient to bring all medications to the visit including over-the-counter medications, alternative, and complimentary therapies
- Review with the patient if he or she is experiencing any side effects associated with any of the medications
- Review the list for duplicative medications
- Evaluate number of times medications may be missed at home
- Determine contributing factors related to missed medications, i.e., memory, cost, inability to open bottles, fear of side effects, or side effects that occur as a result of medication, health beliefs, or the failure to see value in medication

Strategies to improve medication adherence may include the following:

- Collaboration with the patient's care team to eliminate duplicate medications, simplify the regimen, and/or report any noted side effects
- Identification of the patient's potential memory aids, i.e., notes in home, alarms, pill containers, personal journals
- Confirmation that the patient understands the reason for each medication
- Identification of the patient's personal support members, i.e., family members, significant others, visiting nurses

Inconsistent dosing could lead to inappropriate dose adjustments and/or addition of medications that are not necessary, which can lead to additional financial hardships and unnecessary medication side effects.

EDUCATION CONSIDERATION FOR MACROVASCULAR COMPLICATIONS

Coronary Artery Disease

Macrovascular complications include coronary artery disease, cerebrovascular disease, and peripheral arterial disease. These complications can lead to a multitude of other associated complications including myocardial infarctions, heart failure, stroke, and foot and leg ulcers. Modifiable risk factors include hyperglycemia, hypertension, dyslipidemia, smoking, obesity, poor eating habits and food choices, and a sedentary lifestyle *(19)*.

Table 1
Educator Considerations for Patient Self-Care Behaviors
after a Myocardial Infarction and Heart Failure

Medications	• Verify understanding of medications' dosing times • Identify strategies to assure adherence to prescriptions • Review medication list for duplication and completeness • Look for signs and symptoms of drug interactions
Monitoring	• Monitor blood pressure • Monitor lipids to reach even more aggressive goals • Monitor blood glucose * Monitor for signs of fluid overload, i.e., edema, shortness of breath, altered insulin requirements, increased weight
Healthy eating	• Identify weight loss goals • Modify diet plan, which may include recommendations of low sodium, lower saturated fat, and/or decreased calories
Physical activity	• Talk about modification of sexual activity if necessary • Incorporate cardiac rehabilitation if necessary * Adapt physical activity as required
Risk reduction	• Manage medication • Discuss cessation of smoking • Work to achieve LDL and HDL goals • Work to achieve BP goals
Healthy coping	• Be aware of increased risk for depression • Discuss adjustment for newly diagnosed patients • Recognize fears • Discuss potential need for support systems, i.e., family, friends, counselor, spiritual advisor
Problem solving	• Assist individual in identification of fears and potential barriers • Help patient identify when to call health care provider with signs and symptoms, including potential medication interactions • Prioritize goals with patient

The self-care behaviors provide a framework for the prevention or management of all macrovascular complications. Improved health can occur if the individual increases physical activity, modifies his or her eating plan utilizing the DASH meal plan, and follows a low-fat/reduced calorie meal plan to result in weight loss if needed. Tobacco cessation and using alcohol in moderation and taking prescribed medications at the appropriate times also reduce one's risk for complication progression. Monitoring is required for hypertension and dyslipidemia to assure that the individual is meeting their goals for blood pressure and blood lipids.

Additional challenges become apparent when an individual has suffered a myocardial infarction or has developed heart failure as a result of their cardiovascular disease. Table 1 identifies specific goals for self-care behavior areas for patients who have had myocardial infarction; additional considerations for those with heart failure are delineated in the table by an *.

CEREBROVASCULAR DISEASE

Hypertension is the most important risk factor for having a stroke. Smoking more than doubles the risk for having a stroke and increases the incidence of extracranial arterial disease. Risk reduction includes smoking cessation, management of hypertension, and medication management for lipids, blood pressure, and anticoagulation. Assessing the patient's capabilities after a stroke and identifying resources for the individual and family will be important. If hemiperesis has resulted from a stroke, the educator will need to assist the patient and family in identifying adaptive tools. Opening a medication bottle may be impossible and even the tab on a "daily pill box" may not be accessible. Glucose monitoring and insulin administration may require physical assistance or adaptation to collect the blood sample and place it on the glucose strip. Insulin administration may require use of an insulin pen, pre-drawn syringe, or other adaptive device. Consistency of food may need to be adapted which may alter the oral diabetes medication doses or insulin requirements.

Physical activity likely will be altered and options to maintain some level of activity will need to be addressed. A physical or occupational therapy consult may be appropriate for assistance in determining the most appropriate physical activity. Coping and adapting to a new health state may require assistance from our mental health colleagues. Helping the individual identify positive relationships and activities will assist the individual as they adjust following their stroke. Identifying every opportunity possible for the patient to control his or her environment and life will be valuable.

PERIPHERAL ARTERIAL DISEASE

Peripheral arterial disease is a manifestation of atherosclerosis character-ized by atherosclerotic occlusive disease of the lower extremities and is a marker for atherothrombotic disease. In the Framingham Heart Study, 20% of the patients with peripheral arterial disease had diabetes *(20)*. The most common symptom of peripheral arterial disease is intermittent claudication, defined as pain, cramping, or aching in the calves, thighs, or buttocks that appears reproducibly with walking exercise and is relieved by rest. Resting pain, tissue loss, or gangrene are the most severe symptoms of peripheral arte-rial disease. These limb-threatening manifestations of peripheral arterial disease are collectively termed critical limb ischemia and are a major risk factor for lower-extremity amputation. Peripheral arterial disease is a marker for systemic vascular disease involving coronary, cerebral, and renal vessels. The strongest risk factors for peripheral arterial disease are diabetes, smoking, as well as advancing age, hypertension, and hyperlipidemia. Peripheral arterial disease in diabetes adversely affects quality of life and contributes to long-term dis-ability and functional impairment. A slower walking speed (generally <2 mph) and a limited walking distance is noted in patients who have intermittent clau-dication. This may result in a progressive loss of conditioning and loss of function *(21)*.

The medication considerations have been noted previously. Medication may be used to decrease platelet aggregation. There are no special dietary consid-erations with peripheral arterial disease, but one would continue to encourage healthy eating to reduce hypertension, dyslipidemia, and hyperglycemia, which are all risk factors associated with peripheral arterial disease. Adaptation will need to be considered for physical activity. Many randomized trials have demon-strated the benefits of supervised exercise in individuals with peripheral arterial disease *(22)*. In all the studies the best benefit was from supervised exercise. Studies of unsupervised activity showed limited efficacy in improving func-tional capacity. Physical activity recommendations should be prescribed by an exercise specialist or physician.

Compression stockings are often used as treatment for peripheral arterial dis-ease. Patients may have difficulty getting these stockings on and off. Family members may need to be identified to assist, stockings with zippers ordered, or other adaptive tools identified to assist with this task.

Preventive foot care is a risk reduction behavior that will minimize the risk of developing foot complications and limb loss. According to the American Dia-betes Association position statement, the "neuroischemic *(23)*" foot is more prone to traumatic ulceration, infection, and gangrene. The primary aim for footwear is to protect the foot from pressure and shear. A shoe that is suffi-ciently long, broad, and deep is recommended. A referral to a podiatrist or other foot specialist may be appropriate. Daily examination of the foot would be considered an important monitoring function by the individual with diabetes and peripheral arterial disease.

Amputation may be a result of peripheral arterial disease and neuropathy. Opportunities for physical activity likely will change. The educator will need to problem solve with the individual to identify strategies to obtain physical activity such as upper body exercises, swimming, and other adaptive opportunities. Providing opportunities for the individual to express his feelings related to the loss of the limb will be important. Referral to an exercise specialist, physical therapist, and mental health expert may be appropriate. Diligent foot care of the remaining limb on the part of the individual and knowing when to seek attention with any change in integrity are important limb preservation strategies.

DIABETIC EYE DISEASE

Approximately 4.1 million US adults 40 years and older have diabetic retinopathy; 1 of every 12 persons with diabetes in this age group has advanced, vision-threatening retinopathy *(24)*. Age-related macular degeneration is the leading cause of blindness and visual disability in patients 60 years or older in the Western hemisphere *(25)*. Visual impairment will require adaptation to carry out self-care whether it is related to diabetes or other complications or comorbidities. Table 2 identifies specific considerations for self-care areas as they relate to individuals with visual impairments.

NEPHROPATHY

Diabetic nephropathy is the leading cause of kidney disease in patients requiring renal replacement therapy and affects $\sim$ 40% of type 1 and type 2 patients with diabetes. It increases the risk of death, mainly from cardiovascular causes. Hyperglycemia, hypertension, and genetic predisposition are the main risk factors for the development of diabetic nephropathy. Elevated serum lipids, smoking habits, and dietary protein also contribute to the development of renal disease *(26)*.

In diabetic chronic kidney disease patients on routine hemodialysis, poor glycemic control is an independent predictor of prognosis. This finding indicates the importance of careful management of glycemic control even after initiation of hemodialysis *(27)*. Because the human kidney normally takes up and releases glucose, patients with end-stage renal disease are prone to hypoglycemia *(28)*. Progression in renal disease may lead to more variable glucose control.

Table 2
Educator Considerations for Self-Care Behaviors for patients with Visual Impairment

Medications	• Identify adaptive tools for insulin administration, i.e., pens, magnifiers • Suggest tactile day of the week pillboxes for oral meds
Monitoring	• Recommend regular eye exams • Identify a glucose meter that is useable by individual, i.e., talking meter or one with large display, easy blood dosing
Healthy eating	• Help patient to achieve optimal levels of glucose, BP, and lipids • Help patient to identify foods and discover techniques to prepare foods
Physical activity	• Suggest limited lifting and bending if proliferative retinopathy is present • Help patient identify safe activities with reduced visual ability
Risk reduction	• Discuss smoking cessation • Help patient to obtain euglycemia • Help patient to manage hypertension
Healthy coping	• Be aware of increased risk for depression • Discuss adaptation to visual loss • Recognize fears and explain treatments
Problem solving	• Use adaptive tools for medication administration • Use talking glucose meter • Identify resources • Identify support systems • Talk to patient about when to call eye professionals

Hemodialysis or peritoneal dialysis may increase the risk for hypoglycemia and even hyperglycemia if the insulin doses are not managed optimally. During hemodialysis glucose is removed during the dialysis but insulin remains active. Insulin doses may need to be different on dialysis days versus non-dialysis days. Glucose monitoring will need to be increased to determine the most appropriate insulin doses. Many times insulin is withheld due to the fear of hypoglycemia during dialysis which then leads to post-treatment hyperglycemia. During peritoneal dialysis, the dialysis solution, which remains in the peritoneal cavity, may have variable glucose concentration to create ultrafiltration of excess fluid. This level of glucose in the solution is determined by the patient under the guidance

Table 3
Educator Considerations for Self-Care Behaviors for Patients with Kidney Disease

Medications	• Relay understanding that time actions of medications may be prolonged due to decreased renal function and medication clearance
Monitoring	• Monitor blood pressure • Monitor blood glucose due to increased risk of hypoglycemia • Daily weights if on dialysis
Healthy eating	• Alter diet to reduce protein consumption • Discuss alterations in appetite
Physical activity	• Discuss fatigue associated with renal disease • Relay importance of maintaining physical activity • Recommend that patients exercise caution due to increase in osteodystrophy with increased risk of fractures and pain
Risk reduction	• Manage hypertension • Manage dyslipidemia • Work toward optimal glucose control
Healthy coping	• Be aware of increased risk for depression • Recognize fears with declining health
Problem solving	• Assist individual in identification of fears and potential barriers

of their nephrologist and is determined by their weight and blood pressure prior to the treatment. Glucose monitoring will be important including pre- and post-treatment blood glucose levels, amount of insulin taken throughout the day, and amount placed in the dialysis solution *(29)*. See additional self-care educator considerations for patients with kidney disease in Table 3.

DIABETIC NEUROPATHIES
Peripheral Neuropathies

The most common of the neuropathies are chronic sensorimotor distal symmetric polyneuropathy (DPN) and the autonomic neuropathies. Up to 50% of DPN may be asymptomatic. Patients are at risk of insensate injury to their feet and as many as 80% of amputations follow a foot ulcer or injury. Early recognition of at-risk individuals, patient education, and appropriate foot care may result in a reduced incidence of ulceration and consequently amputation *(29)*. Peripheral neuropathy is one of the most painful, debilitating complications of diabetes. Managing pain and addressing the fears and frustrations of living with peripheral neuropathy will be necessary. Research has shown that reducing the excursions in the blood glucose levels can reduce pain. Medications likely will be required to alleviate moderate to severe pain. Neuropathy not only leads to changes in sensation but can lead to muscle wasting and reduced dexterity.

These changes may contribute to a higher risk for falls. Opening and closing medicine bottles or drawing up insulin doses may be a challenge. See

Table 4
Educator Considerations for Self-Care Behaviors for Patients with
Peripheral Neuropathies

Medications	• Verify understanding of time of medications dosing • Identify strategies to assure adherence to prescriptions • Review medication list for duplication and completeness • Discuss signs and symptoms of drug interactions • Discuss adaptation to medicine bottle/insulin delivery devices
Monitoring	• Monitor blood glucose to reduce glucose variability • Discuss use of meter with cartridge or drum • Encourage daily foot inspection
Healthy eating	• Adapt healthy meal plan to optimize glucose control
Physical activity	• Discuss adaptations for physical activity • Discuss strategies to prevent falls • Encourage appropriate footwear
Risk reduction	• Help patient work toward optimal diabetes control with limited glucose variability • Discuss strategies to prevent falls • Encourage appropriate footwear
Healthy coping	• Be aware of increased risk for depression • Recognize fears of living with chronic pain
Problem solving	• Discuss strategies to aid the patient with painful neuropathy to attain restful sleep, e.g., sheets off feet, timing of neuropathy, and analgesic medication

Table 4 for additional self-care considerations for patients with peripheral neuropathies.

Autonomic Neuropathies

Autonomic neuropathy may involve every system in the body and increases morbidity and mortality, particularly if it is cardiovascular autonomic neuropathy *(29)*. Sexual dysfunction, bladder dysfunction, sudomotor dysfunction (gustatory sweating), abnormal pupillomotor response, gastroparesis, nocturnal diarrhea, and hypoglycemia unawareness are all associated with autonomic dysfunction as well.

The educational needs related to medication have previously been discussed and apply to medications that may be administered for any of the symptoms of autonomic neuropathy. The one peril that may be different is in patients who have gastroparesis; both the patients and providers need to consider the effects of gastric delay on the medication action. For example, an antibiotic or a thyroid medication that is directed to be given on an empty stomach. There may not be hours in the day when the stomach is completely empty; thus in this situation, the goal would be to give the medications consistently.

The patient's need to monitor will depend on the organ affected by autonomic neuropathy. For cardiac autonomic neuropathy, the patient may need to be taught to monitor their blood pressure due to the risk of hypotension. To prevent orthostatic hypotension, these patients should be instructed to not stand up from a supine position, without first sitting, and then slowly rising while holding on to something. They may need to monitor their heart rate/pulse especially with exercise. The individual will need to be taught the symptoms of a silent myocardial infarction including nausea, diaphoresis, shortness of breath, and/or fatigue *(30)*. For gastroparesis, glucose monitoring premeal and postmeal will be necessary to determine appropriate timing of insulin. A patient with bladder dysfunction will need to know the signs and symptoms of a urinary tract infection. Individuals with hypoglycemia unawareness will need to know the importance of identifying subtle symptoms of hypoglycemia, and family members and friends should be taught to identify warning symptoms of hypoglycemia. Fissures on the feet may be a result of sudomotor dysfunction; daily foot inspection will be important as well as foot care, i.e., cream application. Monitoring for a change in symptoms will be important for all of the autonomic neuropathies.

For the individual with gastroparesis, food choices may be altered to reduce the fiber and fat content in the meal plan. Small, frequent meals may be suggested. Buccal treatment of hypoglycemia may be more effective than oral ingestion of carbohydrates. Improving gastric emptying may lead to resolution of constipation which may be a sign of gastroparesis. If not, a higher fiber meal plan may be indicated in addition to an increase in fluid intake to decrease the firmness of the stool.

Those with cardiac autonomic neuropathy may have reduced exercise tolerance. A clearance from the patient's cardiologist should be obtained prior to any significant change in physical activity. Armchair activities may be the most appropriate for an individual with cardiac autonomic neuropathy. For the individual with hypoglycemia unawareness, it will be important to stress the importance of glucose monitoring before, immediately after, and up to 24 h after exercise, to reduce the risk of severe hypoglycemia.

Optimal glucose control will not only help to prevent the development of autonomic neuropathy but may also improve autonomic neuropathy *(31)*. Reducing risks includes optimal control of blood glucose levels, blood pressure, and taking safety precautions like glucose monitoring prior to driving, not driving at night (pupillomotor response delay), and rising slowly to prevent dizziness if one has cardiac autonomic neuropathy. Assisting the patient to cope with any of the neuropathies will include listening to their fears, providing positive reinforcement, directing them to support groups if available, and referring to mental health experts if appropriate.

Each patient is unique and thus his or her needs will be different. The neuropathies are a challenge, but the educator can assist the patient in problem solving by helping the individual identify when to call the health care provider, identify key information to share, and in developing the right questions to ask their medical provider. Guiding the patient to appropriate resources is important.

COMORBIDITIES

Individuals with diabetes are at risk of developing any other medical condition. Most medical problems complicate the self-management of diabetes whether it is depression, arthritis, cancer, or influenza. Depression can be acute or chronic. Arthritis and chronic obstructive lung disease are examples of chronic conditions that may create significant barriers to physical activity. The medications used to treat these diseases may cause significant variation in blood glucose levels and blood pressure. Regardless of the comorbidity, the educator can adapt the self-care behavior model to assist in identifying barriers to self-care potentially created by the comorbidity and develop strategies to overcome the barriers. As examples, depression and arthritis present different barriers.

Depression

Major depression as a chronic or recurrent condition has been reported in as many as 11–15% in patients with type 2 diabetes *(32)*. As many as two-thirds of patients with diabetes and major depression have been ill with depression for ≥ 2 years *(33)*. Poorer self-management (i.e., following diet, exercise regimens, and checking blood glucose) and lapses in refilling oral hypoglycemic, lipid-lowering, and antihypertensive medications have been reported in patients with diabetes and depression *(34)*. They are also more likely to have three or more cardiac risk factors (i.e., smoking, obesity, sedentary lifestyle, HbA_{1c} [AIC] > 8.0%) compared with those with diabetes alone *(35)*.

Individuals with diabetes and comorbid major depression have higher odds of functional disability compared with individuals with either diabetes or major depression alone. Additional studies are needed to establish a causal relationship *(36)*. If the diabetes educator believes that an individual is depressed and this is interfering with their ability to perform self-care, they should refer the individual to the appropriate mental health expert.

Arthritis

Arthritis can lead to physical disabilities, cause discomfort when exercising, and lead to decreased exercise capacity. To promote physical activity, the educator can assist the individual in identifying activities that they can comfortably pursue such as swimming in a warm swimming pool or chair exercises. The educator encourages the individual to join a support group for individuals with arthritis. Some medications used in the treatment of arthritis may alter the blood glucose levels. The educator will want to reinforce the importance of monitoring and problem solving.

RESOURCES

Every year in January, the American Diabetes Association publishes a supplement to Diabetes Forecast that identifies resources for people with diabetes. A section is devoted to "aids for people who are visually or physically handicapped *(37)*." The Resource Guide lists tools for insulin administration, glucose monitoring, and other helpful resources. Many organizations have tools and resources that can be identified on the internet. Collaborating with other health professionals including physical therapists, occupational health experts, and mental health colleagues will be of benefit as the educator guides the individual who is striving to live their lives to their optimal potential with diabetes.

ADAPTING GROUP EDUCATION

The educator not only will need to consider the best setting for the patient for learning, i.e., group or individual, but must also consider if adaptations will need to be made for the individual if they have complications or comorbidities. Some considerations may include

- Preferential setting for those with hearing or low-vision problems
- Non-visual note-taking options such as tape recorders, voice recognition software, use of Braille
- Consider how to use non-disabled senses or abilities to convey information and skills
- Choose adaptive tools and techniques to enhance self-management skills such as

  o Arm chair exercises for an individual with Charcot's arthropathy
  o Simplified meal plan for an individual with profound depression
  o Non-visual method for glucose monitoring
  o Availability of tools to examine and try during education
  o One-handed insulin administration using an insulin pen for an individual with hemiparesis

- Accessible location, i.e., near public transportation for those who are visually impaired and do not drive
- Accessible for those with physical handicaps, i.e., those with amputations, wheelchair bound

SUMMARY

Managing diabetes complications and/or comorbidities can seem overwhelming to the individual already living with diabetes and can threaten their independence in providing self-care. The diabetes educator has the opportunity using the AADE 7™ Self-Care Behaviors as a framework to assist the individual to set realistic, attainable goals. Assisting the individual to identify barriers, prioritize needs, and develop strategies to overcome those barriers can break an overwhelming task into smaller more manageable steps and move the individual closer to the goal of optimal self-care and improved quality of life.

REFERENCES

1. www.diabetes.org/uedocuments/NationalDiabetesFactSheetRev.pdf, accessed October 29, 2007
2. Wolfe JL, Starfield B, Anderson G; Prevalence, expenditures, and complications of multiple chronic conditions in the elderly. Arch Intern Med 2002; 62: 2269–2276.

3. Krein SL, Heisler M, Piette JD, Makkie F, Kerr EA. The effect of chronic pain on diabetes self management. Diabetes Care 2005;28:65–70.
4. Aljasem LI, Peyrot M, Wissow L. Rubin R. The impact of barriers and self efficacy on self-care behaviors in type 2 diabetes. Diabetes Educ 2001; 27:393–404
5. Safford MM, Russell L, Suh DC, Roman S, Pogach L. How much time do patients with diabetes spend on self care? J Am Bd Fam Pr 2005; 18:262–270.
6. Bayliss, EA, Steiner JF, Fernald DH, Crane LA, Main DS. Description of barriers to self-care by persons with comorbid chronic diseases. Ann Fm Med, 2003; 1: 15–21,
7. Childs BP. Glucocorticoid use in diabetes. In: Childs, BP, ed, Complete nurse's guide to diabetes care. Alexandria, VA: Am Diabetes Assoc, 2005; 28:320–322.
8. Piette JD, Kerr EA. The impact of comorbid chronic complications on diabetes care. Diabetes Care 2006; 29:725–731.
9. American Association of Diabetes Educators. Position statement: individualization of diabetes self-management education. Diabetes Educ, 2007; 33: 45–49.
10. American Diabetes Association. Standards of medical care in diabetes-2007. Diabetes Care 2007; 30:s4–s41.
11. Degli Esposito L, Degli Esposito E, Valpiani G, Di Martino M, Saragoni S, Buda S, Baio G, Capone A, Sturani A: A retrospective, population-based analysis of persistence with anti-hypertensive drug therapy in primary care practice in Italy. Clin Ther 2002; 8:1347–1357.
12. Collins R, Armitage J, Parish S, Sleigh P, Peto R, Heart Protection Collaborative Group. Heart Protection Study of cholesterol-lowering with simvastatin in 5,963 people with diabetes: a randomized placebo-controlled study. Lancet 2003; 361:2005–2016.
13. Parris RD, Lawrence DB, Mohn LA, Long LB. Adherence to statin therapy and ldl cholesterol goal attainment by patients with diabetes and dyslipidemia. Diabetes Care 2005; 28:595–599.
14. Boccuzzi SJ, Wogen J, Fox J, Sung JCY, Shah AB, Kim J: Utilization of oral hypoglycemic agents in a drug-insured U.S. Population. Diabetes Care 2001;24:1441–1445.
15. Bakris GL: The role of combination anti-hypertensive therapy and the progression of renal disease hypertension: looking toward the next millenium. Am J Hypertens 1998;11: 158S–162S.
16. Grant RW, Devita NG, Singer DE, Meigs JB. Polypharmacy and medication adherence in patients with type 2 diabetes. Diabetes Care 2003; 26,1408–1412.
17. Paes AH, Bakker A, Soe-Agnie CJ: The impact of dose frequency on patient compliance. Diabetes Care 1997; 20:1512–1517.
18. Najm W, Reinsch S, Hoehler F, Tobis J: Use of complementary and alternative medicine among the ethnic elderly. Altern Ther Health Med 2003; 9: 50–57.
19. Lorber D. Macrovascular disease. In Mensing C, ed The art and science of diabetes self-management education. Chicago: Am Assoc Diabetes Educ, 2007; 21:475–501.
20. Murabito JM, D'Agostino RB, Silbershatz H, Wilson WF: Intermittent claudication: a risk profile from the Framingham Heart Study. Circulation 1997: 96:44–49.
21. American Diabetes Association, Peripheral arterial disease in people with diabetes. Diabetes Care 2003: 26:3333–3341.
22. Leng GC, Fowler B, Ernst E. Exercise for intermittent claudication (Cochrane Review). Cochrane Database Syst Rev 2:CD000990, 2000
23. American Diabetes Association: Preventive foot care in people with diabetes (Position Statement). Diabetes Care 26 (Suppl. 1)2003:S78–S79.
24. Kempen JH, O'Colmain BJ, Leske MC, Haffner SM, Klein R, Moss SE, Taylor HR, Hamman RF, the Eye Diseases Prevalence Research Group: The prevalence of diabetic retinopathy among adults in the United States. Arch Ophthalmol 2004; 122:552–563.
25. Klein R, Klein BE, Jensen SC, Meuer SM. The five-year incidence and progression of age-related maculopathy: the beaver dam eye study. Ophthalmology. 1997;104:7–21.

26. Gross JL, de Azevedo MJ, Silveiro SP, Canani LH, Caramori ML, Zelmanovitz T. Diabetic Nephropathy: diagnosis, prevention, and treatment. Diabetes Care 28:164–176, 2005
27. Oomichi T, Emoto M, Tabata T, Morioka T, Tsujimot Y, Tahara H, Shoji T, Nishizawa Y. Impact of glycemic control on the survival of diabetic patients on chronic regular dialysis: a 7-year observational study. Diabetes Care 2006;29: 1496–1500.
28. Meyer C, Dostou JM, Gerich J. Role of the human kidney in glucose counter-regulation. Diabetes 1999, 48: 943–948.
29. Ossman SS. Diabetic nephropathy: where we have been and where we are going. Diabetes Spectr 2006;19:153–156.
30. Vinik AI, Vinik EJ. Diabetic nephropathies. In Mensing C, ed The art and science of diabetes self-management education. Chicago: Am Assoc Diabetes Educ, 2007; 21:561.
31. Boulton AJM, Vinik AI, Arezzo JC, Bril V, Feldman EL, Freeman R. Malik RA, Maser RE, Sosenko JM, Ziegler D. Diabetic neuropathies. Diabetes Care 2005;28:956–962.
32. Anderson RJ, Freedland KE, Clouse RE, Lustman PJ: The prevalence of comorbid depression in adults with diabetes: a meta-analysis. Diabetes Care 2001; 24:1069–1078.
33. Katon W, von Korff M, Ciechanowski P, Russo J, Lin E, Simon G, Ludman E, Walker E, Bush T, Young B: Behavioral and clinical factors associated with depression among individuals with diabetes. Diabetes Care 2004; 27:914–920.
34. Lin EH, Katon W, Von Korff M, Rutter C, Simon GE, Oliver M, Ciechanowski P, Ludman EJ, Bush T, Young B: Relationship of depression and diabetes self-care, medication adherence, and preventive care. Diabetes Care 2004; 27:2154–2160.
35. Katon WJ, Lin EH, Russo J, Von Korff M, Ciechanowski P, Simon G, Ludman E, Bush T, Young B: Cardiac risk factors in patients with diabetes mellitus and major depression. J Gen Intern Med 2004;19:1192–1199.
36. Egede LE. Diabetes, major depression and functional disability among u.s. adults. Diabetes Care 2004; 27:421–428.
37. http://diabetes.org/diabetes-forecast/RG07/RG07insulindelivery.pdf accessed October 29, 2007

8

Role of Culture and Health Literacy in Diabetes Self-Management and Education

Andreina Millan-Ferro and Enrique Caballero, M.D.

CONTENTS

INTRODUCTION
ACCULTURATION
CULTURAL COMPETENCE
LANGUAGE
HEALTH LITERACY
EDUCATIONAL LEVEL
KNOWLEDGE ABOUT THE DISEASE
SOCIOECONOMIC STATUS
JUDGMENT AND BELIEFS ABOUT THE DISEASE
MYTHS
FEARS
OTHER TYPES OF MEDICINE (ALTERNATIVE)
NUTRITIONAL PREFERENCES
PHYSICAL ACTIVITY
BODY IMAGE
WORK ENVIRONMENT
DEPRESSION
RELIGION AND FAITH
GENERAL FAMILY INTEGRATION AND SUPPORT
QUALITY OF LIFE

From: *Contemporary Diabetes: Educating Your Patient with Diabetes*
Edited by: K. Weinger and C. A. Carver, DOI 10.1007/978-1-60327-208-7_8,
© Humana Press, a part of Springer Science+Business Media, LLC 2009

INDIVIDUAL AND SOCIAL INTERACTION
CONCLUSION
REFERENCES

ABSTRACT

To educate patients with diabetes in a multicultural society presents educators with the challenge of becoming culturally sensitive in order to understand and convey the meaning of untranslatable education messages for patients of all health literacy levels. The goal of this chapter is to raise awareness about the most common cultural and social factors that may influence diabetes self-care management and education in patients from culturally diverse populations.

Key Words: Culture, Health literacy, Diabetes, Cultural competence, Minority groups.

INTRODUCTION

We all are the result of a combination of biological, spiritual, psychological and social elements, which makes each one of us unique. But at the same time many of us share enough characteristics such as history, language, traditions, nationality, religion, food preferences, health beliefs, genetics, and cultural heritage that we can live together as societies with distinct cultures.

In the United States white Americans represent three quarters of the population of a country where increasing numbers of other racial and ethnic groups collide to form a multicultural society. Most of these minority groups have an increased risk of developing diabetes, and, as in many other countries, minority groups usually lag behind the predominant group in many health aspects *(1)*. The Institute of Medicine reported that clear health-care disparities exist when a large number of outcomes are compared, including some related to diabetes care, between the white population and the minority groups *(2)*.

The minority groups with the highest numbers of people in the United States are Latinos/Hispanics, African Americans, American Indians, Alaska natives, Asian Americans, Pacific Islanders, and Arabs *(1)*. With such heterogeneity in the population, the need for cultural competence among educators is imminent. The goal of this chapter is to raise awareness about the most common cultural and social factors that may influence diabetes self-care management and education in patients from culturally diverse populations.

ACCULTURATION

Culture refers to the behavior patterns, beliefs, arts, and all other products of human work and thought, as expressed in a particular community *(3)*. *Acculturation* refers to the adoption of some specific elements of one culture by a different cultural group *(4)*. For immigrants to the United States, it relates to the integration of multiple preferences and behaviors from mainstream culture. No uniform instrument to assess acculturation exists. Throughout the literature, various categories of acculturation can be identified: assimilation (abandonment of native cultural identity and adoption of the values and norms of the larger society), integration (maintenance of ethnic cultural integrity at the same time as becoming an integral part of a larger society), separation (self-imposed withdrawal from the larger society while preserving the native culture), and marginalization (being out of cultural contact with both the traditional culture and the larger society) *(4)*.

Self-identification, behavior, and language skills are common elements often used as criteria for classifying individuals into the preceding categories. Many reports consider language preference a good estimate of the degree of acculturation of any given individual *(4)*. Results are conflicting as to whether high acculturation translates into better or worse health-care behaviors, but some reports highlight the fact that groups with low acculturation are more likely to be without a routine place for health care, have no health insurance, and have low levels of education *(4)*. These factors are clearly related to health-care outcomes. A recent report of the 1999–2002 National Health and Nutrition Examination Survey showed that Hispanic individuals with low acculturation, measured using the Short Acculturation Scale (that consists of five questions that can be answered as "only Spanish," "more Spanish than English," "both equally," "more English than Spanish," or "only English"), were more likely to have diabetes and more likely to have diabetic peripheral neuropathy as a chronic complication even after controlling for a variety of demographic characteristics, including health insurance and education *(5)*.

A high acculturation level can be associated with higher rates of diabetes, perhaps through the adoption of a more "diabetogenic" lifestyle—that is, by eating higher portions of foods richer in carbohydrates and fats and by becoming more sedentary. However, the acculturation process may also lead to the adoption of a healthier lifestyle. Ultimately, individuals choose which behaviors and preferences to adopt *(6,7)*.

Cultures also differ in their belief systems about health and illness, methods of communication, in the meanings of words and gestures, and even what is considered appropriate to discuss about family history and health. For example, patients are routinely told about medications and possible side effects in order to help them recognize possible side effects. Imagine discussing side effects with a Navajo patient who believes that events that are verbalized will happen *(8)*.

CULTURAL COMPETENCE

Cultural competence is defined by the American Medical Association as the knowledge and interpersonal skills that allow providers to understand, appreciate, and work with individuals from cultures other than their own *(9)*. It involves an awareness and acceptance of cultural differences, self-awareness, knowledge of the patient's culture, and adaptation of skills.

Although no randomized clinical trial has been conducted to demonstrate that diabetes control and/or complications are improved by a group of health-care providers with higher cultural competence compared with a group with a lower level, that cultural competence can lead to a much more pleasant and productive health-care provider–patient interaction is clear *(10)*. In the field of diabetes, cultural competence may be particularly relevant because disease control is greatly determined by effective lifestyle and behavior modification. Due to the growing number of minorities in the United States, the fact that they suffer from higher rates of diabetes and its complications, and lower quality of diabetes care, the need to improve the skills of health-care providers in the area of cultural competency has been more recognized than ever before.

Cultural competence is integral to the patient–provider relationship *(11)*. For example, a study of Mexican Americans found that knowledge of cultural factors per se and exposure to Mexican Americans in practice did not directly facilitate culturally competent care *(12)*. Rather, such care is most strongly predicted by recognition that cultural factors and awareness of personal biases are important. This finding supports the notion that both providers and patients should be aware of their cultural differences (perceptions, attitudes, cultural customs, and beliefs) and should be ready to listen and acknowledge the other person's agenda.

Both educators and patients need to raise their cultural awareness. Patients should feel comfortable in receiving care from a provider who has a different cultural background. Raising awareness among patients can be a more challenging task, and it may happen naturally as a result of a better and more culturally oriented interaction with educators of different cultures.

LANGUAGE

Language is central to social life. It is a characteristic of a culture and is a way to acquire cultural knowledge. The most obvious "cultural" barrier in a clinical and educational encounter is the inability to communicate in the same language.

It may limit the patient's ability to ask questions, to verbalize important information and concerns, and to establish a natural and spontaneous relationship with the educator. Language has been shown to affect clinical outcomes and may be a serious barrier to effective patient care *(13)*.

In general, patients prefer health-care providers who have a similar ethnic background. It may improve compliance and follow-up *(13)*. However, there is currently a pronounced discrepancy between the number of physicians who can communicate in both English and an additional language and the number of non-English-speaking patients. For instance, in 1999, Latino physicians accounted for $\sim$ 3.3% of practicing physicians in the United States, however, 13.9% of the patient population is of Latino origin *(14)*.

The proper use of interpreters is essential. A word of caution is necessary concerning the common circumstance in which a family member acts as an interpreter during routine clinical encounters. The advantage to this scenario is that the family member may be able to provide additional helpful information to the health-care provider. The disadvantage is that the family member may not be objective about translating all information, may not put aside his or her emotional attachment to the patient, and may communicate only what he or she considers important.

Educators should find the best translating option(s) for their patients. Although speaking the same language facilitates the clinician–patient interaction, other elements (e.g., trust, genuine interest, honesty) have no language barriers.

HEALTH LITERACY

The term "health literacy" is relatively new; it was first used in 1975, and The National Library of Medicine defines health literacy as "the degree to which individuals have the capacity to obtain, process, and understand basic health information and services needed to make appropriate health decisions" *(8)*. Many adults are unable to understand the complex printed materials needed to perform routine tasks. Health-related materials are included, and over 800 studies conducted during the past 25 years have shown that many health materials are written at reading levels above the reading skills of an average high school graduate *(15)*.

Scope of the Health Literacy Problem

The results from the 2003 National Assessment of Adult Literacy (NAAL) reported that the majority of adults (53%) had intermediate health literacy levels. In total, 14% of adults had Below Basic health literacy, 22% had Basic health literacy, and only 12% had proficient health literacy levels. On average, women had higher health literacy levels than men. Adults 65 years and older had lower average health literacy levels than adults in other groups *(16)*. Results by race and ethnicity showed that Hispanic adults had lower average health literacy than adults in any other racial/ethnic group. Whites and Asian/Pacific Islanders had higher average health literacy than Blacks, Hispanics, and American Indian/Alaksa Natives *(16)*.

Regarding languages spoken, adults who live in the United States who spoke only one language other than English had lower average health literacy levels than those who spoke only English before beginning school. Adults living in the United States who spoke only Spanish before starting school had the lowest average health literacy levels, corresponding to Below Basic health literacy *(16)*.

Inadequate health literacy skills have been associated with worse diabetes outcomes *(18)*, limited access to health-care services, poor self-reported health, low levels of adherence to treatment, higher rates of emergency room visits, hospitalization and re-hospitalization, lack of confidence on providers, lower patient satisfaction, and quality of care *(8,15,17)*. Patients with diabetes who have trouble reading are almost twice as likely to have worse glycemic control and higher prevalence of retinopathy compared to those with diabetes who have no difficulty reading *(18)*.

The problem of health literacy in America is not only a consequence of the education system. Society today places high health literacy demands on everybody. Clinicians, educators, and the health-care system ask patients to assume more responsibilities to self-manage their disease in a complex structure and not all patients are able to assume such tasks. These tasks include seeking information, making health decisions, reading warning or food labels, understanding rights and responsibilities, calculating timing and dosage, making decisions about participating in a research study, and using medical devices for personal or family care, among others. Patients may have an adequate understanding of topics that are familiar to them, but they struggle to comprehend new information and concepts. The daily challenge that educators face is to identify this group of patients and educate them to successfully manage their disease *(8,15)*.

Ideally, specific patient educational programs and materials regarding low health literacy should be developed for each racial and ethnic group *(19)*. Educators should evaluate their patients' health literacy levels when implementing a diabetes educational program or when providing patient educational materials. Table 1 shows the more common instruments used to evaluate health literacy *(8,20)*.

Educators in busy health-care settings could consider the use of informal ways to assess health literacy. For example, educators can ask questions during any educational encounter such as: "How do you learn best?" or "What would

Table 1

Measures of health literacy

Name of the instrument, abbreviation and publication year	Description	Language and time of administration	Strengths and weaknesses
Test of Functional Health Literacy in Adults **TOHFLA** 1995 Short Test of Functional Health Literacy in Adults **S-TOHFLA** 1999 A Brief Test of Functional Health Literacy in Adults **Brief TOHFLA** 1999	The content of this test was developed using real hospital medical textbooks.	English and Spanish TOHFLA: 22 minutes S-TOHFLA: approximately 7 minutes Brief TOHFLA: Up to 12 minutes	TOHFLA: Too long to be used in medical settings Appropriate for clinical research S-TOHFLA: Assesses only the patient's ability to read and comprehend In research it can only be used as a descriptive variable
Rapid Estimate of Adult Literacy in Medicine **REALM** 1993 Rapid Estimate of Adult Literacy in Medicine, Revised. **REALM-R** 2006 Rapid Estimate of Adolescent Literacy in Medicine. **REALM-Teen** 2006	This is a medical-word recognition and pronunciation test. All the words for this test were chosen from written materials commonly used in primary care.	English Under 3 minutes REALM-Teen can take up to 5 minutes	Patients with visual limitations may have difficulties with this test. Versions in other languages are not possible because this is a reading test based on pronunciation. This is not a measure of health literacy in itself. It does not directly assess comprehension.
Newest Vital Sign **NVS** 2005	This test uses one scenario that consists of a nutrition label from an ice cream container.	English and Spanish 3 minutes	This test is newer and is not as well studied.

121

help you most as you learn about your illness and how to take care of yourself?" or they can simply ask patients where and how they seek for medical information *(8)*.

Vocabulary and Understanding

The most frequent approach to making health information available to different cultures and other linguistically diverse groups is the use of readily available materials written in English and to translate them without taking into account literacy issues and cultural factors that play a prominent role in the target population's views about the disease in question. The problem with this approach is that it assumes that original materials written at low-reading levels are translatable into easy-to-read language and that low literacy individuals will be able to read and comprehend them. Another problem with that approach is that it assumes that individuals from different cultural backgrounds view and conceive a specific disease in universal terms. Also, patients from different cultures might have different ways to name diabetes. For example, while doing a diabetes screening in the Dominican Republic, we observed that the common name for diabetes on the island is "sugar," which is used as a synonym for diabetes.

Alternative Ways to Deliver Messages

Individuals who have difficulty reading or understanding written materials (printed materials or websites) are less likely to read than those individuals who experience no reading difficulties. Moreover, an individual can read materials without clearly comprehending the intended messages *(15)*. In addition to this, written materials on their own are not as effective as when they are accompanied by other mechanisms such as encouragement from health providers to read them and to ask questions. Also, when written materials are provided as reinforcement for the information already delivered by a provider, patients are more motivated to read them.

To illustrate the differences of culture regarding diabetes-related materials we can use this example: Hispanics seem to prefer to receive information from sources other than written materials. Research marketing has shown that Hispanics have a preference for information through forms of media other than written materials. In fact, mediums such as *fotonovelas* (a print form of a drama or short story told in captioned photographs), radio, or television shows with Hispanic media celebrities maybe more powerful communication tools *(21)*. Through the use of materials such as *fotonovelas*, individuals learn about the topic in question through the experiences of the individuals involved in the plot.

In addition, our group conducted an observational and feasibility pilot study among Spanish-speaking Latinos with type 2 diabetes to assess the acceptance of the storytelling method in an audio format (audiotape) alone or in conjunction with a brochure depicting a story of a Latino patient with type 2 diabetes, in comparison to a traditional, written educational piece. The storytelling method when used in conjunction with the brochure resulted in more positive changes regarding exercise, diet, and physical activity, as well as general information recall about diabetes and diabetes knowledge *(22)*.

EDUCATIONAL LEVEL

Some interesting data show that a higher educational level may be associated with better diabetes-related outcomes *(23)*. For instance, the association of educational level with either type 2 diabetes or cardiovascular disease was examined in a sample of second-generation Japanese American men living in King County, Washington. Men with a grade-school education showed higher frequencies of both diseases compared with men with any college education or high school diplomas. The association of educational level with risk of type 2 diabetes was not explained by other factors, such as occupation, income, diet, physical activity, weight, insulin, lipids, and lipoproteins, whereas the association with cardiovascular disease was explained in part by the larger average body mass index (BMI), higher total and very-low-density lipoprotein, triglycerides, and lower high-density lipoprotein (HDL) and HDL_2 cholesterol observed in men with technical school educations compared with the other men *(23)*. Therefore, a low educational level may not be the direct cause of worse outcomes in patients with type 2 diabetes, but rather a "marker" of multiple socioeconomic and cultural factors that may influence adherence to treatment and the course of the disease.

Educators need to consider patients' educational level when implementing any educational activity, whether in a one–one encounter or through a group diabetes educational program because it may lead to the identification of other important social and cultural factors that may influence diabetes care.

KNOWLEDGE ABOUT THE DISEASE

Patients' knowledge of diabetes is usually associated with self-management behaviors but not necessarily or directly associated with diabetes-related outcomes *(24)*. However, because improving self-management behaviors is likely to lead to better diabetes control, and hence, a lower risk of diabetes complications, general knowledge of diabetes will continue to be an important aspect of diabetes educational programs.

Regarding self-management behaviors in some racial/ethnic groups, data from the 2001 Behavioral Risk Factor Surveillance System (BRFSS) showed that certain diabetes management factors (including participation in diabetes education; medicinal regimen; physical activity level; frequency of eye exams; monitoring of feet; and frequency of checking blood glucose, A1c levels, and cholesterol levels) varied across study groups *(25)*. Some of these differences persisted after adjusting for current age, age at diagnosis, sex, marital status, income, and education. Specific culturally oriented programs to improve self-management behaviors are therefore necessary *(9,26,27)*.

SOCIOECONOMIC STATUS

Poverty influences not only the development of type 2 diabetes but complications of diabetes as well *(28–30)*. A recent study found that family poverty accounts for differences in diabetic amputation rates among blacks, Hispanic Americans, and other persons aged ≥ 50 years *(29)*. From a practical perspective, educators should always consider their patients' socioeconomic status when implementing diabetes self-care management and education programs.

JUDGMENT AND BELIEFS ABOUT THE DISEASE

Every social group shares beliefs about health and illness. Groups and individuals may have a particular explanatory model of illness. Knowledge and understanding of these health beliefs and explanatory models are essential for effective clinical encounters and educational programs. Some beliefs related to the development of diabetes include heredity, eating sweets, stress, emotional instability, and, sometimes, even an acute episode of fear or anxiety.

A recent study explored some health-related beliefs and experiences of black, Hispanic/Latino, American Indian, and Hmong people with diabetes *(31)*. The investigators found that many participants attributed their loss of health to the modern American lifestyle, lack of confidence in the medical system, and the general lack of spirituality in everyday life. Interestingly, participants recommended improvements in the areas of health care, diabetes education, social support, and community action that emphasized respectful and knowledgeable health-care providers, culturally responsive diabetes education for patients and their families, and broad-based community action as ways to improve diabetes care and educational programs *(31)*.

Educators should explore beliefs about the development and course of diabetes with their patients. A simple question to start with is: "Why do you think that you developed diabetes?" This initial evaluation may guide the provider on what important factors to address with that patient.

MYTHS

Myths, which are generally not explicit and are usually interwoven with values and beliefs, are commonly believed among patients with diabetes. There are many possible myths that diabetes occurs from eating a lot of sweets, is the result of destiny, is caused by lack of faith, or is punishment for a particular action. Certain myths and fears have developed in relation to insulin use *(32)*. Educators should ask patients about possible myths and be respectful of patients' answers. Understanding what myths patients believe can help clinicians develop specific strategies to dispel them.

FEARS

Patients can have multiple fears that may influence their adherence to a diabetes treatment plan. Many patients fear the presence of diabetes and its complications. This fear, expressed by a sense of hopelessness, may be due to lack of adequate information about the disease. Conversely, in some patients, a sense of fear may lead to a more responsible attitude toward the disease and may improve self-management behavior *(33)*.

Another common fear in patients with type 2 diabetes, particularly in some ethnic groups, is related to the consequences of insulin use. This medication is considered by many to be a treatment of last resort that leads to the development of severe diabetes-related complications, such as going blind and ultimately dying of the disease. It is perceived as basically a death sentence and decreases patients' likelihood of following a good treatment plan *(34)*.

Our experience in the Latino Diabetes Initiative at the Joslin Diabetes Center confirms that this fear is common among Latinos. We studied 120 patients who attended a first visit in the Latino Diabetes Initiative at the Joslin Diabetes Center in Boston. The group had 53 males and 67 female patients, average age 55 ± 10 years, duration of diabetes 11 ± 9 years. These patients were asked if the use of insulin causes blindness. They could answer: (a) true, (b) false, (c) do not know. Forty-three percent of patients responded true and 25% responded do not know *(26)*. In the group of patients who believed that insulin causes blindness, patients were more likely to change drug dosages on their own, forget insulin shots, have higher scores of emotional distress, and have perceptions of poor health. Ninety-one percent of Latino patients who were seen for the first time in our program were not familiar with the term hemoglobin A1C and were not aware of the importance of tight glycemic control. Because 90% of the patients included in this survey had health insurance coverage and a higher-than-average educational level compared with the general population, it would be expected that such barriers to insulin therapy would be more pronounced in other Latino subgroups *(26)*.

The basic implication of fear regarding diabetes care is quite obvious. Educators should openly ask patients if they have any particular fears about taking insulin or any other diabetes medications.

OTHER TYPES OF MEDICINE (ALTERNATIVE)

Many patients with diabetes combine alternative and traditional medicine. Alternative medicine has long been part of most cultures throughout the world. A recent report showed that of 2,472 adults with diabetes included in the study, 48% used some form of alternative medicine *(35)*. Interestingly, this study found that the use of alternative medicine was associated with the increased likelihood of receiving preventive care services and increased emergency department and primary care visits. This association does not necessarily represent causality. In other words, alternative medicine use may represent a factor that leads to more proactive health-care behavior and use of conventional medical services in adults with diabetes; conversely, high use of conventional medical services may lead to increased use of alternative medicine.

Whatever the true directionality of this association, alternative medicine use is common and appears to be even more frequent in certain minority groups *(36)*. It is estimated that one third of patients with diabetes use some type of dietary supplement *(36)*. Dietary supplements have active pharmacologic ingredients that may cause not only their theorized mechanisms in lowering blood glucose levels but adverse effects and drug interactions as well. Both educators and patients should be aware of alternative medicines currently being used in diabetes care and their adverse effects and monitoring parameters *(37)*.

Research is being conducted on the effect of all different modalities of alternative medicine on diabetes control and diabetes-related outcomes, and some studies have shown encouraging results. For instance, a recent study found that yoga may have a short-term positive influence on blood glucose and lipid levels in some patients with diabetes *(38)*. Obviously, research on alternative medicine use in patients with diabetes is needed. Educators should not forget to ask patients if they are using any form of alternative medicine. This question should be asked in a sensitive and respectful manner so that patients do not feel threatened or embarrassed.

NUTRITIONAL PREFERENCES

Although similarities between racial and ethnic groups exist, different groups have different food and nutritional preferences. In fact, foods may be so diverse that considerable discrepancies may exist in subgroups in each general racial/ethnic group, such as in Asians (i.e., Japanese, Chinese, Korean, Hawaiian) or Hispanics/Latinos (i.e., Caribbean, Mexican American, Central American, South American). Food preferences even vary by country or region in each of these subgroups. For instance, food preferences in Venezuela may differ from those in Colombia, and those in the Dominican Republic may differ from those in Puerto Rico *(9)*.

Food is usually at the core of family and social interaction. In fact, affection is often manifested through the gift of food and socialization revolves around copious eating. Extensive education is required to address healthy eating as a sound choice for any family or social event. An additional challenge resides in the fact that a common pattern of meals is served at any given home. When one family member has been encouraged to modify his or her meal plan, the whole family may be affected, particularly if it is the cook who has type 2 diabetes. Our experience at the Joslin Diabetes Center is consistent with this scenario. Some Latino women have a hard time modifying their meal plans because they usually cook at home, and what they make is what the entire family eats. Generally, not everyone in the family welcomes a change in meal patterns.

Educators must identify local educational resources to help their patients receive culturally oriented medical nutritional therapy. In addition, patient educational materials in this important area of nutrition may be identified through national organizations such as the American Diabetes Association, the National Institutes of Health, and the National Diabetes Education Program. Some specific programs, such as the Latino Diabetes Initiative and the Asian American Initiative at the Joslin Diabetes Center, can also provide some helpful information.

PHYSICAL ACTIVITY

Physical inactivity is associated with increased risk for obesity, type 2 diabetes, and cardiovascular disease, among other conditions. Data in all 50 states and the District of Columbia from the Behavioral Risk Factor Surveillance System for 1994 through 2004 showed that overall, the prevalence of leisure-time physical inactivity declined significantly ($P < 0.001$) from 29.8% in 1994 to 23.7% in 2004 (39). Leisure-time physical inactivity was defined as a "no" response to the survey question, "During the past month, other than your regular job, did you participate in any physical activities or exercise, such as running, calisthenics, golf, gardening, or walking for exercise?" Therefore, clinicians should remember that this question only identifies people who do not exercise at all and not those who may exercise irregularly.

The Behavioral Risk Factor Surveillance System surveys showed that the proportion of men who were inactive decreased from 27.9 to 21.4% and women from 31.5 to 25.9% (39). Among racial/ethnic groups, between 1994 and 2004, leisure-time physical inactivity was lowest among non-Hispanic white men (decreased from 26.4 to 18.4%). Among non-Hispanic black men, inactivity decreased from 34.2 to 27.0%, and among Hispanic men, it decreased from 37.5% in 1994 to 32.5%. The proportion of physical inactivity decreased from 45.7 to 33.9% in non-Hispanic black women, from

44.8 to 39.6% in Hispanic women, and from 28.3 to 21.6% in non-Hispanic white women. Asians/Pacific Islanders, American Indians/Alaska natives, and other multiracial groups did not have sufficient sample sizes to assess trends.

These data demonstrate that adults living in the United States are becoming more active during leisure time. However, a substantial number of people do not engage in regular vigorous physical activity that contributes to reducing the risk of developing type 2 diabetes and to controlling the disease. Additional data show that > 30% of older adults aged ≥ 70 years are inactive.

Physical activity preferences may vary among racial and ethnic groups. For instance, older white Americans may prefer jogging or going to the gym; older Latinos may prefer activities such as walking or dancing (40). When recommending an exercise program for a patient, clinicians and patients should discuss preferred physical activities to enhance a higher chance of continuity (41).

Further research is needed to identify attitudes toward, and barriers to, physical activity in specific ethnic and racial groups. This type of research may help the development of community culturally oriented programs that, in combination with the availability of accessible facilities and transportation options, may motivate people from certain racial/ethnic populations to engage in regular physical activity.

BODY IMAGE

The concept of ideal body weight may vary among individuals within and across racial and ethnic groups. Although it would be erroneous to assume that some people prefer to be overweight, people's conceptualization of an ideal weight may be different. In some groups, being robust and slightly overweight has been considered equivalent to being well nourished and financially success-ful (9). As an example, a study in black women with type 2 diabetes found that most participants preferred a middle-to-small body size but indicated that a middle-to-large body size was healthier. They also said that a large body size did result in some untoward social consequences (42). When discussing weight-loss strategies, it is therefore crucial that educators ask patients about their personal goals.

WORK ENVIRONMENT

Minority groups often works in low-wage and physically active jobs. A project evaluating whether the work environment of adults with diabetes treated with insulin impacts their care showed that work environment variables (such as work pressure, managerial control, involvement, coworker cohesion, supervisor support, and perceptions of support at the work place) are not directly related to glycemic control. The study also notes numerous work-related modifications patients need to accommodate in their diabetes care regimens (43). Efforts to make the workplace more sensitive to people with diabetes is important as well as thinking about this issues is an important aspect to take into account when establishing meal, exercise, blood glucose testing, and medication regimens for working patients.

DEPRESSION

Depression is more prevalent in patients with diabetes than in the general population, and particularly among minority groups (44). Depression is a powerful predictor of poor health outcomes in people with diabetes, which has been demonstrated in Mexican Americans (45).

The presence of depression also influences adherence to any diabetes treatment plan (46). Some immigrants to the United States may be more likely to develop stress and depression because of the need to live in, and adapt to, a completely different social and cultural environment. A recent study showed that Puerto Rican elders in Massachusetts were significantly more likely to have a physical disability, depression, cognitive impairment, diabetes, and other chronic health conditions than non-Hispanic white elders living in the same neighborhoods (47).

Depression is one of the most frequently missed diagnoses in clinical practice (48). Educators should become familiar with various ways of assessing the presence of depression in their patients. Specific questions such as "Have you felt depressed or sad much of the time this past year?" may provide insight into whether a patient may be depressed (49).

Cross-cultural studies have shown some particular differences regarding depression in some racial/ethnic groups. For instance, Hispanic patients may interpret symptoms of depression more benignly, are more likely to use prayer and other non-medical therapies, and are less likely to receive treatment in the mental health specialty setting than non-Hispanic white patients (49).

RELIGION AND FAITH

Religion and faith influence daily life. Religious traditions are expressions of faith in—and reverence for—specific conceptions of ultimate reality. They express one's place in, and relation to, this reality. Ultimate reality may be known as God, Allah, Atman, or Nirvana or by many other names, and it is understood and experienced differently by people of each religious tradition. The forms of faith and reverence of a tradition may be expressed and experienced through sacred stories; sacred symbols and objects; sacred music, art, and dance; devotion; meditation; rituals; sacred laws; philosophy; ethics; calls to social transformation; relationship with spirits; and healing *(50)*.

Some of these expressions may affect the health-care arena. In diabetes care, a clear example of one important influence is the fasting during the daylight hours that Muslims practice during 1 month each year. This practice requires the educators to show cultural sensitivity and understanding by adjusting any treatment strategies during this time *(51)*.

For an educator to address the topic of religion and faith, two sets of skills are indispensable. The first involves cultivating self-awareness and reflecting on the components of one's own identity. The second involves learning strategies for talking with patients about this topic and for responding to what patients say.

GENERAL FAMILY INTEGRATION AND SUPPORT

Although family is important for virtually all human beings, the level of closeness and dependence between family members may differ in various populations. In general, some groups (e.g., Latinos) often exhibit a collective loyalty—often referred to as *familismo*—to the extended family or group that supersedes the needs of the individual. The benefit of this loyalty is that more members in any given family may provide support to Latino patients. At the same time, it may be more difficult for some patients to make their own independent decisions. It is not unusual to see some patients who have to discuss decisions about their diabetes treatment, such as a new meal plan or the use of certain medications, with several members in the family before making a decision *(9,52,53)*.

Educators should recognize the importance of this particular value for some groups. Rather than seeing it as a cultural barrier, this close relationship to many family members brings a unique opportunity to address some important aspects of diabetes care and prevention that may be applicable to the extended family *(54)*. Some research suggests that structural togetherness in families is positively related to diabetes quality of life and satisfaction among patients with this disease *(55)*.

QUALITY OF LIFE

Various measures of quality of life have been assessed in people with diabetes. Several studies have demonstrated significant reductions in health status compared with other chronic disease populations and healthy controls *(56)*. The effect of diabetes on reducing health-related quality of life has also been evaluated and confirmed in multiethnic populations *(57)*. Some factors, such as family structure and support, may improve quality of life in patients with diabetes, as shown in a study of blacks *(55)*.

Although a patient's quality of life is difficult to routinely assess in clinical practice, educators should try to explore how diabetes and its complications have affected this factor. Quality of life clearly influences patients' behavior, receptiveness to treatment, and adherence to a treatment plan.

INDIVIDUAL AND SOCIAL INTERACTION

Every individual has a unique character and personality and different approaches to interacting with other people. There is no right or wrong way for how various cultures approach this issue. Each group may just be different. For example, many Latino patients expect to develop a warm and personal relationship with their health-care team. This type of patient–provider relationship would be characterized by interactions that occur at close distances and emphasize physical contact, such as handshakes, a hand on the shoulder, and even hugging under certain circumstances *(9,54)*. Even though health-care providers may not be able to switch behaviors as they interact with patients with diverse backgrounds and cultures, keeping in mind that certain groups prefer particular approaches may facilitate clinical encounters and help establish a more trusting and effective relationship with patients.

CONCLUSION

Patients and educators often have a different "agenda" in their mind in any given clinical encounter. Both must become more open and receptive to the other person's point of view regarding the disease process and treatment strategies. Any therapeutic plan is an agreement or "contract" between the patient and the educator where culture and health literacy may play and important role.

All these factors should be applied in the context of the standards of diabetes care. However, improving cultural competence among educators may help improve the quality of care and education provided to minority populations in the United States and around the world to reduce and eliminate health-care disparities in patients with diabetes.

REFERENCES

1. US Census Bureau, 2004. US Interim Projections by Age, Sex, Race, and Hispanic Origin. Available at: http://www.census.gov/ipc/www/usinterimproj/. Accessed January 18, 2005.
2. Institute of Medicine of the National Academies. Unequal treat ment confronting racial and ethnic disparities in health care. Available at: http://www.iom.edu. Accessed April 19, 2004.
3. Office of Minority Health, U.S. Department of Health and Human Services. Teaching Cultural Competence in Health Care: A Review of Concepts, Policies and Practices. Washington, DC: U.S. Department of Health and Human Services: 2002.

4. Lara M, Gamboa C, Kahramanian MI, et al. Acculturation and Latino health in the United States: A review of the literature and its sociopolitical context. Annu Rev Public Health. 2005;26:367–397.

5. Mainous AG III, Majeed A, Koopman RJ, et al. Acculturation and diabetes among Hispanics: Evidence from the 1999–2002 National Health and Nutrition Examination Survery. Public Health Rep. 2006;121:60–66.

6. Cortes DE, Rogler LH, Malgady RG, et al. Biculturality among Puerto Rican adults in the United States. Am J Comm Psychol. 1994;22:707–721.

7. Arcia E, Skinner M, Bailey D, Correa V. Models of acculturation and health behaviors among Latino immigrants to the US. Soc Sci Med. 2001;53:41–53.

8. Committee on Health Literacy, Institute of Medicine. Nielsen-Bohlman LN, Panzer AM, Kindig DA (eds). Health Literacy: A Prescription to End Confusion. Washington, DC: The National Academies Press, 2004.

9. Caballero AE. Diabetes in the Hispanic or Latino population: Genes, environment, culture, and more. Curr Diab Rep. 2005;5:217–225.

10. Betancourt JR. Cultural competence—marginal or mainstream movement? N Engl J Med. 2004;351:953–955.

11. Burgess D, van Ryn M, Davidio J, Saha S. Reducing Racial Bias Among Health Care Providers: Lessons from Social-Cognitive Psychology. J Gen Intern Med. 2007; 22:882–887.

12. Reimann JO, Talavera GA, Salmon M, et al. Cultural competence among physicians treating Mexican Americans who have diabetes: A structural model. Soc Sci Med. 2004;59: 2195–2205.

13. Hornberger JC, Gibson CD Jr, Wood W, et al. Eliminating language barriers for non-English-speaking patients. Med Care. 1996;34:845–856.

14. Huerta EE, Macario E. Communicating health risk to ethnic groups: Reaching Hispanics as a case study. J Natl Cancer Inst Monogr. 1999;25:23–26.

15. Rudd, RE. Health Literacy Skills of U. S. Adults. Am J Health Behav. 2007;31(Suppl 1): S8–S18.

16. Kutner M, Greenberg E, Jin Y, Paulsen C. The Health Literacy of America's Adults: Results From the 2003 National Assessment of Adult Literacy. National Center for Education Statistics, U.S. Department of Education.

17. Baker DW, Parker RM, Williams MV et al. The health care experience of patients with low literacy. Arch Fam Med 1996;5: 329–34.

18. Schillinger D, Grumbach K, Piette J, et al. Association of health literacy with diabetes outcomes. JAMA. 2002;288:475–482.

19. Rosal MC, Goins KV, Carbone ET, Cortes DE. Views and preferences of low-literate Hispanics regarding diabetes education: Results of formative research. Health Educ Behav. 2004;31: 388–405.

20. Weiss BD, Mays MZ, Martz W et al. Quick Assessment of Literacy in Primary Care: The Newest Vital Sign. Ann Fam Med. 2005;3(6):514–522.

21. Lalonde B, Rabinowitz P, Shefsky ML, Washienko K. La Esperanza del Valle: alcohol prevention novelas for Hispanic youth and their families. Health Educ Bahav. 1997, Oct; 24(5):587–602.

22. Millan-Ferro A, Cortes DE, Weinger K, Caballero AE: Development of a culturally oriented educational tool for low health literacy Latino/Hispanic patients with type 2 diabetes and their families. Diabetes, 2007, 56 (Suppl 1): A89.

23. Leonetti DL, Tsunehara CH, Wahl PW, Fujimoto WY. Educational attainment and the risk of non-insulin-dependent diabetes or coronary heart disease in Japanese-American men. Ethn Dis. 1992;2:326–336.

24. Norris SL, Engelgau MM, Narayan KM. Effectiveness of self-management training in type 2 diabetes: A systematic review of randomized controlled trials. Diabetes Care. 2001;24: 561–587.

25. Thackeray R, Merrill RM, Neiger BL. Disparities in diabetes management practice between racial and ethnic groups in the United States. Diabetes Educ. 2004;30:665–675.
26. Caballero AE, Montagnani V, Ward MA, et al. The assessment of diabetes knowledge, socio-economic and cultural factors for the development of an appropriate education program for Latinos with diabetes. Diabetes. 2004;53(Suppl 2):A514.
27. Brown SA, Blozis SA, Kouzekanani K, et al. Dosage effects of diabetes self-management education for Mexican Americans: The Starr County Border Health Initiative. Diabetes Care. 2005; 28:527–532.
28. Robbins JM, Vaccarino V, Zhang H, Kasl SV. Socioeconomic status and diagnosed diabetes incidence. Diabetes Res Clin Pract. 2005;68:230–236.
29. Wachtel MS. Family poverty accounts for differences in lower-extremity amputation rates of minorities 50 years old or more with diabetes. J Natl Med Assoc. 2005;97:334–338.
30. Diez Roux AV, Detrano R, Jackson S, et al. Acculturation and socioeconomic position as predictors of coronary calcification in a multiethnic sample. Circulation. 2005;112:1557–1565.
31. Devlin H, Roberts M, Okaya A, Xiong YM. Our lives were healthier before: Focus groups with African American, American Indian, Hispanic/Latino, and Hmong people with diabetes. Health Promot Pract. 2006;7:47–55.
32. Meece J. Dispelling myths and removing barriers about insulin in type 2 diabetes. Diabetes Educ. 2006;32(Suppl 1):9S–18S.
33. Glasgow RE, Hampson SE, Strycker LA, Ruggiero L. Personal-model beliefs and social-environmental barriers related to diabetes self-management. Diabetes Care. 1997;20:556–561.
34. Hunt LM, Valenzuela MA, Pugh JA. NIDDM patients' fears and hopes about insulin therapy. The basis of patient reluctance. Diabetes Care. 1997;20:292–298.
35. Garrow D, Egede LE. Association between complementary and alternative medicine use, preventive care practices, and use of conventional medical services among adults with diabetes. Diabetes Care. 2006;29:15–19.
36. Dham S, Shah V, Hirsch S, Banerji MA. The role of complementary and alternative medicine in diabetes. Curr Diab Rep. 2006; 6:251–258.
37. Shane-McWhorter L. Botanical dietary supplements and the treatment of diabetes: What is the evidence? Curr Diab Rep. 2005;5:391–398.
38. Bijlani RL, Vempati RP, Yadav RK, et al. A brief but comprehensive lifestyle education program based on yoga reduces risk factors for cardiovascular disease and diabetes mellitus. J Altern Complement Med. 2005;11:267–274.
39. Centers for Disease Control and Prevention (CDC). Trends in leisure-time physical inactivity by age, sex, and race/ethnicity—United States, 1994–2004. MMWR Morb Mortal Wkly Rep. 2005;54:991–994.
40. Wood FG. Leisure time activity of Mexican Americans with diabetes. J Adv Nurs. 2004;45:190–196.
41. Clark DO. Physical activity efficacy and effectiveness among older adults and minorities. Diabetes Care. 1997;20:1176–1182.
42. Liburd LC, Anderson LA, Edgar T, Jack L Jr. Body size and body shape: Perceptions of black women with diabetes. Diabetes Educ. 1999;25:382–388.
43. Trief P, Aquilino C, Paradies K, Weinstock RS. Impact of the work environment on Glycemic Control and Adaptation to Diabetes. Diab Care. 1999 Apr; 22(4):569–74.
44. Caballero AE. Diabetes in minority populations. In: Kahn CR, Weir G, King GL, et al, eds. Joslin's Diabetes Mellitus. ed 14. Philadelphia: Lippincott Williams & Wilkins; 2005:505–524.
45. Black SA, Markides KS, Ray LA. Depression predicts increased incidence of adverse health outcomes in older Mexican Americans with type 2 diabetes. Diabetes Care. 2003;26:2822–2828.

46. Lerman I, Lozano L, Villa AR, et al. Psychosocial factors associated with poor diabetes self-care management in a specialized center in Mexico City. Biomed Pharmacother. 2004;58: 566–570.
47. Tucker KL. Stress and nutrition in relation to excess development of chronic disease in Puerto Rican adults living in the Northeastern USA. J Med Invest. 2005;52(Suppl):252–258.
48. Saver BG, Van-Nguyen V, Keppel G, Doescher MP. A qualitative study of depression in primary care: Missed opportunities for diagnosis and education. J Am Board Fam Med. 2007;20:28–35.
49. Williams JW Jr, Mulrow CD, Kroenke K, et al. Case-finding for depression in primary care: A randomized trial. Am J Med. 1999;106:36–43.
50. Hall DE. Medicine and religion. N Engl J Med. 2000;343:1340–1341; author reply 1341–1342.
51. Al-Arouj M, Bouguerra R, Buse J, et al. Recommendations for management of diabetes during Ramadan. Diabetes Care. 2005;28:2305–2311.
52. Wen LK, Parchman ML, Shepherd MD. Family support and diet barriers among older Hispanic adults with type 2 diabetes. Fam Med. 2004;36:423–430.
53. Fisher L, Chesla C, Skaff MM, et al. The family and disease management in Hispanic and European-American patients with type 2 diabetes. Diabetes Care. 2000;23:267–272.
54. Caballero AE. Bridging cultural barriers: Understanding ethnicity to improve acceptance of insulin therapy in patients with type 2 diabetes. Ethn Dis. 2006;16:559–568.
55. Chesla CA, Fisher L, Mullan JT, et al. Family and disease management in African-American patients with type 2 diabetes. Diabetes Care. 2004;27:2850–2855.
56. Luscombe FA. Health-related quality of life measurement in type 2 diabetes. Value Health. 2000;3(Suppl 1):15–28.
57. Wee HL, Cheung YB, Li SC, et al. The impact of diabetes mellitus and other chronic medical conditions on health related quality of life: Is the whole greater than the sum of its parts? Health Qual Life Outcomes. 2005;3:2.

9 Technology in Self-Care: Implications for Diabetes Education

William C. Hsu, MD
and Howard A. Wolpert, MD

CONTENTS

INTRODUCTION
INSULIN PUMP THERAPY
REAL-TIME CONTINUOUS GLUCOSE MONITORING
REFERENCES

ABSTRACT

New diabetes technologies, such as insulin pump therapies and continuous glucose monitors (CGM), have become important tools for helping control hypoglycemia and achieving glycemic targets. There are, of course, advantages and disadvantages to the adoption of these technological tools, and patients require mastery of new skills in order to use these tools successfully. For the patient, use of the new technologies can be overwhelming or extremely helpful, which often depends on one's level of knowledge about the new tools. Therefore, this chapter provides the basic foundation for educating patients about these new diabetes technologies.

Key Words: Continuous Glucose Monitors (CGM), Continuous Subcutaneous Insulin Infusion (CSII), Diabetes Technology.

From: *Contemporary Diabetes: Educating Your Patient with Diabetes*
Edited by: K. Weinger and C. A. Carver, DOI 10.1007/978-1-60327-208-7_9,
© Humana Press, a part of Springer Science+Business Media, LLC 2009

INTRODUCTION

The daily challenges of managing diabetes are inseparable from the complexities of life. Finding a balance between the demands of maintaining quality of life and managing diabetes becomes a daily struggle for people with diabetes. Diabetes technologies, such as insulin pumps and continuous glucose monitors (CGM), have opened up unprecedented possibilities for improved diabetes self-care and intensification of glycemic control. While the adoption of these technological tools has been increasingly popular, successful outcomes can only come about by the skillful application of these tools. A comprehensive review on this topic is beyond the scope of this chapter. Instead, the focus will be on a selection of clinical issues that are often overlooked in patient education.

INSULIN PUMP THERAPY

An insulin pump, also known as continuous subcutaneous insulin infusion (CSII) device, is designed to mimic physiologic insulin delivery. A meta-analysis of published studies demonstrates that continuous subcutaneous insulin infusion therapy lowers A1c (0.5%) compared to multiple daily injections and is associated with reduced insulin requirements (14%) (1). Some studies where the average duration of pump therapy was less than 1 year did not observe an A1c improvement, suggesting a steep learning curve may be required for mastery (2). Arguably, the greatest clinical benefit is in the reduction of nocturnal hypoglycemia and glycemic variability and elimination of the Dawn phenomenon (3). Due to the pump's precise delivery of insulin with multiple basal and bolus patterns, this form of insulin replacement has a special utility for patients who require small increments of insulin doses, want to control weight, have different levels of physical activity throughout the day, eat out frequently, or simply want to eliminate the hassle of multiple insulin injections. In addition, helping patients regain hypoglycemic awareness and facilitate insulin administration in severe gastroparesis are some of the important clinical applications of pump therapy. Contrary to common belief, those with "brittle diabetes" often have underlying physiologic or psychosocial barriers, and therefore glycemic control cannot be improved simply by a switch to insulin pump therapy (4); this illustrates that technology alone cannot improve diabetes control. Further, a focus group study of insulin pump users found that patients who were in better glycemic control described being actively involved in their self-care and were able to view the pump simply as another tool to help them manage their diabetes compared to those in poor glycemic control (5).

Some of the disadvantages for pump therapy are real and significant, such as high financial cost and physical attachment to a pump. Other disadvantages such as increased risks for infection and diabetic ketoacidosis can be minimized with adequate patient education. Diabetic ketoacidosis occurs not infrequently in patients transitioning from multiple daily injections to pump therapy when insulin delivery is accidentally interrupted. One of the common misconceptions new pumpers have is that ketonemia can only occur with hyperglycemia. Therefore, they do not think of testing for ketones when glucose levels are not very high. The mechanism of ketogenesis is distinct from hyperglycemia, thus ketones can reach significant levels without the presence of hyperglycemia. Training pump patients to get into the habit of checking ketones when they do not feel well regardless of blood glucose levels and to identify mechanical causes for unexplained hyperglycemia can prevent serious complications of diabetic ketoacidosis. Insulin pumps bring their unique causes for hyperglycemia and diabetic ketoacidosis, including kinked or blocked catheters, pump site infection, or air bubbles in catheters. While modern pumps have built in alarms that inform patients in case of insulin non-delivery, an important teaching point is that malfunctions caused by electrostatic interference, pump failure, and dislodged catheters can only be picked up by patients through vigilant visual inspection.

Insulin is a powerful hypoglycemic agent with a narrow therapeutic window. Stacking of insulin doses is one of the most common causes for hypoglycemia associated with insulin pump therapy. When faced with hyperglycemia, the ease of giving a second bolus via a pump before the initial bolus completes its biologic action can lead to serious hypoglycemia. Some patients may not understand that larger insulin doses have longer pharmacodynamic profiles, which makes dose stacking even more a potential problem. The risk for dose stacking can be considerably reduced with use of the "insulin on board" feature in the bolus calculators of modern so-called smart pumps. Many patients do not fully grasp the importance of this pump feature. Pumpers who use the "insulin on board" function on their pumps yet continue to experience hypoglycemia from dose stacking should have the "active insulin time" in the pump software increased to a longer duration.

Another clinical issue that deserves attention in patient education is choosing infusion sites. The amount of subcutaneous fat is important in determining the rate of insulin absorption. Catheters placed in areas with more fat such as in the buttock will have different rates of insulin absorption compared to the abdomen, and this can result in otherwise unexplained differences in glycemic responses with infusion site changes. Patients who are runners should not place catheters in the thighs due to faster insulin absorption while exercising. Teaching patients to identify and avoid placing catheters in areas of insulin-induced lipohypertrophy and scar tissue from repeated catheter insertions will minimize inconsistency in insulin absorption.

REAL-TIME CONTINUOUS GLUCOSE MONITORING

Real-time continuous glucose-monitoring (RT-CGM) devices are portable, minimally invasive systems that provide continuous information on glucose patterns and trends, and have alarms that alert the patient when the glucose level crosses preset hyper- and hypoglycemic thresholds. Current glucose sensors consist of a subcutaneous electrode and are based on the glucose oxidase electrochemical reaction used in fingerstick glucose monitors. The information derived is communicated through a sensor-coupled wireless transmitter to a monitor, which displays real-time glucose values or trends. In contrast to traditional fingerstick glucose monitoring that only offers glucose values a few times each day, this technology offers substantially more glucose information to patients and promises to be a major advance in diabetes care. While long-term health outcome data are not yet available, studies performed to date indicate that patients using real-time continuous glucose monitoring have less hypo- and hyperglycemia and spend more time within the target glucose range *(6,7)*. In addition, patients who intensify glucose control while on real-time continuous glucose monitoring experience less hypoglycemia than those who use traditional fingerstick glucose monitoring to guide therapy *(6)*. The safe and optimal use of real-time continuous glucose monitoring in diabetes management rests on patient's understanding of several technological as well as physiological issues.

The current continuous glucose-monitoring devices measure glucose concentration in the interstitial fluid of subcutaneous tissue, whereas traditional fingerstick devices measure capillary blood glucose. When the glucose level is changing, there is a physiologic lag in the equilibration of glucose between the blood and the interstitial fluid that can be up to 30 minutes in duration. Because of this delay, rapid increases or decreases of the glucose concentration in the blood will generally not be evident in the interstitial fluid until minutes later. In some rare situations however, if the sensor is close to a large muscle group then exercise may cause the glucose level to initially decrease in the interstitial fluid before this change is reflected in capillary blood.

The physiologic lag has important implications for patient education in regards to the detection and treatment of hypoglycemia. When blood glucose is falling rapidly into the hypoglycemic range, the interstitial glucose as detected by the sensor could still be within target range *(8,9)*. Some patients find it helpful to use the trend graph on the sensor display or rate of change arrows to help them decide what action to take. However, it is important to note that physiologic lag can also lead to underestimation of the rate of change indicator on the continuous glucose-monitoring device *(10)*. Therefore, the important message to communicate to patients is that whenever they suspect hypoglycemia or are in situations where hypoglycemia is prone to happen, they should perform a fingerstick glucose measurement even if the continuous glucose-monitoring results show the glucose level to be normal.

Because interstitial glucose lags behind blood glucose during recovery from hypoglycemia, patients who rely on the sensor may overtreat hypoglycemia. During the recovery from hypoglycemia the blood glucose may have already normalized at a time when the interstitial glucose may still be in the low range *(11)*; patients who do not understand physiologic lag may mistakenly assume that they need to take in more carbohydrates, resulting in overtreatment of hypoglycemia.

Just as use of continuous glucose monitoring can lead to overtreatment of hypoglycemia, there is also a risk that some patients confronted by the postprandial spikes revealed by the sensor will take excessive boluses of insulin leading to overtreatment of hyperglycemia. This problem is, in part, related to patients not understanding the pharmacodynamic action profile of insulin. Because of the ease of bolusing with a pump overtreatment of hyperglycemia tends to be more common among pump users. Reducing this tendency for over-bolusing is an important focus of patient education.

The physiologic lag also has important implications for sensor calibration when glucose levels are changing. If the continuous glucose-monitoring device is calibrated using capillary glucose measurements obtained when the glucose level is rising, this will give the sensor an upward bias and affect accuracy of the device in detecting hypoglycemia. Therefore, the important issue in patient education is to emphasize that continuous glucose monitoring should be calibrated only under stable glucose levels when capillary and interstitial glucose levels are in equilibrium. In practice, this means calibration should take place at least 3 h after a meal or bolus, and calibration should be avoided during exercise or anytime glucose levels are fluctuating. Because any compromise in the accuracy of the calibration glucoses will be amplified, it is important that accurate glucose-monitoring measurements be used. Proper fingerstick technique and meter coding should be followed, and alternate site testing should be avoided. In addition, glucose measurements used for calibration should be immediately entered into the continuous glucose-monitoring device. Although some advocate performing calibration only twice daily in order to optimize accuracy, calibration may need to take place 3–4 times a day. Initially after the sensor is inserted, trauma can interfere with fluid flow to the sensor, leading to inaccurate readings. It can take up to 12–24 h for the sensor to settle and give accurate readings. Unlike pump infusion sets, sensor function tends to improve with time.

Setting alarm threshold is a trade-off between sensitivity and specificity and needs to be individualized. For people suffering from hypoglycemic unawareness, the priority is for the alarm to go off whenever potential hypoglycemia occurs. As discussed earlier, when the alarm goes off the blood glucose levels will generally be lower than the sensor measurement; therefore, physiologic lag needs to be taken into consideration in setting alarm thresholds. For those who fear hypoglycemia, the low threshold should be set at 80 mg/dl or higher. Although patients will be warned of most lows at this threshold, they may also experience many false alarms. This can be particularly disturbing during sleep and can become a source of frustration not only to patients but to family members as well. In many instances, this can lead to emotional burnout and a tendency to ignore sensor alarms or even discontinue use of the RT-CGM device. Alternatively, when the lower threshold is set at 60 mg/dl or below, the alarm will be highly specific, and there will be fewer false alarms; however, patients will not always be warned of every hypoglycemic event. Similarly, setting high alarms at levels too close to target range, such as 180 mg/dl, can lead to frequent nuisance alarms.

For individuals on real-time continuous glucose monitoring whose primary goal is to track glucose excursions and who are not looking specifically for alarm functions, it is reasonable to set the alarms with a low threshold at 55–60 mg/dl, and a high threshold at 250 mg/dl or greater. For those who do not have a history of severe hypoglycemia, this setting ensures that there will not be too many intrusive and false alarms while they are initially learning how to apply the sensor information to minimize glucose fluctuations. As the patient's comfort level increases, threshold settings can be further tightened closer to the target glucose ranges. Discussing these considerations in setting alarm thresholds with the patient can be crucial in ensuring successful use of continuous glucose monitoring.

Real-time continuous glucose monitoring creates clearer pictures of glucose patterns but can also present a potential danger for information overload, reminding patients on a minute by minute basis of the unrelenting challenge of living with diabetes. As one patient expressed it, in the past she had to deal with the results from glucose monitoring only a few times a day, but "now, since using real-time, diabetes has become a full time job." While there has not been extensive literature on the psychological impact of continuous glucose-monitoring use, preventing user burnout is a clinical priority. Some of the common frustrations stem from seeing the discrepancies between fingerstick glucose and sensor glucose values, getting overwhelmed by the glucose fluctuations and relating it as a personal failure, and feeling trapped by the constant deluge of glucose data. Setting realistic patient expectations and being attentive to the emotional responses to using continuous glucose monitoring are the keys to effective use. Given the appealing features of real-time continuous glucose monitoring, it is tempting for health-care providers to think that a continuous glucose-monitoring device is the universal solution for any patient with difficult to control diabetes. In reality, the proficient use of this device requires an in depth understanding of physiology and pharmacodynamics and a certain degree of technological savviness. A rule of thumb is if a patient does not have the motivational and intellectual capacity to go on a pump, then he/she is not likely to be a good candidate for real-time continuous glucose monitoring.

In summary, technology brings about new capacity for patients to gather glucose information and expand their options for intensive diabetes therapy. Health-care providers and patients alike must have realistic expectations of pumps and sensors and prepare for a steep learning curve during training. Successful use of technology ultimately depends on the patients acquiring adequate knowledge and mastering the diabete self-care skills. The foundation for successful adoption of technologies still rests on comprehensive patient education.

REFERENCES

1. Pickup J, Mattock M, Kerry S. Glycaemic control with continuous subcutaneous insulin infusion compared with intensive insulin injections in patients with type 1 diabetes: meta-analysis of randomised controlled trials. BMJ. 2002 Mar 23;324(7339):705–711.
2. Weissberg-Benchell J, Antisdel-Lomaglio J, Seshadri R. Insulin Pump Therapy: A meta-analysis. Diabetes Care 2003;26: 1079–1087.
3. Hirsch IB, Bode BW, Garg S, Lane WS, Sussman A, Hu P, Santiago OM, Kolaczynski JW for the Insulin Aspart CSII/MDI Comparison Study Group. Continuous Subcutaneous Insulin Infusion (CSII) of Insulin Aspart Versus Multiple Daily Injection of Insulin Aspart/Insulin Glargine in Type 1 Diabetic Patients Previously Treated With CSII. Diabetes Care 2005;28: 533–538.
4. Pick up J, Keen H. Continuous Subcutaneous Insulin Infusion at 25 Years: Evidence base for the expanding use of insulin pump therapy in type 1 diabetes. Diabetes Care 2002;25:593–598.
5. Ritholz MD, Smaldone A, Lee J, Castillo A, Wolpert H, Weinger K. Perceptions of psychosocial factors and the insulin pump. Diabetes Care 2007;30(3):549–54.
6. Garg S, Zisser H, Schwartz S, Bailey T, Kaplan R, Ellis S, Jovanovic L. Improvement in Glycemic Excursions with a Transcutaneous, Real-Time Continuous Glucose Sensor: A randomized controlled trial. Diabetes Care 2006;29:44–50.
7. The Juvenile Diabetes Research Foundation Continuous Glucose Monitoring Study Group. Continuous Glucose Monitoring and Intensive Treatment of Type 1 Diabetes. New England Journal of Medicine 2008; epublished ahead of print.
8. Moberg E, Hagstrom-Toft E, Arner P, Bolinder J: Protracted glucose fall in subcutaneous adipose tissue and skeletal muscle compared with blood during insulin-induced hypoglycaemia. Diabetologia 1997;40:1320–1326.
9. Steil GM, Rebrin K, Hariri F, Jinagonda S, Tadros S, Darwin C, Saad MF: Interstitial fluid glucose dynamics during insulin-induced hypoglycemia. Diabetologia 2005;48:1833–1840.
10. Wilson DM, Beck RW, Tamborlane WV, Dontchev MJ, Kollman C, Chase P, Fox LA, Ruedy KJ, Tsalikian E, Weinzimer SA; DirecNet Study Group. The accuracy of the FreeStyle Navigator continuous glucose monitoring system in children with type 1 diabetes. Diabetes Care. 2007;30(1):59–64.
11. Cheyne E, Cavan D, Kerr D: Performance of a continuous glucose monitoring system during controlled hypoglycaemia in health volunteers. Diabetes Technol Ther 2002;4:607–613.

10 Deciphering the Blood Glucose Puzzle with Pattern Management Skills

Donna Tomky, MSN, RN, C-ANP, CDE

CONTENTS

INTRODUCTION
DEFINITION OF PATTERN MANAGEMENT
WHAT SKILLS AND KNOWLEDGE ARE REQUIRED?
CONSIDER GUIDELINES AND ESTABLISH
  INDIVIDUAL BLOOD GLUCOSE TARGETS
GATHER AND ORGANIZE BLOOD GLUCOSE DATA
DETECTING TRENDS AND PATTERNS
  AND CONSIDERING CAUSES
IDENTIFYING DESIRED CHANGES
  AND CONSIDERING STRATEGIES
DEVELOP A PLAN
IMPLEMENT PLAN
EVALUATE RESPONSE TO PLAN
  AND REVISE PLAN IF NECESSARY
CONCLUSIONS
REFERENCES

ABSTRACT

Diabetes educators are expected to educate patients in many aspects of self-care. Often blood glucose records are the end results of self-care behavior, which is multi-factorial. When evaluating blood glucose records, multiple aspects of patient

From: *Contemporary Diabetes: Educating Your Patient with Diabetes*
Edited by: K. Weinger and C. A. Carver, DOI 10.1007/978-1-60327-208-7_10,
© Humana Press, a part of Springer Science+Business Media, LLC 2009

behaviors are essential for assessing patterns and explanations of abnormal glucose results. Too often providers focus on just one aspect, typically medication dose, instead of considering all the other factors that affect the glucose level. Asking questions about what, how, and when the patient is eating, exercising, or taking their medications may lead the diabetes educator to discover the missing link in self-care. Using a systematic approach to evaluate your patient's blood glucose records is critical in determining the appropriate therapeutic options for diabetes care.

Key Words: Self-monitoring of blood glucose, Glucose patterns, Pattern management, Pattern recognition of blood glucose results.

INTRODUCTION

Diabetes affects nearly 200 million people worldwide and is expected to reach 350 million by 2030 *(1)*. With the growing epidemic of diabetes, the role of the diabetes educator in providing diabetes self-management education is a critical element of care for all people with diabetes and is necessary in order to improve patient outcomes *(2)*. Patient outcomes improve as individuals are taught to successfully self-manage their chronic condition. A critical component of successful self-management of glycemic control is pattern recognition of blood glucose data with the added attention to details that require a change by the patient or provider. Both diabetes educators and patients alike are expected to recognize data trends and apply appropriate interventions for improving blood glucose levels. Pattern recognition or management is difficult unless the diabetes educator understands the essential skills and knowledge that are requisite of patients.

Behavior change is the measurable outcome of diabetes self-management education *(3)*. The aim for the diabetes educator is to facilitate change with the patient for optimal clinical and health outcomes. For this to occur, one must understand the definition of pattern management for those involved. Pattern management can be a simple or complex process in reviewing clinical data. Most of the techniques and skills of diabetes pattern management are similar to the framework used in information management, where data are collected and organized in a systematic manner that is useful to the user for interpretation of that information *(4)*. Furthermore, that process is the transformation of data into information that then makes the recipient more knowledgeable for making decisions or new discoveries. Once data are organized into trends, then providers can recognize patterns and focus on appropriate educational, therapeutic, or behavioral interventions. Pattern management is further defined for both the diabetes educator and the patient with diabetes.

DEFINITION OF PATTERN MANAGEMENT

For the diabetes educator, pattern management includes blood glucose data that provide "a system to organize, sort, and process blood glucose data that links to patient self-care behaviors and reveals blood glucose trends or patterns" *(6)*. It is used to (1) determine targeted strategies and therapies, (2) discuss and negotiate strategies and goals with the patient, and (3) bring the patient back to the blood glucose goal *(6)*.

Pattern management is equally important for the person with diabetes. It provides a way for patients to look at their blood glucose records in relationship to food, activity, stress, and medication. The purpose is to give immediate feedback, which allows them to reflect on what makes their "blood sugar go up and down." Together, the patient and diabetes educator can formulate a plan to improve glycemic control as well as improve health-related outcomes, e.g., reduce illness and missed work or school days *(6)*.

WHAT SKILLS AND KNOWLEDGE ARE REQUIRED?

When interpreting self-monitoring of blood glucose records for patterns and then applying interventions, a systematic approach can be followed by using seven basic steps adapted from Pearson and Bergenstal *(7)*:

1. Consider guidelines and establish individual blood glucose targets
2. Gather and organize blood glucose data
3. Find patterns by detecting trends and consider causes
4. Identify desired changes and consider strategies for bringing blood glucose back to target ranges
5. Develop a plan of action
6. Implement plan
7. Evaluate response to plan and revise plan if necessary

CONSIDER GUIDELINES AND ESTABLISH INDIVIDUAL BLOOD GLUCOSE TARGETS

Professional diabetes organizations (ADA, IDF, AACE, and AADE) frequently review the evidence and develop guidelines for establishing glycemic targets for patients. Diabetes educators and health care providers need to discuss proposed guidelines with their medical and health care colleagues to reach a consensus for implementation into practice. Key concepts in setting glycemic goals for your patients who are children, adolescents, adults with limited life expectancy, and geriatric individuals *(8,9)* include the following:

1. Goals should be individualized, and lower goals may be reasonably based on benefit–risk assessment.

2. Blood glucose goals should be higher than those listed in individuals with frequent hypoglycemia or hypoglycemia unawareness.
3. Post-prandial blood glucose values should be measured when there is a disparity between pre-prandial blood glucose values and A1C levels.
4. A lower goal (< 7.0%) is reasonable if it can be achieved without excessive hypoglycemia.

GATHER AND ORGANIZE BLOOD GLUCOSE DATA

Gathering blood glucose data is easy if the patient is already monitoring their blood glucose. If the patient is not, then you must get started by establishing a patient profile. Asking basic questions related to eating, exercise, and daily routine are important for establishing a safe and basic treatment plan with a new patient (6). All of these questions assess patient knowledge and behavior related to self-management.

Pattern management starts with accurate and sufficient blood glucose data to begin viewing meaningful records. Examining the patient's technique and reviewing unique features of his or her meter and strips assure accuracy of blood glucose data. Sufficiency and frequency of blood glucose data are determined by (1) type of therapy, (2) degree of glycemic control, (3) risk of hypoglycemia, (4) need for short-term adjustment of therapy, and (5) special situations (pregnancy, intercurrent illness, or hypoglycemia unawareness) (5).

The time to monitor blood glucose is an intensely debated issue among experts. There are potentially seven points within a 24-h glucose profile including pre-meals, post-meals, and at bedtime (10,11). Monnier et al. found that the contribution of fasting plasma glucose measurements approached 70% of overall glucose mean as A1C neared 10%. It was also found that post-prandial glucose contributes about 70% to the overall glucose profile when the A1C values approach around 7% (12). Both monitoring and targeting pre- and post-prandial blood glucose treatment depend on A1C and individualized assessment or patient glycemic goals. So targeting fasting plasma glucose is more beneficial when hemoglobin A1C results are very high, whereas targeting post-prandial glucose is more effective when A1C results are lower (13). Furthermore, monitoring and targeting treatment of fasting blood glucose are important as it is a determinant of post-prandial glucose and more reproducible. It is important to monitor and target post-prandial glucose when A1C is not to goal. Also post-prandial glucose is frequently the earliest abnormality of type 2 diabetes as well as represents an independent risk for cardiovascular disease (13,14), shown to be important in gestational diabetes (15), and helps detect post-prandial hypoglycemia (16).

Another approach for monitoring blood glucose in non-insulin-treated patients is described by Schwedes and colleagues as well as Guerci and co-workers as a blood glucose "weekly profile" *(17,18)*. In these randomized controlled trials the study group was asked to monitor a weekly profile consisting of self-monitoring their blood glucose six times a day (pre- and 1 or 2 h post-main meals) on 2 or 3 days per week that included one or two weekdays and a weekend day. Study subjects kept diaries of blood glucose, eating habits, and feelings of well-being. They were taught how to use the blood glucose monitoring data for applying a counseling algorithm. Subjects increased self-perception by keeping a diary on eating, self-monitoring of blood glucose data, and their overall well-being. The weekly profile approach promoted self-reflection and regulation by patients asking themselves questions about what did or did not work well. Results showed that subjects increased their self-regulation by giving them ideas on how to use self-monitoring of blood glucose data results to improve metabolic control by guiding changes in eating and physical activity behaviors as well as lowering hemoglobin A1C by $1.0 \pm 1.08\%$ in the study group compared with $0.54 \pm 1.41\%$ ($P = 0.0086$) in the control group *(17,18)*.

Organizing blood glucose data depends on type of format used by patients. The methods of viewing the data are in either written format such as a logbook or in electronic data management format generated by a computer. Optimally, blood glucose data are organized into time slots throughout the day so that data trends can be evaluated. The next step is arranging the data into pre- or post-meal or bedtime time slots. You want to find out what the patient is doing regarding eating, activity, medication taking, and stressful events in relation to the data. It is very important to assess the patient's current behaviors. A helpful framework to use is the AADE7[TM] Self-Care Behaviors labeled as healthy eating, being active, monitoring, taking medications, problem solving, coping, and reducing risks *(19)*. Correlating the self-monitoring of blood glucose patterns to clinical indicators such as A1C, weight changes, or random blood glucose testing in the clinic are helpful to validate the self-monitoring of blood glucose data.

Strategies for Organizing Self-Monitoring of Blood Glucose Data

1. If the patient brings in serial self-monitoring of blood glucose data, organize the serial data into columns by times of day. Of note, computer-generated data management records automatically organize data. You will still need to clarify with patients about where their data falls within the pre-determined columns.
2. Establish patient's target blood glucose range pre- and post-meals.
3. Look for blood glucose data that fall out of the target range.
4. Use "highlighter" method to easily identify out-of-target levels (see Table 1).
5. Calculate meaningful statistics into percentages, averages, and range of blood glucose data (see Table 2).

Table 1
"Highlighter Method" for Detecting SMBG Pattern (Reprinted with permission from the New Mexico Department of Health)

For the Educator

Purpose of highlighting:

Highlighters are an ideal way to assist your patient with seeing which blood glucoses (BG) fall above and below the targets you have set with them.

Tools needed: Two highlighter pens (not opaque-colored pens) to mark numbers without obscuring them. Best colors: yellow, green, orange, pink.

How to mark the BG:

- List patients target BG in the front of logbook or top of the page for easy reference.
- Start with records from the last 2 weeks.
- A succinct and most recent block of time is most useful.
- Pick one color for blood glucose above target and another for blood glucose below target, e.g., yellow for below and pink for above targets.
- As you highlight and discuss them with patient encourage patient to discuss why they might be out of target (use SMBG Assessment Tool).
- Calculate? (Percentages, averages and ranges over the last 2 weeks. Data management software does this for you.) Write down percentage of BGs in target on patient logbook so they can see improvement over time.
- Suggest that patient might want to try this on a weekly basis at home and bring to next visit.

For the Patient

Purpose of highlighting:

Highlighters are an ideal way to mark your blood sugars logbook to see blood sugars that are higher or lower than your targets. You can quickly see what is working or not working in your diabetes plan. You may need to change something to bring your blood sugar levels closer to target (see SMBG Assessment Tool).

Tools needed:

- Two highlighter pens in different colors. One for blood sugars above target and one for below target numbers, e.g., yellow for below and pink for above targets.
- Do not use a regular colored pen; it will cover up your records!
- Best colors: yellow, light green, orange, pink.

How to mark your book:

- Ask what your BG targets are (if you do not know). Now write them at the top of each page in your logbook.
- At the end of each week, get out your highlighter pens to mark blood sugars that are *not* in target.

(Continued)

Table 1 *(Continued)*

- Notice how many blood sugars were marked, and how many are not marked (because they are in target).
- Bring logbook with your highlighted numbers to your next clinic visit and discuss with your diabetes educator.

Developed by Sue Perry, PhD, CDE and Donna Tomky, MSN, RN, CNP, CDE for New Mexico Department of Health • Diabetes Prevention and Control Program • Version 2006

Table 2
Example of Highlighter Method with Statistical Calculations

Patient is on glyburide 5 mg twice a day and metformin 500 mg twice a day. He eats three meals a day and a "small" bedtime snack.

- Target BG pre-meal: 80–120 pre-meal
- Total # of BGs? 28
- Total # above target? 17 (BGs highlighted in light gray indicate above target values)
- Total # below target? 3 (BGs highlighted in dark gray indicate below target values)
- Total # in target? 8
- Percent in target? $(8/28) \times 100 = 29\%$
- Percent above target? $(17/28) \times 100 = 61\%$
- Percent below target? $(3/28) \times 100 = 10\%$

Benefits of "highlighter method" are (1) quick visualization of above, below, and in target blood glucoses, (2) quick calculations of percentages, (3) quick view of patterns for further probing of the causes

"Highlighter Method" Not Used				"Highlighter Method" Used				
Day	AM	Noon	PM	HS	Day	AM	Noon	PM	HS
M	101	150	70	102	M	101	150	70	102
T	142	160	112	86	T	142	160	112	86
W	125	142	108	97	W	125	142	108	97
Th	121	131	157	50	Th	121	131	157	50
F	146	160	69	210	F	146	160	69	210
Sat	125	132	141	110	Sat	125	132	141	110
Sun	160	171	111	131	Sun	160	171	111	131

DETECTING TRENDS AND PATTERNS AND CONSIDERING CAUSES

A pattern is a series of blood glucose readings taken at the same testing time each day *(7)*. Even missing blood glucose data can form a pattern. Most pattern management resources focus on medications, specifically adjusting insulin, versus considering other variables that may cause problems. There is much more to the picture once you organize and review the trends. Pattern recognition requires reviewing self-monitoring of blood glucose data over a period of time. At least 3 days or more of data are required to confidently identify patterns for recommending therapy changes. Some basic questions to ask when evaluating blood glucose monitoring results are

1. Is there enough data throughout the day or at meaningful times (e.g., fasting, pre-meal, bedtime, etc.) to evaluate?
2. Is the patient consistent about their self-care behaviors, including weekend versus weekdays?
3. Are there emerging patterns that happen consistently upon reviewing at least 3 days or more?
4. Are there any problems of low or high blood glucoses occurring at the same time of day?
5. Are there blood glucose results representing "peak" times of each medication, physical activity, or food intake?
6. Have there been any changes in a typical day such as illness, stress, travel, etc.?
7. Are there any physiological changes or new medications that might be occurring (pregnancy, weight gain or loss, puberty, steroids, thyroid medications, etc.)?

The diabetes educator must consider the patient's current self-care behavior that may include multiple factors or causes for out-of-target blood glucoses. Patients need to know what and how to successfully self-manage their diabetes. Some key components in diabetes self-management include consistent timing of monitoring blood glucose, amount of food or carbohydrate to be eaten at meals and snacks, medication dosing and administration, and level of physical activity, particularly if the patient is on set doses of oral medications or insulin (20). More frequent self-monitoring of blood glucose is required if implementing an intensive insulin therapy regime, allowing for flexibility in meal timing and food amounts (21). Diabetes educators and patients need to be detectives when assessing possible causes of high or low blood glucoses while considering strategies for bringing blood glucoses back to target ranges (see Table 3).

IDENTIFYING DESIRED CHANGES AND CONSIDERING STRATEGIES

Diabetes education consists of diabetes self-management knowledge and skill training as well as behavior change strategies like goal setting, problem solving, and enhancing motivation. Assessing the patient's current behavior along with barriers to changing or enhancing behavior is critical to understanding possible interventional strategies to improve blood glucose results

Table 3

Self-monitoring of Blood Glucose. Assessment of possible causes for out-of-target Blood Glucose (BG) and interventional strategies to improve BG

Behavior		Reasons for BG to be too high	Reasons for BG to be too low	Strategies to bring BG back to target range
Eating	*Patient*	Ate more food? Ate out or special occasion? Snacking or nibbling on food? Drank alcohol? Type of food?	Ate less food? Drank alcohol? Missed snack? Delayed or missed meal? Inconsistent carb intake? Inaccurate carb counting? Alcohol consumption? High fat meal with rapid insulin absorption and slow digestion	• Consistent carbohydrate intake and timing of meals and snacks • Choose low carb snacks. • Minimize alcohol consumption • Teach how to accurately count carbohydrates and encourage consistent intake if on fixed doses of insulin • Consider timing of insulin in relation to slow digestion related to high fat foods or delayed gastric emptying
	Educator	Gastroparesis? Inaccurate carb counting? Snacking? Large or high fat meal with slow digestion?		
Activity	*Patient*	Got less exercise? Changed schedule?	Changed schedule? Got more exercise? Exercise was more intense? Injection site near active extremity? Timing of med or insulin in relationship to activity? Weight loss?	• Consider consistent timing and intensity of exercise • Consider snack prior to exercise session • Consider adjusting insulin or medications in anticipation of exercise or if weight loss occurred • Teach patient to monitor BG before, during, and after exercise
	Educator	Insufficient insulin with counterregulatory hormones release? Intense workout with elevated BG		

(Continued)

Table 3 (*Continued*)

Behavior		Reasons for BG to be too high	Reasons for BG to be too low	Strategies to bring BG back to target range
Blood glucose monitoring	*Patient*	Missed checking? Got off schedule? Not enough blood? Integrity of strips? Meter/technique? Data accuracy? Insufficient data? Somogyi or dawn phenomenon?	Missed checking? Got off schedule? Not enough blood? Data accuracy? Integrity of strips? Meter/technique? Insufficient data	• Need to check BG on time especially if dosing insulin • Review SMBG supplies, technique, and meter accuracy • Compare meter results with lab results • Encourage more SMBG based on medication regime • Consider medication adjustment
	Educator			
Taking medication	*Patient*	Took after eating? Missed? Problems drawing up insulin? Took too little? Need more medication? Lipohypertrophy? Timing of meds/insulin? Absorption of meds or insulin? Insulin integrity? Not enough meds/insulin? No access to medication?	Problems drawing up insulin? Took too much? Need less medication? Took at wrong time? Timing of insulin? Wrong med? Inconsistent taking of meds/insulin?	• Get medication or insulin on time. • Consider using reminder system, e.g., alarm, pill reminder • Adjust dose of medication or insulin based on patterns • Rotate injection sites • Match timing of insulin in relationship with food intake • Adjust basal insulin if fasting blood glucoses are not to target • Adjust bolus insulin if pre- or post-meal BG out of target • Check medication carefully before taking
	Educator			

152

		Patient	Educator	
Coping (feelings, e.g., stress, anger, sadness)	*Patient*	Stressed out? Family problems? Financial problems? I'm depressed? Work problems? Stress hormones? Memory loss/forgetfulness Untreated psych disorder?	*Educator* — Stressed out? Inconsistent taking of meds/insulin? Depression? Anxious? Memory loss/forgetfulness Untreated psych disorder?	• Consider timing, type of medication in relationship to food or other medication • Consider options for affordable medications • Consider changing insulin regime • Teach appropriate coping skills • Consider behavioral health counseling • Consider referral to behavioral health or social worker • Consider appropriate pharmacological therapy • Consider strategies for getting medication on time • Discuss strategies for working through problems
Problem solving (cough, fever, pain, vomiting)	*Patient*	I've been sick? Got a sore? Over treated low blood sugar? Recent infection? Silent infection? Oral or injection of steroids? Pubertal or growth hormones? Hyperthyroidism?	*Educator* — Over treated high blood sugar? Irregular eating? Hypoglycemia unawareness? Missed other meds, i.e., steroids? Hypothyroidism?	• Triage patient's problems, treat or refer to appropriate provider • Review appropriate sick day rules • Review appropriate detection, prevention, and treatment of low and high blood sugars • Consider medication adjustments

(Continued)

153

Table 3 (*Continued*)

Behavior		*Reasons for BG to be too high*	*Reasons for BG to be too low*	*Strategies to bring BG back to target range*
Complications or risks (related health problems, e.g., heart, eyesight, pregnancy, kidneys)	*Patient*	Stomach problems? Chest pain? Hard to draw up insulin with poor vision? Pregnant? Second or third trimester of pregnancy? Recent myocardial infarction? Visual acuity? Dexterity problems?	Stomach problems? Kidneys are failing? Hard to draw up insulin with poor vision? First trimester of pregnancy	• Triage patient's problems, treat or refer to appropriate provider • Consider appropriate tools for safe and effective dosing of insulin • Consider medication adjustments • Consider timing of insulin dosing
	Educator		Gastroparesis? Visual acuity? Dexterity problems? Renal insufficiency?	

154

and overall health. Diabetes educators must discuss with the patient and mutually determine safe and desired patient behavioral and clinical goals before recommending interventional strategies. The American Association of Diabetes Educators 7 Self-Care Behaviors[TM] provide a framework for assessment, problem solving, barrier identification and resolution, and goal setting in identifying desired changes and appropriate interventions to deal with out-of-target blood glucose patterns. Considering the patient's readiness, conviction, and confidence to make changes are also important in recommending therapeutic changes. Table 3 addresses possible causes for high and low blood glucoses and gives suggestions on possible interventional strategies to consider. Table 4 offers recommendation for adjusting insulin based on type of insulin regime, blood glucose patterns and levels, diet history, and lifestyle. Diabetes educators and patients alike may determine other causes and strategies that are not listed but need attention in identifying desired changes and therapeutic strategies.

DEVELOP A PLAN

A plan of action for patients should be based on individualized assessment for determining (1) the frequency of blood glucose monitoring, (2) appropriate recommendations based on a framework such as self-care behaviors, (3) safe and effective target blood glucoses considering national guidelines, and (4) readiness and ability to make changes. Important questions to ask while interpreting blood glucose records:

- What does the A1C level tell you? Does it correlate with the self-monitoring of blood glucose records?
- What does the history tell you? Ask questions about what the patient is doing versus assuming that they are doing what they were told to do.
- What do the self-monitoring of blood glucose records tell you? Look for patterns or lack of patterns to determine if the patient has accurate and sufficient blood glucose data to recommend a safe and effective therapeutic plan.
- What's your approach? Consider all approaches including behavioral goals and medical management strategies.

Diabetes educators can negotiate and set goals that are specific, measurable, achievable, and compatible with the patient in recommending self-management strategies to improve glycemic control. The plan of action should be documented in the patient's record with a written plan of action given to the patient. An example of a patient "diabetes management plan" form (English and Spanish versions) to be used for documentation of patient goals and plan of action can be downloaded from the New Mexico Diabetes Control and Prevention Program's web site at http://www.diabetesnm.org/education/forms.htm

Table 4
Recommended Adjustments based on SMBG Patterns and Other Variables (adapted from Hirsch et al.)

Type of Insulin	Pattern	Adjustments made based on blood glucose levels	Diet history	Lifestyle
Basal-only Insulin w/oral agents	High FBG w/minimal glucose rise during day	Fasting	Small, regular meals	Reluctance to do MDI, requires oral agents
Rapid-acting analog or intermediate basal insulin	Any FBG or BG rise during day	Fasting and pre-supper with timing of injection (if insulin is administered twice daily)	Large suppers/small lunches	Consistent daily routine, reluctance to do MDI
Regular/NPH	Any FBG or BG rise during day	Fasting and pre-supper with timing of injection (if insulin is administered twice daily)	Isocaloric meals or larger lunches	Consistent daily routine, reluctance to do MDI
Basal and bolus insulin (MDI)	Any FBG or BG rise during day	Minimum before each meal and bedtime	Regimen can be matched to any diet to achieve glycemic control	Erratic schedule, motivated to achieve tight glycemic control

IMPLEMENT PLAN

Once a plan of action is agreed upon by team members, then clear goals, steps, and expectations are mapped out for the patient. It is important to allow the patient to "practice" the specified steps for accomplishing the identified goals. Provide contact information in case problems arise such as multiple and consistent hyperglycemia or hypoglycemia events to avoid frustration and concerns the patient might experience.

EVALUATE RESPONSE TO PLAN AND REVISE PLAN IF NECESSARY

It is essential to set up short-term follow-up visits for evaluating the patient's response to action plan. Short-term follow-up may be defined in days, weeks, or months for evaluating the patient's progress or lack of improvement. It is critical to understand your patient's barriers or facilitators in changing behaviors that lead to improved diabetes outcomes. If necessary, the plan can and should be revised if goals continue to be unmet.

CONCLUSIONS

Diabetes self-management is very complex and involves multiple factors affecting the diabetes education and treatment plan. National guidelines provide diabetes educators and health care providers a framework for diabetes self-management education and care in clinical practice with guidance to further individualized blood glucose goals. Accurate and sufficient self-monitoring of blood glucose data is necessary for determining patterns, problem solving, and developing a plan of action for patients. Documentation is critical to satisfy legal, financial, and self-management care issues. When interpreting blood glucose records always ask yourself the following questions: (1) What does the A1C level tell you? (2) What does the history tell you? (3) What do the self-monitoring of blood glucose records tell you? (4) What is your approach for developing a plan of action with the patient?

REFERENCES

1. Wild S, Roglic G, Green A, Sicree R, King H. Global Prevalence of Diabetes: Estimates for the year 2000 and projections for 2030. *Diabetes Care*. May 1, 2004 2004;27(5):1047–1053.
2. Funnell M, Brown T, Childs B, Haas L, Hosey G, Jensen B, Maryniuk M, Peyrot M, Piette J, Reader D, Siminerio L, Weinger K, Weiss M. National Standards for Diabetes Self-Management Education. *Diabetes Care*. June 1, 2007 2007;30(6):1630–1637.
3. Mulcahy K, Peeples, M.,Tomky, D., Weaver, T. National Diabetes Education Outcomes System: Application to Practice. *Diabetes Educ*. November 1, 2000 2000;26(6):957–964.

4. Graves JR, Corcoran S. The Study of Nursing Informatics. *Image: Journal of Nursing Scholar.* Winter 1989;21(4):227–231.
5. Bergenstal R, Gavin, J. The role of self-monitoring of blood glucose in the care of people with diabetes: report of a global consensus conference. *Am J Med.* Sep 2005;118 (Suppl 9A):1S–6S.
6. Perry S, Tomky D. Definition of blood glucose pattern management. Pattern management: Deciphering the blood glucose testing puzzle workshop: New Mexico Dept of Health Diabetes Control and Prevention Program; 2006.
7. Pearson J, Bergenstal R. Fine-Tuning Control: Pattern Management Versus Supplementation: View 1: Pattern Management: an Essential Component of Effective Insulin Management. *Diabetes Spectr.* April 1, 2001 2001;14(2):75–78.
8. Endocrinology. American College of Endocrinology Consensus Statement on Guidelines for Glycemic Control. *Endocr Pract.* 2002;8(Suppl 1):5–10.
9. American Diabetes Association. Standards of Medical Care for Patients With Diabetes Mellitus. *Diabetes Care.* 2003;26(90001):33S–50.
10. Service F, O'Brien P. Influence of glycemic variables on hemoglobin A1c. *Endocr Pract.* 2007 Jul–Aug(13(4)):350–354.
11. McCarter R, Hempe J, Chalew S. Mean Blood Glucose and Biological Variation Have Greater Influence on HbA1c Levels Than Glucose Instability: An analysis of data from the Diabetes Control and Complications Trial. *Diabetes Care.* February 1, 2006 2006;29(2):352–355.
12. Monnier L, Lapinski H, Colette C. Contributions of Fasting and Postprandial Plasma Glucose Increments to the Overall Diurnal Hyperglycemia of Type 2 Diabetic Patients: Variations with increasing levels of HbA1c. *Diabetes Care.* March 1, 2003 2003;26(3):881–885.
13. Schrot R. Targeting Plasma Glucose: Preprandial Versus Postprandial. *Clin Diabetes.* October 1, 2004 2004;22(4):169–172.
14. Soonthornpun S, Rattarasarn C, Leelawattana R, Setasuban W. Postprandial plasma glucose: a good index of glycemic control in type 2 diabetic patients having near-normal fasting glucose levels. *Diabetes Res Clin Pract.* Oct 1999;46(1):23–27.
15. de Veciana M, Major C, Morgan M, Asrat T, Toohey J, Lien J, Evans A. Postprandial versus preprandial blood glucose monitoring in women with gestational diabetes mellitus requiring insulin therapy. *N Engl J Med.* Nov 9 1995;333(19):1237–1241.
16. American Diabetes Association. Postprandial blood glucose (Consensus Statement). *Diabetes Care.* Apr 2001;24(4):775–778.
17. Schwedes U, Siebolds M, Mertes G. Meal-Related Structured Self-Monitoring of Blood Glucose: Effect on diabetes control in non-insulin-treated type 2 diabetic patients. *Diabetes Care.* November 1, 2002 2002;25(11):1928–1932.
18. Guerci B, Drouin P, Grange V, Bougneres P, Fontaine P, Kerlan V, Passa P, Thivolet C, Vialettes B, Charbonnel B. Self-monitoring of blood glucose significantly improves metabolic control in patients with type 2 diabetes mellitus: the Auto-Surveillance Intervention Active (ASIA) study. *Diabetes Metab.* Dec 2003;29(6):587–594.
19. Austin M. Diabetes educators: partners in diabetes care and management. *Endocr Pract.* Jan-Feb 2006;12 Suppl 1:138–141.
20. Linekin PL. Diabetes pattern management: the key to diabetes self-management and glycemic control. *Home Healthc Nurse.* Mar 2002;20(3):168–177.
21. Tomky D. Intensifying insulin therapy: Multiple daily injections to pump therapy. In: Mensing C, ed. *The Art and Science of Diabetes Self-Management Education: A Desk Reference for Healthcare Professionals.* Chicago: American Association of Diabetes Educators; 2006:821.

11 Measuring Diabetes Outcomes and Measuring Behavior

Malinda Peeples, MS, RN, CDE

CONTENTS

INTRODUCTION
SCIENCE ON MEASURING
   DIABETES SELF-CARE BEHAVIOR
WHAT TO MEASURE
APPLICATION TO PRACTICE
CASE STUDY
CONCLUSION: THE JOURNEY
ACKNOWLEDGMENT
REFERENCES

ABSTRACT

During the last decade much progress has been made in national measurement for health care, which includes both quality and costs of care. National organizations have worked with stakeholder groups, professional organizations, researchers, and policy makers to adopt measurements that are based on science and expert consensus. The current measures primarily address health plan performance and provider level performance. The development of patient-centered measures is slower. This chapter provides an overview of standards and application for self-care outcomes in diabetes education practice. Measurement of self-care behaviors can be applied at the individual educator level to guide interventions and at the program level for quality improvement efforts. These evidence-based approaches support

From: *Contemporary Diabetes: Educating Your Patient with Diabetes*
Edited by: K. Weinger and C. A. Carver, DOI 10.1007/978-1-60327-208-7_11,
© Humana Press, a part of Springer Science+Business Media, LLC 2009

educators to more effectively integrate self-care behavior assessment, intervention, and measurement into their practices and their programs.

Key Words: Diabetes Self-Management Education, Outcomes, Diabetes Education Outcomes, Behavior Change, Self-care Behavior Outcome.

INTRODUCTION

During the last decade much progress has been made in national measurement for health care, which includes both quality and costs of care. Efforts to provide effective and meaningful measurement for providers, payers, and health care consumers (or patients) have proliferated. National organizations have worked with these stakeholder groups as well as professional organizations, researchers, and policy makers to adopt measurements that are based on science and expert consensus. The current measures primarily address health plan performance and provider level performance. The development of patient-centered measures is slower. Quality measurement and reporting, still an evolving process, is transforming health care delivery and outcomes.

Diabetes, cardiac conditions, asthma, congestive obstructive pulmonary disease (COPD), uncontrolled hypertension, and acute low back pain account for 50–60% of all direct medical costs *(1)*. Also, people with chronic conditions typically do not have one condition but may have as many as three to five of these costly (in both resources and human terms) conditions *(2)*. This presents challenges for care coordination, disease management, and quality measurement.

Primarily diabetes care measures focus on the provider and what measures their patient population is achieving. These measures focus on metabolic indicators such as A1c and process measures such as eye exams. They are primarily influenced by what medications and tests are ordered. They are measured and monitored through claims reporting with health plans or, in some practices, with patient registries for the goal of promoting quality diabetes care. Currently the most commonly measured aspects of diabetes care are directed by quality organizations such as Health Effectiveness Data and Information Set (HEDIS) and National Committee on Quality Assurance (NCQA)/American Diabetes Association (ADA) Provider Recognition Program. In 2006, The Joint Commission Certificate of Distinction for Inpatient Diabetes Care was introduced as the first measurement effort for hospitals on diabetes inpatient care *(3)*. For public health practitioners, the state-based Diabetes Prevention and Control Programs (DCPC) direct collection of surveillance, epidemiology, and program evaluation data *(4)*.

A challenge for diabetes educators is what measures do they capture, how are these reported, and how do they apply them to their practice. Depending on the practice setting and whether the educator is providing educational interventions only or if he/she is engaged in clinical co-management, the outcomes of interest can vary. Educators may be involved in capturing data for multiple customers, and the primary customer for that practice setting will drive much of the data capture and reporting. In Table 1, the current diabetes measurement sets are identified with the practice setting where they are most often implemented These measurements primarily address metabolic and process measures.

In 2000, the Institute of Medicine Report advanced patient-centered care as one of the characteristics of the future of health care (5). This public announcement shifted the attention from a provider-centric system to one that acknowledges the values and interests of the patient. While many providers have always put the patient at the center of the interaction, the health care systems are now directed to include the patient in health care measurement and redesign. Additionally, as the epidemic of chronic diseases burdens the health care system, much effort is being focused on redesigning an essentially "acute care" health care system to one that supports chronic disease care. This systems approach addresses the health care system as well as integrates self-management support and community health resources into a comprehensive view of health care (6). In this environment, the issues of patient lifestyle and self-management of disease and complications are gaining attention with providers, health system administrators, researchers, and policy makers.

The National Standards for Diabetes Self-Management Education were established in 1985 and are revised approximately every 5 years to reflect the current knowledge base and state of the science of diabetes education (7). Standards serve to provide guidance for the profession and measurements are developed to monitor progress toward standards achievement. The American Diabetes Association Education Recognition Program (8) and Indian Health Service (9) certify diabetes education programs using criteria based on the National Standards.

During the last decade, in response to the increasing emphasis on outcomes of care, the Diabetes Self-Management Education Outcome Standards were developed to provide specificity to the measurement of the impact of diabetes education on program participants. These standards focus on the outcomes of diabetes education in the context of the overall diabetes care system (10). The standards direct measurement of self-care behavior and behavior change for individual patients and populations. Measures of diabetes self-care are different from measures of diabetes care as they are reported by the patient. These patient-centered measures and specific process measures about diabetes education are absent from the current national measurement sets (11). The remainder of this chapter will focus on self-management, self-care behavior, and behavior change as a key outcome of diabetes education.

Table 1
A Diabetes Measurement Sets or Certifications for Practice Settings

Setting	Measurement sets or certification	Customers	Measures
Physician practice	– NCQA HEDIS – Diabetes Physician Recognition Program (DPRP) (http://web.ncqa.org)	– Health plans – CMS	– Diabetes care measures – HbA1c control >9.0% – HbA1c control <7.0% – Blood pressure control <140/90 mm Hg – Blood pressure control <130/80 mm Hg – Eye examination – Smoking status and cessation advice or treatment – Complete lipid profile – LDL control <130 mg/dl – LDL control <100 mg/dl – Nephropathy assessment – Foot examination (monofilament)
Hospital inpatient	– JCAHO Disease Specific Certification for Inpatient Diabetes (http://www.jointcommission.org/)	– JCAHO – Hospital administration	– Staff education requirements – Blood glucose monitoring protocols – Treatment plans for hypoglycemia and hyperglycemia – Data collection of incidences of hypoglycemia – Patient education on self – management of diabetes – An identified program champion or program champion team

(Continued)

162

Table 1
(Continued)

Setting	Measurement sets or certification	Customers	Measures
Outpatient education program	– ADA Education Recognition Program (ERP) (http://diabetes.org/ for – health – professionals – and – scientists/recognition) – Indian Health Service (IHS) http://www.ihs.gov/MedicalPrograms/diabetes/recognition/recog_index.asp – Payer driven	– Health Plans – Facility Administration – ADA/ERP or HIS (if program recognized)	– At least 2 outcomes must be tracked: 1. Patient defined goals & measures 2. Program measures (metabolic, clinical, quality of life, processes)
Diabetes educator in private practice	– NCQA or ADA/ERP depending on billing structure	– Dependent on business model	Any or all of following – Clinical and behavioral – Patient and program measures – HEDIS measures
Public health	Diabetes Prevention & Control Program (DCPC): state based	– State and national governments	Surveillance, epidemiology, and program evaluation http://www.cdc.gov/diabetes/statistics/didit/index.htm

ADA – American Diabetes Association; JCAHO – Joint Commission on Accreditation of Hospital Organizations; NCQA HEDIS – National Committee for Quality Assurance – Health Effectiveness Data and Information Set.

SCIENCE ON MEASURING DIABETES SELF-CARE BEHAVIOR

Diabetes self-management is a key responsibility of the person with diabetes. Unlike an acute medical problem that can be "fixed" with a procedure, medication, or therapy, chronic diseases require ongoing and often extensive self-care by the individual. Self-care is defined as the daily tasks (or behaviors) that the individual performs to manage diabetes (12). These self-care behaviors are complex in terms of treatment regimen, costly in terms of time, energy, and resources, and are relentless in terms of the 24/7 commitment. Behavior change is defined as modifying old behaviors or adapting new ones (13). Behavior change is not simply related to knowledge of how to perform the behavior but is influenced by the motivation and self-efficacy of the individual health belief system, and the social and community resources and support (14).

Most survey instruments address one to three self-care behaviors necessary for successful self-management. Most frequently studied are eating, activity, blood glucose monitoring, and medication adherence (15). Increasingly, psychosocial, problem-solving, and risky behaviors such as smoking are being included as areas of self-care behavior related to diabetes.

Self-report measurement has many difficulties. Most methods have been used as part of research studies and involve multi-item questions that are not practical for assessing all self-care behaviors related to diabetes care. The Self-Care Inventory-Revised (SCI-R), developed as SCE by La Greca and colleagues and modified by Weinger and colleagues, has been evaluated to be a sound measure of perceptions of adherence to recommended self-care behaviors of adults with type 1 and type 2 diabetes (16). The Diabetes Problem-Solving Interview (DSPI) has been found in research to be a predictor of self-management behaviors, to be sensitive to self-management training interventions, and to mediate behavior change (17). The Diabetes Self-Management Assessment Report Tool (D-SMART) is an instrument that assesses self-management behaviors and supports the patient in identifying areas of interest for behavior change and goal setting (18). The state of science is evolving as research is focusing on developing practical, simpler self-report instruments that can be applied at the point of service. Also, most quality data using patient self-report has been cross-sectional and not longitudinal which would be more helpful in assessing processes of care that lead to particular outcomes (19).

Additional problems exist because most methods to assess self-care behaviors rely on patients memory to recall activities over a specific time period of 24 h, 1 week, or the previous week (20,21). Patients' reports of frequency of specific self-care behavior may be collected but analysis may not account for the individual treatment plan (22).

Self-reported behaviors may not represent actual behaviors. Some studies suggest that over time, as the appropriate behaviors are learned, patients may tend to respond as expected rather than with actual behavior – especially those who are not well controlled (23). The most rigorous evaluation of self-care requires concurrent measurement with biometric devices and at this time is intensive and costly for both patients and providers. This approach to validating self-care behaviors can also impact trust for the provider–patient relationship.

The American Diabetes Association Clinical Standards for Diabetes Care states that a psychological assessment and treatment should be a part of routine care (24). The National Standards for Diabetes Self-Management Education state that patient outcomes should be evaluated at regular intervals (25). The American Association of Diabetes Educators position statement directs educators to measure behavior change pre- and post-program (26). While there is increasing recognition of the importance of assessment of self-care behaviors, this has yet to be integrated into national measurement sets.

WHAT TO MEASURE

Self-report measures can provide information to the patient about their progress toward meeting behavioral goals. For the diabetes educator and other health care providers, patient self-report provides feedback on the effectiveness of their interventions with the patient and also information about how to modify the interventions to improve outcomes.

Self-management support is an evidence-based intervention for diabetes (27). However, measuring the effectiveness of this intervention is quite challenging. First, determining what behaviors to measure, what instruments to use, the frequency of measurement, and the application to practice is evolving. The American Association of Diabetes Educators Diabetes Education Outcomes Standards published in 2003 (28) and incorporated into the 2007 revision of the National Standards for DSME provide direction for beginning to address some of the problems related to measurement of self-care behavior:

Standard 1. Behavior change is the unique measurement for diabetes self-management education.

Standard 2: Seven self-care behaviors determine the effectiveness of diabetes education at the individual and population participant levels.

Standard 3: Diabetes self-care behaviors should be evaluated at baseline and then at regular intervals after the educational program.

Standard 4: The continuum of outcomes including learning, behavioral, clinical, and health status should be assessed to demonstrate the interrelationship between diabetes self-management education and behavior change in the care of individuals with diabetes.

Standard 5: Individual patient outcomes are used to drive the intervention and improve care for the patient. Aggregate population outcomes are used to guide programmatic services and for continuous quality improvement activities for the diabetes self-management education and the population services.

Health Care Outcomes Continuum

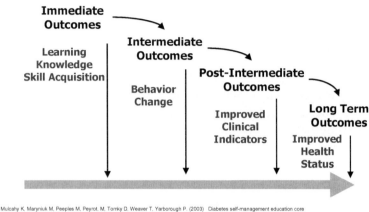

Mulcahy K, Maryniuk M, Peeples M, Peyrot, M, Tomky D, Weaver T, Yarborough P. (2003) Diabetes self-management education core outcome measures *The Diabetes ducator* **29**,768-803.

Fig. 1. Health Care Outcomes Continuum.

These standards provide guidance and specificity for the educator in the work with patients and programs and specify behavior change as the primary outcome of the educational intervention. Standard 4 acknowledges the importance of other outcomes and conceptualizes these outcomes as part of a continuum from immediate to long term (see Fig. 1). Prior to the development of the standards, learning outcomes were often thought of as a primary outcome of diabetes education. With the identification of behavior as the primary educational outcome, learning goals were re-conceptualized as important only to the degree that they contribute to behavior change; learning which does not help patients better manage their diabetes is irrelevant. Clinical and health outcomes also had been proposed in the past as primary outcomes of diabetes education. The national outcome standards acknowledge the importance of these goals, but regard them as a consequence of achieving the primary outcome; patients who improve their self-care behavior should experience improved clinical and health outcomes. However, these outcomes can be influenced by factors that are not subject to the direct impact of diabetes education (e.g., prescribed medication regimens, lack of financial resources to purchase medication, equipment and supplies).

As a feasible, practical way to conceptualize behavior change for diabetes education practice, seven self-care behaviors were identified as essential in effective self-management practices of people with diabetes. The seven self-care behaviors are *healthy eating, being active, monitoring, taking medication, problem-solving, healthy coping, and reducing risks*. These behaviors have been

Table 2
Self-Care Behaviors: Assessment and Measurement

AADE7[TM] behavior	Measures[1]	Methods of measurement[1]	Relationship to National[2] Standards for DSME
			Standard 6: content areas
Healthy eating	– Type and amount of food – Timing of meals – Alcohol intake – Special situations	– Food and BG records – 24 h recall, food frequency questionnaires	Incorporating *nutritional* management into lifestyle

Being active	– Activity
	  Type
	  Frequency
	  Duration
	  Intensity
		– Lifestyle log
		– Pedometer
			Incorporating *physical activity* into lifestyle

Monitoring	– Frequency and schedule of monitoring (e.g., times/day, days/wk) – # Unplanned testing – # Missed testing	– Log book review – Meter memory review or printout – Demonstration of technique – Pharmacy strip refill rate	*Monitoring blood* glucose and other parameters, interpreting and using the results for self-management decision making
Medication taking	– Adherence to medication regimen – Dose and schedule accuracy	– Patient self-report – Pill count – Review of pharmacy refill record – Demonstration – BG and medication records	Using *medication* safely and maximum therapeutic effectveness

(Continued)

Table 2
(Continued)

AADE7[TM] *behavior*	*Measures*[1]	*Methods of measurement*[1]	*Relationship to National*[2] *Standards for DSME*
Problem-solving	– BG testing results – Checking meter and strips for function – #BG results/month that require assistance – # Ketones tested when appropriate – # Missed days from work, school, or related activities	– Review of log book – Meter memory or printout – Medical chart review – Frequency of medication adjustment	Preventing, detecting, and treating *acute complications*
Reducing risks	– Measures per ADA Clinical standards of care – Diabetes education visits	– Patient self-report – Personal health record – Chart or claims data	– Preventing detecting and treating *chronic complications* – Developing personalized strategies to promote *health and behavior change*
Healthy coping	– Depression score, stress – Quality of life – Functional measurement – Treatment self-efficacy	– Validated instruments: – SF-36/SF12, PAID – Zung/Beck Depression Scale, D – SMART	Developing personalized strategies to address *psychosocial issues and concerns*

[1] Mulcahy K, Maryniuk M, Peeples M, Peyrot, M, Tomky D, Weaver T, Yarborough P. (2003) Diabetes self-management education core outcome measures *The Diabetes Educator* **29**,768–803.

[2] Funnell, M., Brown, T., Childs, B., Haas, L., Hosey, G., Jensen, B., Maryniuk, M., Peyrot, M., Piette, J., Reader, D., Siminerio, L., Weinger, K., Weiss, M. (2007). National standards for diabetes self-management education *Diabetes Care* **30**,1630–1637.

standardized into a nomenclature – AADE 7 Self-Care Behaviors[TM] – that reflects patient-centered self-management and provides a common language for communication for both providers and patients. Table 2 links these behaviors with the education content areas of the national standards and suggest measures and measurement methods.

This framework of seven self-care behaviors provides a foundation for a model for measuring self-care behavior that includes assessing current behaviors, identifying barriers, and facilitating problem-solving for barrier resolution. The model supports targeted behavioral interventions and goal setting with patients. On follow-up visits, measuring and monitoring of behavior change and clinical indicators supports educator evaluation of outcomes. A simple method of tracking, measuring, and documenting the self-care behavior goals is available in paper format (AADE7 Goal Sheet) and has been incorporated into an electronic web-based tracking system – IMPACT[TM] (www.aadenet.org).

The seven behaviors are addressed in an earlier chapter of this book, so each will not be reviewed here. Also, a systematic review of each of the seven behaviors has been completed by researchers and provides a solid foundation for integrating the behaviors into educator practice (29).

As further evidence is accumulated on the seven behaviors, measurement methods will be refined. Currently, the framework provides a "behavioral review" of self-care behaviors just as the "head to toe" method provides a structured process for the review of systems for a physical exam. The standardized approach to the physical exam allows for brief review of the systems of the body with a more in-depth review for the system that relates to the symptom or concern of interest. So applying this concept to the "behavioral review," the seven areas of self-care provide a structured approach for the educator to assess. Then based on discussion with the patient, review of other assessment data – including metabolic data, the educator can collaborate with the patient to focus on the behaviors of interest. This process is incorporated in the case study at the end of this chapter.

APPLICATION TO PRACTICE

Measurement of self-care behaviors can be applied at the individual educator level to guide interventions and at the program level for quality improvement efforts. Traditionally diabetes education programs focused on delivery of content about diabetes disease, the treatment skills, the complications, and lifestyle challenges. Clearly, this is an acute care focus. Over the last 10 years, increasing evidence has supported the movement to viewing diabetes as a chronic disease and that individuals who deal with diabetes daily make decisions about how to integrate treatment strategies into their lives. With the increased attention on self-care and behavior change, diabetes education programs have integrated more behavioral interventions into their program design. Challenging to programs has been the desire to incorporate behavioral strategies while the state of evidence is evolving for interventions that are practical, feasible, and patient-centered. The population level of data on self-care behaviors can inform program curriculum design, educator intervention strategies, community resource identification, and organizational support. The continuous quality improvement process is addressed in other chapters, so the remainder of this chapter will focus on the diabetes education process at the individual educator and patient levels from assessment though outcomes.

The diabetes education process typically involves assessment, intervention (including planning and implementation), and outcomes (or evaluation). It is an iterative process that includes skill training, behavioral interventions, and clinical management. Outcomes impacted vary on the intervention. Depending on the scope of practice, the level of clinical management can vary from making recommendations for medication changes to ordering medications based on protocol or prescriptive authority.

The 2007 National Standards for Diabetes Self-Management Education (DSME) address outcome measurement at the patient level and direct programs to measure patient goal attainment.

Standard 9

The DSME entity will measure attainment of patient-defined goals and patient outcomes at regular intervals using appropriate measurement techniques to evaluate the effectiveness of the educational intervention.
In addition to program-defined goals and objectives (e.g., learning goals, metabolic and other health outcomes), the DSME entity needs to assess each patient's personal self-management goals and his/her progress toward those personal goals. The AADE7 self-care behaviors provide a useful framework for assessment and documentation. Diabetes self-management behaviors include physical activity, eating, medications, monitoring of blood glucose, diabetes self-care related problem solving, reducing risks of acute and chronic complications, and psychosocial aspects of living with diabetes. The intervals for assessment of patient level outcomes depend on the outcome itself and the timeframe provided within the defined goals. For some areas of assessment, the indicators, measures, and timeframes may be based on guidelines from professional organizations or government agencies (30).

For the practical application of this standard, educators and programs can work with tools already developed. For others who already have electronic records, these goal categories can be integrated into the data collection process. Within each goal category or behavior, there can be many individualized goals, ranging from simple to complex. When following patients at the individual level, progress in the specific goal is important, but at a program level, the goal category is what can be tracked. As electronic records become more ubiquitous, this record keeping will become more seamless. The use of standardized goal categories is beneficial for comparisons across programs and communication among providers.

CASE STUDY

The processes of education and clinical management for the diabetes educator have been addressed in Chapter 4 and elsewhere *(31)*. However, it is important to note that the process(es) addressed are based on patient need, educator assessment, educator scope of practice, and education program design. In the following section, integrating a behavior approach into the diabetes education intervention will be explained and applied to a case study.

This case study applies the behavior approach for a patient who is referred by his primary care physician to a diabetes educator. The process can also be applied in a group class setting by thinking about the education process from the patient perspective and integrating it into the class discussion to guide participants in thinking about behavior change.

Case Study for Behavior Change and Outcomes Measurement

Background: Leo is a 57-year-old male who schedules an appointment to see the diabetes educator on referral from his primary care physician who has been following Leo for a number of years. At his last visit, Leo's A1c was 7.5% and Dr. Janus was considering adding some bolus insulin to the medication regimen of Metformin 1000 mg bid and Lantus 20 units hs. Leo was resistant to the idea of daytime injections because of challenges he perceived that he would have at his work site. Dr. Janus referred Leo to John, the diabetes educator affiliated with his practice.

Assessment: At the initial visit, John performs a general assessment of Leo's knowledge and skills, self-care behaviors, and clinical treatment plan so that he has a baseline assessment of Leo's self-care knowledge, behavior, and the integration of his treatment plan into his lifestyle. He determines that Leo is knowledgeable about diabetes and his treatment plan. He is skilled in the techniques of monitoring and insulin administration. So he decides to focus on the self-care behaviors. In a facilitated discussion, John finds out from Leo that Dr. Janus wants to add additional daytime insulin to the treatment plan and Leo is resisting because of his work demands. John, knowing that Leo has the knowledge and skills of insulin administration, continues the discussion. As he evaluates Leo's "medication-taking behavior," Leo states that he often forgets the bedtime insulin and so the main diabetes medication that he is using is the

Metformin. John understands that if Leo can modify his "medication taking behavior," the daytime insulin may not be needed.

Intervention: Leo states that he is missing his bedtime insulin at least 3 days a week. Starting today, Leo wants to administer his bedtime insulin every night as ordered by Dr. Janus. With discussion, John found out that Leo did not have a consistent time to administer the bedtime insulin. However, Leo always watched the 11 p.m. news as part of his nightly ritual. Collaboratively Leo and John agreed that taking the insulin at the beginning of the news would be doable. Leo filled in the goal sheet with the goal to "Improve my medication-taking by administering the bedtime insulin at the beginning of the 11 p.m. news. I will enter the insulin dose on my diabetes cellphone after taking my injection. I want to do this every night until my return visit to Dr. Janus in 1 month. By doing this I hope to control my blood sugars with 1 insulin injection a day." John communicated this goal to Dr. Janus so that he would have the information at the return visit.

In 1 month, Leo returned to Dr. Janus. Dr. Janus reviewed the electronic logbook with Leo and found the blood sugars to be within target range. So he determined that the bedtime insulin was working well and there was no need to add additional injections. Dr. Janus discussed ways of Leo continuing to get reinforcement for this activity. They talked about how Leo's wife was typically supportive of his diabetes care and that she would continue to encourage/remind him about that bedtime dose of insulin. However, Leo said that feeling better and seeing those good numbers were strong motivators for him to continue effective "medication-taking behavior." Two months after the visit with Dr. Janus, John contacts Leo by phone for evaluation of his medication-taking. He completes the outcomes evaluation as follows.

OUTCOME MEASUREMENT

- Initial visit: baseline assessment for outcomes

  - *Behavior*: identified "medication-taking" behavior as area of interest –

    - reported missing bedtime dose of insulin at least 3 days a week – 45% of doses

  - *Clinical*: A1c 7.5%

- Intervention – goal setting for bedtime insulin administration
- Follow-up visit (3 months later): outcomes evaluation

  - *Behavior*: medication-taking behavior re-evaluated – no missing medications
  - *Clinical*: A1c improved to 6.8%. No additional insulin injections were added to the treatment plan.

CONCLUSION: THE JOURNEY

Diabetes educators support patients in their journey toward successful self-management, a better quality of life, and the best health possible for them. Diabetes educators are participating in a journey toward improving the science and practice of diabetes education through quality measurement of learning, behavioral, and clinical outcomes. This chapter has provided educators with evidence-based approaches to more effectively integrate self-care behavior assessment, intervention, and measurement into their practices and their programs. Diabetes educators, as part of the overall diabetes care system, will support the health care system journey toward quality, cost-effective health care for chronic disease.

ACKNOWLEDGMENT

Ms Peeples is Past President of the American Association of Diabetes Educators (AADE) and acknowledges the contributions of those involved in the AADE Outcomes Project and the AADE/University Pittsburgh Medical Center Outcomes Project.

REFERENCES

1. Online. http://www.ncqa.org/Communications/SOHC2006/SOHC_2006_Executive_Summary. pg 11. Accessed October 27, 2007.
2. Wolff, J.L., Starfield, B., Anderson, G. (2002) Prevalence, expenditures, and complications of multiple chronic conditions in the elderly *Archives Internal Medicine* **162**, 2269–76.
3. Online. http://www.jointcommission.org/HTBAC/DSC/InpatientDiabetes.htm. Accessed October 27, 2007.
4. Online. http://www.cdc.gov/diabetes/statistics/didit/index.htm. Accessed January 18, 2008.
5. Institute of Medicine, Committee on Quality of Health Care in America. Crossing the quality chasm: A new health system for the 21st Century. Washington, DC: National Academy Press; 2001.
6. Wagner, E.H. (1998) Chronic Disease Management: What Will It Take to Improve Care for Chronic Illness? *Effective Clinical Practice* **1**, 2–4.
7. Funnell, M., Brown, T., Childs, B., Haas, L., Hosey, G., Jensen, B., Maryniuk, M., Peyrot, M., Piette, J., Reader, D., Siminerio, L., Weinger, K., Weiss, M. (2007). National standards for diabetes self-management education *Diabetes Care* **30**, 1630–1637.
8. Online. http://www.diabetes.org/for-health-professionals-and-scientists/recognition/faqs.jsp# benefits-recognition Accessed October 22, 2007.
9. Online. http://www.ihs.gov/MedicalPrograms/diabetes/recognition/recog. Accessed October 22, 2007.
10. American Association of Diaetes Educators. Standards for outcomes measurement of diabetes self-management education (2003) *The Diabetes Educator* **29**, 804–816.
11. Peeples M, Tomky D, Mulcahy K, Peyrot M, Siminerio L on behalf of AADE Outcomes Project and AADE UPMC Diabetes Education Outcomes Project. Evolution of the American Association of Diabetes Educators' diabetes education outcomes project (2007) *The Diabetes Educator.* **33**, 794–817.

12. Weinger, K., Butler, H.A., Welch, G. W., La Greca, A.M. (2005) Measuring diabetes self-care: a psychometric analysis of the self-care inventory-revised with adults *Diabetes Care* **28**, 1346–52.
13. Peyrot, M. (1999) Behavior change in diabetes education *The Diabetes Educator* **25**, 62–73.
14. Fisher, E.B., Brownson, C.A., O'Toole, M.L., Shetty G., Anwuri, V.V., Glasgow, R.E. (2005) Ecological approaches to self-management: The case of diabetes. *Am J Public Health* **95**, 1523–35.
15. Bradley C. Measures of perceived control (1994) In *Handbook of Psychology and Diabetes*, ed. Clare Bradley. Harwood Academic Publishers: Amsterdam.
16. Weinger, K., Butler, H.A., Welch, G. W., La Greca, A.M. (2005) Measuring diabetes self-care: a psychometric analysis of the self-care inventory-revised with adults *Diabetes Care* **28**, 1346–52.
17. Glasgow, R. E., Fisher, L., Skaff, M., Mullan, J., and Toobert, D.J., (2007) Problem solving and diabetes self-management: investigation in a large, multiracial sample *Diabetes Care* **30**, 33–37.
18. Peyrot, M., Peeples, M., Tomky, D., Charron-Prochownik, D., Weaver, T. AADE Outcomes Project and AADE/UPMC Diabetes Education Outcomes Project (2007) Development of the American Association of Diabetes Educators' diabetes self-management assessment report tool *Diabetes Educator*. **33**, 818–26.
19. Kahn K.L., Liu H., Adams J.L., Chen W.P., Tisnado D.M., Carlisle D.M., Hays R.D., Mangione C.M., Damberg C.L. (2003) Methodological challenges associated with patient responses to follow-up longitudinal surveys regarding quality of care *Health Serv Res* **38**, 1579–98.
20. Freund, A., Johnson, S.B., Silverstein, J., Thomas, J. (1991). Assessing daily management of childhood diabetes using 24-hour recall interviews: reliability and stability. *Health Psychol* **10** 200–208.
21. Sallis, J.F., Haskell, W.L., Wood, P.D., Fortmann, S.P., Rogers,T., Blair, S.N., Paffenbarger, R.S. Jr. (1985) Physical activity assessment methodology in the Five-City Project. *Am J Epidemiol* **121**, 91–106.
22. Toobert, D.J., Glasgow, R.E. (1994) Assessing diabetes self-management: the summary of diabetes self-care activities questionnaire. In *Handbook of Psychology and Diabetes*. Bradley C, Ed. Chur, Switzerland, Hardwood Academic, p. 351–375.
23. Parchman, M.L., Arambula-Solomon. T.G., Noël, P.H., Larme, A.C., Pugh, J.A. (2003) Stage of change advancement for diabetes self-management behaviors and glucose control The Diabetes Educator **29**, 128–34.
24. American Diabetes Association. Clinical practice recommendations (2007) *Diabetes Care* **1**, 514.
25. Funnell, M., Brown, T., Childs, B., Haas, L., Hosey, G., Jensen, B., Maryniuk, M., Peyrot, M., Piette, J., Reader, D., Siminerio, L., Weinger, K., Weiss, M. (2007). National standards for diabetes self-management education *Diabetes Care* **30**, 1630–1637.
26. American Association of Diabetes Educators. Standards for outcomes measurement of diabetes self-management education (2003) *The Diabetes Educator* **29**, 804–816.
27. Norris, S.L., Engelgau, M.M., Narayan, K.M. (2001) Effectiveness of self-management training in type 2 diabetes: Systematic review of randomized controlled trials Diabetes Care **24**, 561–87.
28. Mulcahy K, Maryniuk M, Peeples M, Peyrot, M, Tomky D, Weaver T, Yarborough P. (2003) Diabetes self-management education core outcome measures *The Diabetes Educator* **29**, 768–803.
29. Boren, S. (2007). AADE7™ Self-care behaviors: systematic reviews. *The Diabetes Educator* **11**(33) 866–871.

30. Funnell, M., Brown, T., Childs, B., Haas, L., Hosey, G., Jensen, B., Maryniuk, M., Peyrot, M., Piette, J., Reader, D., Siminerio, L., Weinger, K., Weiss, M. (2007). National standards for diabetes self-management education *Diabetes Care* **30**, 1630–1637.
31. Peeples, M., Mulcahy, K., Tomky, D., Weaver, T. (2001) The conceptual framework of the national diabetes education outcomes system (NDEOS). *The Diabetes Educator* **27**, 547–562.

12 Diabetes Education Program Evaluation: Ensuring Effective Operations

Melinda D. Maryniuk, MEd, RD, CDE
and Judith E. Goodwin, MBA

CONTENTS

INTRODUCTION
RATIONALE FOR PROGRAM EVALUATION
TYPES OF PROGRAM EVALUATION:
    CLINICAL AND OPERATIONAL
BASELINE OPERATIONAL METRICS
PROGRAM OPERATIONS
CONTINUOUS QUALITY IMPROVEMENT
CONCLUSIONS
REFERENCES

ABSTRACT

The effectiveness of a diabetes education program is evaluated not only in clinical terms but also in operational terms. Each program needs to be routinely assessed in order for it to be considered comprehensive. This chapter will highlight the rationale for program evaluation, recommend how to use a variety of metrics to assess program impact, and provide practical suggestions for ways to help demonstrate the value of a diabetes education program.

From: *Contemporary Diabetes: Educating Your Patient with Diabetes*
Edited by: K. Weinger and C. A. Carver, DOI 10.1007/978-1-60327-208-7_12,
© Humana Press, a part of Springer Science+Business Media, LLC 2009

Key Words: Program Evaluation, Clinical Evaluation, Operational Evaluation, Operational Metrics, Pro Forma, Productivity, Satisfaction, Continuous Quality Improvement.

INTRODUCTION

Evaluating the effectiveness of a diabetes education program is an essential business practice. Just as patient education is not considered complete until outcomes are reviewed and evaluated, a program cannot be considered comprehensive if the overall clinical effectiveness and operational metrics are not routinely assessed. This chapter will highlight the rationale for program evaluation, recommend how to use a variety of metrics to assess program impact, and provide practical suggestions for ways to help demonstrate the value of a diabetes education program. Many of the examples are based on our experience managing the Joslin Diabetes Center Affiliate program, where we have helped guide the operations of over 30 different Joslin affiliates nationwide over the past 15 years.

According to the National Standards for Diabetes Self-Management Education *(1)*, a diabetes education program coordinator needs to have academic preparation and/or experience in the care of persons with chronic disease. Many program coordinators and administrators are excellent educators and clinicians but they have had little training or experience in medical practice management. Although sometimes it seems that good business decisions may be incongruent with the best clinical care, ultimately, good business is good medicine.

RATIONALE FOR PROGRAM EVALUATION

So, why bother? Why measure program effectiveness and impact? Regardless if a program is large or small, new or established, or hospital-based or independent, all programs need to evaluate metrics on a variety of levels. Consider the following four reasons.

Ensure Effectiveness

When most diabetes educators think of evaluating a program's effectiveness, they think immediately in terms of behavioral or clinical outcomes. Did the program lead to increased frequency of glucose monitoring or physical activity? Did it achieve lower A1Cs, increased weight loss, or increased frequency of eye exams? These outcomes are important, but equally important are the metrics related to the business of the diabetes education program. Establishing program operational goals, including budgetary and productivity goals in terms of the number of patients to be seen, is key in being able to measure progress and program effectiveness. If the education program successfully lowers the A1C on every patient seen but if it only sees half the patients it is targeting and the revenues fall far short of projections, one will have to ask if it is truly an effective program.

Allocate Resources

By assessing various operational metrics on a regular basis, the most efficient use of personnel and other resources can be determined. Without adequate operational data, it is difficult to justify the addition of new staff members or the expense of equipment such as practice management software and computers. More in-depth study of how educator time is used can guide the program administrator to ensure their time is put toward patient-centered, billable activities and that non-billable or non-clinical tasks are delegated to others. Ultimately, the goal is to use the right person for the right task.

Widen the Reach

Diabetes is a growing epidemic and there are not enough diabetes education programs or diabetes educators to serve the population. Yet, many programs seem to suffer from slow growth and inadequate revenues. A thorough program evaluation process will help ensure that the education program reaches a wide audience. How are the services being marketed? What is the effectiveness of the different marketing interventions? Tracking and evaluating the results of each type of marketing intervention can help assess their overall effectiveness in reaching the target audience and ideally result in increased visits.

Minimize Risk

If program metrics are not measured, monitored, and managed, the likelihood that the program will not be valued or taken seriously is increased. For many years, offering a diabetes education program was considered a community service and it was not expected to generate revenue (and a loss was even anticipated). Minimize the risk that administrators, perhaps more driven by the bottom line than by community service, might subject the program and staff to drastic cuts and be able to demonstrate the value of the service. This chapter will explore a variety of metrics that will help demonstrate the value of the diabetes education program including numbers of patients seen, numbers of providers referring patients, number of referrals to ancillary hospital services, number of readmissions, and decreased length of stay for an inpatient service.

TYPES OF PROGRAM EVALUATION: CLINICAL
AND OPERATIONAL

Evaluation is an essential part of a comprehensive diabetes education program. Outcomes evaluation should involve the measurement, monitoring, and management of both clinical and operational metrics and outcomes. Two of the 10 National Standards speak of the importance of evaluation, particularly as it relates to educational interventions *(1)* (see Table 1) and it is the position of the American Association of Diabetes Educators (AADE) that measurable behavior change is the desired outcome of diabetes education and the unique domain of diabetes educators *(2)*. The American Diabetes Association (ADA) Education Recognition Program requires the collection and analysis of both behavioral outcomes and an "other" type of outcome (see Table 2). Recognize that clinical outcomes fall along a continuum with outcomes related to knowledge or skill acquisition considered learning outcomes that can be measured immediately, while behavior change, clinical changes, and improved health status represent longer term changes (for more detail, see Chapter 11).

Table 1
Excerpt from National Standards for Diabetes Self-Management Education (DSME)

Standard 9: The DSME entity will measure attainment of patient-defined goals and
   patient outcomes at regular intervals using appropriate measurement techniques to
   evaluate the effectiveness of the educational intervention.
Standard 10: The DSME entity will measure the effectiveness of the education
   process and determine opportunities for improvement using a written continuous
   quality improvement plan that describes and documents a systematic review of the
   entities' process and outcome data.

Table 2
Outcome Measures for ADA Program Recognition *(4)*

Behavioral Outcomes	*Other Program Outcomes*
1. Healthy eating	• A1C
2. Being active	• Lipids
3. Taking medication	• Eye exam
4. Monitoring	• Weight change
5. Problem solving	• Patient satisfaction
6. Healthy coping	• Provider satisfaction
7. Reducing risks	• Quality of life
	• Blood pressure

In order to capture meaningful metrics and document improvement in behaviors, educators need to assess behaviors using tools that facilitate the measurement of change. For example, asking a question that requires a "yes/no" response in an assessment such as "Are you physically active on a regular basis?" is not specific and not useful in setting up a basis for post-program assessment of behavior change. Instead, ask a question that assesses activity level in a way that can better measure progress over time, such as "How many days in the last 2 weeks were you physically active for at least 30 min a day?" Assist each patient in defining his or her own behavioral goals that are specific and measurable as well. An example of such a goal is "I will walk for 30 min at least three times each week for the next 2 weeks," which is a realistic, measurable goal, whereas "I will exercise more" is not specific enough and "I will lose 2 pounds next week" is an outcome, but not a behavior. Tools such as the AADE 7™ IMPACT assessment can facilitate the evaluation of these behavioral outcomes *(3)*.

BASELINE OPERATIONAL METRICS

The results of the National Diabetes Education Practice Survey conducted by the American Association of Diabetes Educators revealed that for the most part, there is much room for improvement in diabetes education practice management. It reported that only 42% of respondents saw more than 1000 patients per year. Assuming 250 work days each year, that is only 4 patient visits a day. Unsurprisingly, the survey also reported only 13% programs operating at a profit *(4)*.

Operational metrics are equally important and often overlooked. This includes having a mission statement, a written plan that defines program goals, a business plan and pro forma, staff productivity goals, and a marketing plan. The whole team should be aware of program goals and the role they each play in helping meet those goals. The following tools and metrics are helpful to establish at the beginning of a diabetes education program so that there is baseline data from which to measure progress.

Mission Statement

Begin by committing to writing a mission statement. It need not be long; it needs to clearly and concisely capture the reason for the existence of the diabetes education program. Ideally, it is recognized as that one set of guiding ideas that is articulated, understood, and supported by the larger organization's stakeholders, administrators, staff, patients, volunteers, and community members. The American Diabetes Association Education Recognition Program offers this example of a mission statement: *The mission of the diabetes team at this facility is to provide quality comprehensive diabetes self-management education. We believe that education is the key to empowering the person with diabetes to better manage his or her disease and avoid the complications of diabetes and achieve an optimum health status (5).* Take time to review the program's mission statement annually with the advisory group or board that has been established for the education program and make modifications as necessary.

Program Goals and Objectives

The next step in establishing your written plan is to identify several measurable objectives that will support the mission. The objectives can include statements regarding the target audience as well as metrics related to the reach and volume of patients to be seen. A review of the program goals and objectives should be conducted annually with the program's advisory board. It is essential to obtain an understanding of the program goals of the various different program stakeholders. For example, do not assume that hospital administrators are only interested in program goals that demonstrate clinical excellence. They may be looking at goals that establish financial return or increased outreach to community providers. Take the time to understand the kinds of goals that are important to all of the stakeholders. Three sample program goals are

- To increase the percent of patients discharged from the hospital who receive follow-up care in the diabetes program from 20 to 40%.
- To increase the number of women with gestational diabetes seen at the center by 10%.
- To increase the number of referring providers by 50%.

Business Plan and Pro Forma

A written business plan including budgets helps establish clear expectations for the program. The term "pro forma" means "as a matter of form" and is applied to the process of presenting financial projections for a specific period in a standardized format. Pro forma statements are used for decision making as well as program management and plans for expected expenses and revenues by which the program can be managed and evaluated. Essential to the development of a useful pro forma is having a set of realistic assumptions in terms of expenses (salary, education materials, and other operating supplies) and revenues (number of patients expected to be seen, expected revenues based on reimbursement rates, etc.).

An important way to measure financial success is to track the direct expenses of the education program, that is, those related to patient care and the revenue associated with those activities. In the case of diabetes education programs, the largest expense is salary. Net revenue is defined as cash that is received once any contract discounts that have been agreed upon are taken. If the revenue is divided by expenses, you have a handy indicator called the return on investment or "ROI." By assessing the ROI, it can be determined if expenses are being covered, and, if something is being returned to the program, hospital, or larger organization. This overage can be used to cover expenses like rent or can be reinvested in improving your operations. For the program to be financially viable, covering direct expenses, it should produce an ROI of at least one. A helpful resource is available online and is listed in the reference section (11).

The written business plan should also include the strategy or plan for how to achieve the objectives – both operational and financial. Following the first sample goal above, the strategy might be to develop an approach to follow-up on all patients with a diabetes diagnosis who have been discharged from the hospital's inpatient service in an effort to have them referred to the outpatient program.

A program should not attempt to achieve more than three to four goals in a year. It is better to do a handful of initiatives well, and evaluate the outcomes, than fail by attempting to do more than is realistically possible. A key part of the plan is establishing how success will be measured against baseline and program objectives. Define these program success metrics carefully and be faithful about measuring them.

Staff Productivity Goals

Each diabetes educator should have a clear understanding of the number of patients that need to be seen. For the Joslin Diabetes Center-Affiliated Programs, the goals have been set for educators to aim for 60% of their time spent in face-to-face diabetes education and to aim to achieve 100% hours billed as a percent of educator paid time *(6)*. Consider this example of a full-time educator who works a 40-h week. If he or she teaches four 1-h classes, each with 10 patients, he or she has achieved 40 h of billable patient care (and thus achieves the 100% goal). However, to an outside administrator who only sees the educator in direct face-to-face contact with patients for 4 h during the week (10% of the time), it may be difficult to justify full-time employment. Additional hours should be spent in some one-to-one visits to bring the "face time" closer to 60% and thus demonstrating a better use of the educator's time.

Marketing Plan

A written marketing plan is essential to establish the program's goals and activities and to create community awareness. A marketing plan should outline the various activities that are planned for the year. Depending on the budget, it can include paid advertising as well as free publicity activities. Aim to design a marketing plan that targets a variety of audiences, including existing patients, people with diabetes who are not patients, family members, and those at risk for diabetes, referring providers, employees of your institution (especially if you work in a hospital), and more. Be prepared to capture the name and address of every new caller as he or she can be a potential patient. Periodically evaluate how those calling for information hear about the diabetes program so the success of different marketing efforts can be evaluated. For example, if your staff spends a day at a health fair, but you are not able to document that it results in any new patient referrals, this kind of marketing effort might be discontinued. On the other hand, if having an educator make visits with local primary care providers to explain the diabetes education program services results in increased referrals from those providers, this activity might be maintained (or even strengthened).

If the diabetes program is part of a hospital or health system, do not discount marketing and communication program within the hospital. Employees and their families are potential patients also. A significant opportunity exists in making inpatients and their admitting physicians aware of the diabetes education program. They already know a good deal about the organization and should be easy to approach.

PROGRAM OPERATIONS

A responsible program manager, no matter what the size of the diabetes education service offered, should be evaluating a variety of metrics to ensure program survival and effectiveness. The evaluation process involves not only collecting the data but taking time to consider possible interpretations and plan strategies for improvement based on the data. Consider the types of metrics that can be measured and monitored as it relates to program growth and satisfaction. When possible, obtain baseline or pre-program measurements in order to report on changes since the implementation of the diabetes education service. Two case studies are included that illustrate the importance of operational program evaluation.

Case Study #1: Low A1C but No ROI

General Hospital has had a community diabetes education program for 5 years. It employed one full-time nurse and one full-time dietitian. The program was recognized by the American Diabetes Association and had been audited with no areas for improvement identified. Both educators were well qualified, both being CDEs, and the dietitian was also a BC-ADM. Resource instructors from the hospital included a pharmacist, exercise physiologist (from the cardiac rehab center), and a social worker. The two full-time educators provided inpatient consult services for 10–20 h/week. The educators had a CQI poster at the last American Association of Diabetes Educators meeting displaying results of two projects: one showing results of high patient satisfaction with the educational classes.

ASSESSMENT

Clinical outcomes measurements revealed that the hospital successfully and consistently lowered A1C for patients seen in the community diabetes education program. However, the hospital was experiencing financial difficulties and had to evaluate each program for financial viability. Expenses for the program were mounting due to the inclusion of additional resource instructors, and the CFO had no basis for evaluating the financial contribution the program was making to the hospital.

PLAN

The Program Manager realized that she and the CFO were not speaking the same language. The Program Manager realized that she needed to

- Obtain salary and other direct expense information from the hospital's monthly profit and loss statements for the Diabetes Education Program. This included the salaries related to additional resources called upon to deliver diabetes education.
- Deduct expenses related to delivering inpatient care, as related revenue is not credited to the outpatient program.
- Determine revenue related to direct billable activities of the department. This may require contacting the billing department of the hospital in order to be sure bills are being paid and not denied by the insurance carriers.
- Compare the expenses to the revenue to determine the shortfall that needs to be made up with productivity improvements. Establish goals and guidelines based on the number of visits required per educator to produce revenue required to cover expenses.
- Identify other measurable ways the diabetes program could be contributing to either cost savings or increased revenue to the hospital such as decreasing length of stay or increasing referrals to ancillary departments such as laboratory services, podiatry, and cardiology.

RESULTS

The Program Manager was able to demonstrate a high utilization of hospital lab services by patients from the diabetes education center. Also, a focused study on one of the medical floors revealed that patients receiving more intensive hyperglycemia management and education had a decreased length of stay. Thus, the CFO was impressed with these contributions of the diabetes program that were not readily apparent from the monthly departmental profit and loss statements.

Case Study #2: the Dilemma of Full Classes and Few 1:1 Appointments

Regional Medical Center has an ADA-recognized program that runs numerous group education classes, each class having an average of nine patients per class (one educator) producing significant revenue for the program. The Program Manager worked hard on this metric and the result was that billable time was in excess of 100% of the educators paid time. The Program Manager was thrilled as she had set this as a goal for the program. The program was so busy she requested additional administrative support to schedule and support all the classes being held. Armed with this data, she approached the CFO who denied her request and further stated he might need to reduce the number of educators as his "labor utilization" report suggested the program was overstaffed. How could this be?

ASSESSMENT

The Program Manager reviewed additional program data and learned that the educators, on average, were spending only 30% of their time in front of patients in billable activities. Therefore, in order to preserve existing staff and resubmit a request for administrative support, a plan needed to be implemented to improve this metric.

PLAN

The Program Manager realized not enough 1:1 visits were being scheduled. A big opportunity to bring patients back in years subsequent to the calendar year in which the 10-h comprehensive program was delivered existed. The goal was to schedule enough 1:1 visits to improve 30% face time to 45% face time by the end of the next quarter to demonstrate improvement to the CFO. Specific steps to executing the plan included

- Review medical records for patients who completed comprehensive program in the last calendar year and are eligible for follow-up DSMT.
- Develop a campaign to contact patients by phone or letter to stress the need for follow-up education and explain the process: making an appointment, getting a referral, etc.
- Schedule 1:1 appointments for follow-up patients.

RESULTS

The Program Manager was able to document an increase in the time spent in 1:1 patient care and thus demonstrated both increased revenues and improved utilization of educator time. She scheduled an appointment with the CFO to share the results.

Growth

PATIENT VOLUME AND PRODUCTIVITY METRICS

Each month, the diabetes program should be evaluating some basic patient volume metrics. Many educators collect data on the number of new and the number of follow-up patients seen. However, this does not always capture the actual time worked (and revenue realized). Thus, many programs find it more informative to calculate the number of billable 1:1 patient hours and the number of billable group hours (5 patients in a 2-h group yields 10 billable group hours) and report it based on a per FTE (full-time equivalent) calculation.

For Joslin Diabetes Center affiliates, we look at "outpatient hours billed as a percent of paid time" as well as "percent of time spent treating billable out-patients." The goal is for educators to achieve 100% each month for the first metric and 60% for the second. For example, consider Lee, a certified diabetes educator who in 1 week saw 20 h of 1:1 appointments and conducted two 2-h classes, each with six patients (resulting in 24 billable hours). Lee kept that same schedule for the 4 weeks in the month resulting in 80 1:1 hours + 96 group hours = 176 h. If that number is divided by the standard for number of working hours in a month (173 h), then Lee is considered to be very productive by the Joslin Affiliate standard – as she is billing for patient care 102% of her time.

Using the same figures, how much time is Lee actually face-to-face with patients? This calculation provides an estimate of educator efficiency and pro-ductivity. The goal is to aim for 60% of an educator's time to be face-to-face with patients, either 1:1 or in a group. Using the figures above, in a typical week, Lee is face-to-face with patients 20 h (1:1) plus an additional 4 h in group each week, for an average of 24 h a week or 96 h per month. This calculates to 55% "face time" (when 96 is divided by the standard of 173 h worked per month), which nearly meets the goal set of 60%. It is clear that by seeing patients in groups, educators can be more productive.

An analysis of diabetes educator productivity in 22 different sites demon-strated that on average, educators were billing 0.55 h of education (1:1 or group) for each hour of salary they were paid (range 0.19–1.21) and spent 25% of their time on billable activities (range 11–46%). Group visits allow educators to bill more hours than they are paid, but they cannot spend more than 100% of their time on billable activities (7).

Aim to have productivity goals for each educator that roll up to support the objectives of the program. Look for continuous improvement each month and identify ways to increase both face time and billable time, as educators need to do what they do best – work with patients. As an administrator of a program, it is key to identify and minimize the non-billable activities.

IMPACT OF DIABETES PROGRAM ON OTHER SERVICES

If the diabetes program is part of a larger business, such as a hospital or a large multi-specialty group practice, consider tracking additional metrics to show that the program benefits other departments. For example, track the number of referrals from the diabetes program to other departments such as podiatry, laboratory services, or other medical specialties. If inpatient services are provided with the goal of improving diabetes care, make sure metrics that will really speak to hospital administrators are tracked, such as length of stay data, to demonstrate cost reduction.

GEOGRAPHIC REACH OF DIABETES PROGRAM

As the reputation of the program grows, patients will be attracted from a wider geographic area. By running a zip code analysis of the patients, it may be possible to demonstrate that patients are coming into the health care system that might not otherwise have come, which also speaks to the value of the diabetes program.

ANALYSIS OF MARKETING EFFORTS

If there are dollars invested into a marketing program, make sure the results of those initiatives are measured so the worth of the marketing initiatives can be evaluated. It is useful to collect data from first time callers to a diabetes program to find out how they heard of the center (Referral? Newspaper article? Radio spot? Word of mouth?). Design a form and use it daily to track the reasons and have it available in the office whenever new appointments are made. After a marketing campaign or a community event is held such as a large health fair or diabetes day, make sure you track calls and inquiries for several weeks afterward to determine if the event helped to generate business. Do not be discouraged if expected targets are not hit in the first few days, as often these types of events take a few weeks to demonstrate the results, as much is also driven by word of mouth.

STAFF TIME – STUDY ASSESSMENT

There is no question that diabetes educators stay very busy. But what percent of time is spent on billable activities? A time study looking at 123 days of educator activities revealed that on average, educators worked 30 min longer than their scheduled day. However, during that day, only an average of 4 h of patient appointments were scheduled and only 3.5 h was spent in actual patient visits (due to cancellations and no-shows.) Nearly 2 h each day was spent in charting and phone work. Over 2 h was spent in "other" activities which included a wide range of things from stuffing educational packets to setting up rooms for classes to looking for and filing medical records to supervising students *(8)*. Conducting a time study over 1–2 "typical" weeks of your own activities or those of your staff can be a useful exercise to see how you can be better allocating your time. It might result in justification for additional support staff to relieve the educators of activities such as chart filing and preparing educational packets when they can be generating more revenue in patient care activities.

Satisfaction

PATIENT SATISFACTION

When evaluating patient satisfaction, it is helpful to have a core of basic assessment questions that are continuously assessed as well as several questions that may be specific for a particular time period or need. For example, the standard patient evaluation assessment tool might always ask for patients to respond on a scale of 1–5 on how satisfied they were with the following:

- Diabetes care overall;
- Ease of reaching someone in an emergency;
- Lab tests reviewed and explained;
- Concern, courtesy, respect, and sensitivity of the provider;
- Would you recommend your diabetes care provider if a family member or friend needed diabetes care?

Questions such as these asked on a consistent basis are valuable for benchmarking progress across time. Many commercial patient satisfaction survey businesses will benchmark results against similar institutions or programs that are also their customers. Optional questions that could be varied based on need might address issues related to parking, time of day for classes, interest in different kinds of support groups, or satisfaction with new educational material being offered. It is valuable to regularly review your satisfaction survey and ensure you are obtaining information that can really help effect program improvement and change as needed.

OTHER CUSTOMER GROUPS

Remember that patients are not the only group to keep satisfied. Think about the other customer groups who influence the business of the diabetes program. Consider surveying referring providers to determine if the education services are meeting their needs. Many of our Joslin Diabetes Center affiliates have been surprised to see that the community physicians really do take time to complete a short questionnaire as they can see it ultimately results in improved service for themselves and their patients. It also serves as a good marketing tool and reminder to the referring providers of the diabetes education program services.

Other customer groups might include inpatient unit managers (Do they know of the diabetes consultation service? Are there improvements that could be made?) or hospital staff nurses and medical office assistants (Are there ways to improve their diabetes knowledge, skills, or awareness of services?).

CONTINUOUS QUALITY IMPROVEMENT

A continuous quality improvement (CQI) process is an essential component of a comprehensive, quality diabetes self-management education program. It is a required element of a diabetes program designed to meet the National Standards of DSME (diabetes self-management education) *(1)* and ADA (American Diabetes Association) program recognition *(5,9)*. Not only is it a mechanism to ensure the delivery of quality clinical and education services, it also is a valuable way to evaluate and improve a program's operational success and thus lead to an improved financial bottom line. A helpful workbook, that is, a step-by-step guide for quality improvement in diabetes education was recently published and is a useful resource for diabetes educators needing additional guidance for conducting CQI projects *(10)*.

As part of the ADA Education Recognition process, programs are asked to respond (yes or no) if in fact, *"there is documentation that the DSME entity uses a formal CQI plan/process to evaluate the effectiveness of the DSME program at the site and whether the results of the CQI evaluation are used to determine opportunities for improving DSME services at the site and that a current project is in progress using the plan/process."* In addition, programs must identify (by check mark) which behavioral outcome areas are tracked and which program outcome measures are evaluated (Table 2). Finally, a "formal CQI plan with a demonstration project" is one of the items requested to be submitted as part of a "random paper audit" when applying for recognition *(5)*.

Implementing a CQI process

Here are some basic steps to get you started. An example of an operational CQI project is illustrated in Table 3.

1. *Select a formal process*
   There are a variety of CQI frameworks. Some of the more common ones include the PDCA cycle (plan–do–check–act) and the AADIE model (assess–design–develop–implement–evaluate) *(10)*. The exact process is not as important as ensuring the model contains the components of obtaining baseline measurements to document the problem, implementing a solution, and remeasuring.
2. *Involve all the staff*
   The CQI process works best when everyone has an understanding of the process, participates in the planning, data gathering, brainstorming for solutions,

Table 3
CQI Case Example: Improving Appointment Scheduling at Diabetes Classes

(1)	Identify the problem	Although patients were encouraged as part of a group class to schedule a 1:1 follow-up appointment, patients seemed to be leaving class before scheduling an appointment
(2)	Collect and analyze data	At the monthly comprehensive class attended by 10 patients, the team determined that only 1 person made a follow-up appointment after class, and 1 more called before the next scheduled class. At the next class, each person was asked individually the reason an appointment was not made. Five of the eight said "forgot" or "did not understand that I was supposed to do it"
(3)	Consider possible solutions	The team brainstormed the following solutions: (1) Ask the secretary to come to class to schedule appointments (2) CDEs will call patients to schedule appointments (3) CDEs will write possible class dates on the board and patients will each select the one they want and turn it in (4) Mount a large piece of paper in front of the class listing date options for follow-up class and invite patients to write their name next to the class they will attend
(4)	Make recommendations	The third choice above was selected for trial as it required not only the least amount of time but also empowered the patient to take the action and potentially join a class he or she saw a classmate/friend sign up for
(5)	Implement	For the next two series of classes, a piece of large poster paper was mounted in the front of the class with options for three different follow-up classes. The CDEs and scheduling staff met to discuss implementation. CDEs introduced the follow-up class sign-up at the beginning of the class and again at the end
(6)	Evaluate	After the first class series, 7 out of 10 class members signed up for class, and 6 actually attended. After the second series, 9 out of 11 signed up, and 8 attended
(7)	Maintenance Plan	The solution demonstrated an excellent improvement, without extra staff time needing to be committed. When class members sign up for a follow-up class, they are given the choice of two different kinds of classes, at two different times. They also can complete a reminder card for themselves to take home with them

and remeasurement. The full team can take pride in seeing specific, measurable improvements. Take turns so that each staff member in a program (from secretary to physician) can be a team leader on a project.

3. *Choose a project*

Although both a behavioral outcome and an "other" outcome must be measured for ADA recognition purposes, do not let that limit your thinking about potential CQI projects that would be helpful to the growth of your program. In addition to doing projects, assess behavioral outcomes and clinical are, do not forget the importance of assessing operational or program management outcomes. For example, such as decreasing wait time, increasing number of physician referrals, or increasing the percent of patients who return for a follow-up visit).

4. *Use data to set targets for performance improvements*

The baseline data collection can be used to set goals for improving performance. Measure after some suggested solutions are implemented and see if additional improvement is shown.

5. *Document, share, and celebrate your findings*

All results are useful, even if they did not yield the conclusion you had hoped for. You always learn from it. Minutes need to document your CQI project for ADA, but better yet, think about sharing your findings (particularly if you were testing a creative solution) in the form of an abstract, poster presentation, or short article.

Additional Tips for CQI Projects

Vary the projects. If something is working well, it does not have to continue being the subject of a study, but can just be periodically reassessed to make sure the quality is not slipping. In addition to measuring behavioral outcomes, aim to vary the type of "other" metrics that are evaluated. Conducting a CQI project is often useful in influencing administrative executives to provide needed equipment, resources, or services to enhance the patient experience. If your diabetes education service or program has an advisory group, use them to discuss the findings and implications of current projects and to generate ideas for future studies. Continuously improving means everyone is working together to achieve ways to do their jobs better, faster, more productively, and more effectively while also delivering the highest quality patient care.

CONCLUSIONS

Diabetes is a disease of epidemic proportions. There is no question that an enormous clinical need exists to equip patients with the tools they need to manage the disease on a daily basis. Our work does not stop there. It is not only our challenge to provide the best care to patients but to provide that care to as many patients as possible and in a way that secures the longevity of our programs. A systematic approach to program evaluation helps put educators in a position to measure what we do in order to manage it against program goals. Just as knowing the specific clinical data are essential in defining the treatment plan for a patient, we must have operational data to best measure and evaluate the health of our diabetes programs and to continuously identify areas for improvement. Providing excellent care requires attention to business details so that we can be available to treat those who need us when they need us.

REFERENCES

1. Funnell MM, Brown TL, Childs BP, Haas LB, Hosey GM, Jensen B, Maryniuk M, Peyrot M, Piette JD, Reader D, Siminero LM, Weinger K, Weiss MA. National standards for diabetes self-management education. Diabetes Care 2007; 30:1630–1637.
2. Mulcahy K, Maryniuk M, Peeples M, et al. Diabetes self-management education core outcomes measures. Diabetes Educ 2003; 29: 768–788.
3. AADE 7™ IMPACT. www.diabeteseducator.org; http://www.diabeteseducator.org/Professional Resources/AADE7/Impact/index.html Accessed November 14, 2007
4. Peeples M, Austin MM. Toward describing practice: The AADE national diabetes education practice survey: Diabetes education in the United States – Who, What, Where and How. Diabetes Educ. 2007; 33:424–433.
5. ADA Program Recognition. www.diabetes.org/recognition Accessed November 14, 2007
6. Sullivan E and Goodwin J. Business Basics: From A1C to ROI. AADE Annual Meeting Presentation. August 2006.
7. Maryniuk MD, Rossi G, Goodwin JE, Hare JW. Diabetes clinician productivity. 1160-P. 66th Scientific Sessions American Diabetes Association. June 2006.
8. Maryniuk MD, Moore T, Weinger K, Blair E, Connor D, Hare J. Diabetes educator productivity: An outpatient time study of daily activities. 300-PP. Diabetes 50 (suppl 2): A75, 2001.
9. Maryniuk MD, Bronzini B, Lorenzi G. Quality Diabetes Self-Management Education: Achieving and Maintaining ADA Education Program Recognition. Diabetes Educ 2004; 30: 467–475.
10. AADE Research Committee. CQI: A Step-by-Step Guide for Quality Improvement in Diabetes Education. 2nd Edition. Chicago, IL: American Diabetes Association, 2008.
11. Kilpatrick KE, Brownson CA. Building the Business Case for Diabetes Self Management: A Hand book for Program Managers. 2008. Diabetes Initiative. A National Program of the Robert Wood Johnson Foundation, Accessed September 19, 2007, www.diabetesinitiative.org

II EDUCATING SPECIFIC POPULATIONS

13 Working with Challenging Patients in Diabetes Treatment

Marilyn D. Ritholz, Ph.D.

CONTENTS

INTRODUCTION
CHALLENGING PATIENT ENCOUNTERS
CHALLENGING PATIENTS
   AND PSYCHOSOCIAL FACTORS
CHALLENGING PATIENTS AND
   CO-MORBID CONDITIONS
CREATING A WORKING ALLIANCE IN
   CHALLENGING PATIENT ENCOUNTERS
SUPPORT AN ACTIVE PROBLEM-SOLVING APPROACH
CONCLUSION
REFERENCES

ABSTRACT

Patients in diabetes treatment sometimes struggle with psychosocial problems that may interact with their abilities to manage diabetes. Health care providers may feel frustrated, ineffective, and helpless because it is difficult to form a working alliance with these challenging patients. This chapter defines the working alliance and presents it as an essential ingredient of patient-centered diabetes treatment and as a salient factor in counteracting challenging patient encounters. It also reviews the literature on fear-based psychosocial problems in relation to hypoglycemia, hyperglycemia, or weight gain as well as co-morbid conditions of diabetes, depression, and other chronic illnesses. This chapter also discusses the

From: *Contemporary Diabetes: Educating Your Patient with Diabetes*
Edited by: K. Weinger and C. A. Carver, DOI 10.1007/978-1-60327-208-7_13,
© Humana Press, a part of Springer Science+Business Media, LLC 2009

ways these conditions contribute to challenging patient encounters and presents clinical vignettes to illustrate the dynamics and complexities of working with these psychosocial difficulties. Finally, suggestions are offered on ways to build a working alliance with patients in challenging patient encounters.

Key Words: Challenging patients, Working alliance, type 1 and type 2 diabetes, Psychosocial problems, Fear of hypoglycemia, Fear of hyperglycemia, Fear of weight gain, Depression, co-morbid chronic conditions.

INTRODUCTION

Diabetes is a time and task-demanding illness that easily can interfere with patients' daily lives. Effective self-care requires a constant need to observe, be aware, and modulate blood glucose, insulin, eating, exercise, and emotional well-being. Psychosocial difficulties often interact with patients' abilities to manage diabetes *(1)*, and diabetes health care providers are reported to have difficulties recognizing and managing patients' psychosocial difficulties *(2)*. At times, these patient–provider interactions contribute to challenging patient encounters and can negatively influence effective ongoing treatment. The creation of a working treatment alliance between patients and health care providers (henceforth called "working alliance") is one of the essential ingredients in addressing challenging patient encounters *(3,4)*. This alliance entails understanding both patients' psychosocial difficulties and health providers' effective reactions to these difficulties.

CHALLENGING PATIENT ENCOUNTERS
The Working Alliance

The working alliance entails the ability of the patient and the provider to establish a relationship where they have shared goals, recognition of the tasks each of them performs, and an emotional bond characterized by liking and trust *(5)*. Patient-centered medicine has reaffirmed the importance of the working alliance in diabetes treatment *(6–8)* and research shows the significance of this construct in optimal medical outcomes for diabetes and other chronic illnesses *(3,9–11)*. The absence of this working alliance between all health care providers and patients in the treatment of diabetes can contribute to challenging patient encounters and perceptions of challenging patients.

To identify the non-adherent patient or the insensitive practitioner as the cause of the non-establishment of the working alliance is counterproductive *(6)*. Building an alliance must entail a position of non-blame and working toward a partnership between health care providers and patients. In order for a working alliance to develop, providers must have a degree of self-awareness so that they monitor and acknowledge how patients affect them and how their responses, in turn, affect patients. The working alliance is minimally a two-person interaction, i.e., patient and provider, and therefore providers of diabetes care need to be aware not only of their patients' beliefs and behaviors but also of their own responses to medical non-adherence, worsening chronic illnesses, and the relational basis of effective treatment. An alliance is of particular importance when patient interactions lead to provider feelings of frustration, helplessness, and a sense of ineffectiveness. In these situations, providers can become angry toward or dismissive of patients (12). Unacknowledged negative feelings on the part of providers can interfere with the establishment of a working alliance.

The lack of both a positive partnership and good communication between provider and patient was associated with poor treatment adherence in patients with diabetes who had dismissing attachment style (avoid seeking support from others, are overly self-reliant, and uncomfortable trusting others) and fearful attachment style (demonstrate approach-avoidance behavior, are hesitant, vulnerable, self-conscious, and have low self-confidence) (13). Another study found that patients valued the relationship with their providers when they listened, empathized, and understood patients' difficulties with non-compliance rather than imposed treatment and communicated recrimination and threat (9). In an effective working alliance, patients and practitioners both pursue treatment goals with a sense of patience and understanding rather than with frustration and recrimination.

The empowerment model of diabetes treatment has greatly supported the partnership approach to diabetes care (7). Providers' awareness of how they can form a partnership with their patients is the building block in establishing the working alliance (6). This awareness reinforces collaborative treatment. In one study, providers recognized and acknowledged that their lack of effective communication skills in making patients partners in diabetes treatment was associated with patients' non-adherence (14). Another study (15) explored partnership in diabetes treatment in terms of physicians' participatory decision-making styles and race/ethnicity and gender of patients and physicians. Findings of this study demonstrated that, on average, African-American patients rated their physician visits as significantly less participatory than whites; and patients in race concordant relationships with their physicians rated their visits as significantly more participatory than race discordant relationships. That we, as diabetes health care providers, be aware of how we interact with our patients is essential. Our attitudes, feelings, interpersonal styles, racial and ethnic awareness, and general self-awareness either contribute to or detract from building a working alliance with our patients.

Health care providers working with diabetes need ongoing training in promoting behavioral change. They need to learn treatment strategies for behavioral change and how to build relational and communication skills. When patients do not meet evidence-based treatment goals, it is important that providers not feel like failures and carry this defeatist sense into their patient encounters *(14)*. Furthermore, ongoing consultation with mental health professionals is useful in allowing providers to process challenging patient encounters in order to dispel patient blame and self-blame and to learn how best to manage these encounters. This kind of consultation can occur individually and/or in a group situation so that learning is interactive and professional.

CHALLENGING PATIENTS AND PSYCHOSOCIAL FACTORS
Defining Challenging Patients

The term "challenging" refers to patients whom health care providers consider difficult to treat. These patients often are spoken of in treatment team meetings, case consultations, and privately among colleagues. Although we do not wish to blame patients for their behaviors or lack of success in following treatment recommendations, challenging patients sometimes make health professionals feel frustrated, ineffective, and helpless regarding achievement of treatment goals and poor provider–patient interactions. In the psychological literature, challenging patients also have been called "difficult patients" and have been seen to display a lack of cooperation and an unwillingness to accept treatment *(16)* and are described as demanding, help-rejecting, and denying the competence and authority of the mental health provider *(17)*. In the nursing literature, MacDonald *(18)* discusses how the term "difficult" patient is commonly used in nursing practice and how this term describes patients who do not assume the expected patient role, have beliefs or personal characteristics that differ from the provider, contribute to the provider's self-doubt, and how most often the difficulty is seen as existing in the patient rather than the interaction between patient and provider. Interestingly, there is no literature looking specifically at diabetes educators in challenging/difficult patient encounters. Therefore, it is useful to describe some characteristics of these encounters and to discuss how to address establishing a working alliance for optimal treatment.

In some cases, the working alliance is difficult to establish because there is a lack of agreement on the goals of treatment. For example, this can easily occur when a provider's main goal is to attain acceptable blood glucose numbers whereas a patient's main goal is to manage fears of hypoglycemia/hyperglycemia or to keep his/her weight at the lowest possible number. These fear-based difficulties can lead to mismanagement of insulin and poor diabetes self-care. Other patients present with diabetes and co-morbid depression and/or chronic complications (kidney disease, peripheral and autonomic neuropathy, and retinopathy). These co-morbid conditions with diabetes also contribute to challenging patient encounters.

Fear of Hypoglycemia

Patients with diabetes live with many fears in terms of having a serious chronic illness, learning how to manage this illness, and risk of developing future complications. There is a high prevalence of clinical anxiety disorders and sub-clinical anxiety-based problems in patients with diabetes *(19–21)*. Maintaining blood glucose within acceptable levels requires that patients self-monitor their blood glucose level in order to make sure that it falls within a designated target range and know what to do when blood glucose levels are not within the expected range. Fear-based problems may develop with regard to managing blood glucose levels and balancing intake of insulin and food.

Hypoglycemia is an aversive event for most patients. They worry about loss of control, appearing stupid, or passing out *(22)*. They also sometimes cannot discriminate between actual anxiety and what they perceive as hypoglycemia *(23)* and may misattribute any manifestation of anxiety for hypoglycemia. During hypoglycemic episodes, patients experience symptoms similar to those manifested during anxiety attacks, i.e., sweating, dizziness, shaking, palpitation, tremors, cognitive confusion, poor concentration, lack of coordination, and slurred speech *(24)*. When blood glucose levels drop too low, patients also may lose consciousness or experience seizures. These symptoms become dreaded events that patients attempt to avoid at all costs. One study showed that the difficulty discriminating between anxiety and hypoglycemia was associated with the development of more serious anxiety disorders *(25)*.

Fear of hypoglycemia occurs when patients become inordinately anxious about the possibility of having a low blood glucose (below 70 mg/dL). They develop an irrational belief that a low blood glucose level is occurring or can occur, and they need to seek safety *(26)* even when evidence of hypoglycemia is to the contrary. For example, the fear may start because a certain amount of time has passed since they have taken their insulin or have eaten. They then begin checking their blood glucose numerous times and treating the imagined low blood glucose despite the fact that glucose readings do not validate their fears. At other times, they may have a low blood glucose value, treat it appropriately with a quick acting carbohydrate but cannot tolerate waiting for hypoglycemic symptoms to subside. Therefore, they overtreat the low blood glucose without waiting for the appropriate passage of time (about 15 min) for symptoms to diminish. Most importantly, patients with fear of hypoglycemia may keep their blood glucose levels higher than recommended as a means of coping with their fear. The end result is poor diabetes control. The following clinical vignette is given to help providers understand the psychological underpinnings of the fear of hypoglycemia, illustrate how high blood glucose levels are used as protection against this fear, and provide some treatment strategies used to address this behavior.

Clinical Vignette #1

Hannah is a 25-year-old, well-educated, married young woman who holds a responsible job. She had HbA1c levels consistently above 10.0% since diagnosed with type 1 diabetes at age 17. Hannah checked her blood glucose about 20 times a day but even when glucose levels refuted the presence or immediate possibility of a low glucose, she would still treat it with a carbohydrate or take less insulin than required to ensure that hypoglycemia did not occur. When asked about this, she said that blood glucose levels were "tricky" and you never could actually trust if the meter reading was a real number or if it was on its way down to lower numbers. Of interest, Hannah had never experienced a serious hypoglycemic episode, which differs from reports in the literature on people with fear of hypoglycemia (23). Hannah also was started on insulin pump therapy and used the continuous glucose monitor for several months; however, these treatments neither greatly decreased her fears nor improved A1C level.

The focus of Hannah's psychological treatment was to learn to distinguish between symptoms of anxiety and symptoms of hypoglycemia and to learn to cope with her anxiety. When the blood glucose number was not in the hypoglycemic range, Hannah learned to trust that she was solely anxious and learned to tolerate this anxiety. We worked to determine a blood glucose number where Hannah felt safe without needing to treat with food or continually checking her blood glucose. She also developed a method of self-talk, i.e., calming and motivating herself by repeating that she was not going to panic or lose control and that she could successfully handle her feelings.

At the present time, Hannah's A1C is at 9.0%, and she feels slightly more confident about allowing her blood glucose numbers to be lower. She reports feeling more able to engage in activities at work and in the social arena. She also is much better able to differentiate symptoms of anxiety from symptoms of hypoglycemia, and she checks her blood sugars fewer times each day. Although great strides in glycemic management have not yet occurred, the working alliance between Hannah and her psychologist, manifested through trust, understanding, patience, and setting collaborative treatment goals, indicates a positive and steady movement of progress.

Fear of Hyperglycemia

Much less has been reported about the fear of hyperglycemia than about fear of hypoglycemia. Fear of hyperglycemia is an extreme preoccupation with keeping blood glucose levels so low that severe hypoglycemia is often experienced. Over time, frequent hypoglycemia can lead to a deficit in the body's secretion of counter-regulatory hormones that defend against low blood glucose levels and lead to hypoglycemia unawareness (27). Clinically, these patients present with excellent A1Cs but with very frequent severe hypoglycemia and a lack of concern about the frequency and severity of these hypoglycemic episodes. They sometimes experience seizures, comas, and periods of unconsciousness but seem to minimize or not acknowledge the danger of these occurrences. They believe that they are engaging in good diabetes control and are avoiding the development of microvascular complications.

In the author's clinical experience, patients with fear of hyperglycemia are hard to treat. They appear to have an impaired cognitive model where avoidance of hyperglycemia is so sought after that frequent severe hypoglycemia is perceived as positive, even with the occurrence of unconsciousness and seizures. They also manifest an extreme concreteness and rigidity of thought and a lack of insight about the seriousness of their behaviors. Because of their difficulty recognizing and acknowledging the danger inherent in frequent severe hypoglycemic episodes, clinicians may wonder if they have impaired reality testing, although they do not clearly fit this diagnosis. They are challenging because their belief system and behaviors can appear irrational and incomprehensible to the provider, while A1c levels are in target.

Clinical Vignette #2

Ethan is a 45-year-old, well-educated man who has had type 1 diabetes for 32 years. He is married and has two children. He reported symptoms of depression, difficulties sleeping, poor concentration, sadness, feelings of hopelessness, and loss of interest and pleasure in many things. Ethan's wife also reported to the endocrinologist that Ethan was having seizures at least three nights a week and that she feared Ethan was taking too much insulin. Ethan's A1C was 6.4% and before his wife's conversation with the endocrinologist there was no indication that his diabetes was problematic in any way. What was most noteworthy was Ethan's passivity about these hypoglycemic events. He reported not liking that he lost consciousness and had seizures, but he also did not make any changes in his diabetes self-care that might affect this hypoglycemia.

Ethan's depression decreased in response to SSRI medication and psychotherapy, but his hypoglycemic episodes remained. When questioned about his frequent hypoglycemia, Ethan declared, "Low blood sugars are better than high blood sugars." He also stated that he did not mind the hypoglycemia because he often was not conscious of what happened or did not remember the reported events. Only when asked about his wife and children's experience did he, for the first time, seem more willing to address the frequency of hypoglycemia. However, Ethan refused to attend a blood glucose awareness training program that helps patients learn to detect and monitor blood glucose fluctuations (28). Yet once Ethan began to have fewer hypoglycemic episodes, he dropped out of therapy. Therefore, it is not known if he was able to tolerate less hypoglycemia and the possible continuing anxiety about hyperglycemia or if his improvement in self-care endured. Ethan's story raised the following clinical questions: Did the patient's improvement in hypoglycemia threaten his individual treatment goals and fears of complications? Were the clinician's goals threatening to Ethan? Was there a working alliance? These questions are useful to consider and demonstrate the tenuous nature of the working alliance.

Fear of Weight Gain

Intensive insulin treatment with tighter control of blood glucose is associated with weight gain *(29,30)*. Therefore women with type 1 diabetes may be especially concerned about weight gain *(31)* and may face a serious obstacle in their attempts to achieve target glucose levels and desired body weights. One means that some patients with type 1 diabetes (notably women) use to handle their concern about weight is intentional insulin restriction or insulin under-administration as a means of weight loss *(32–34)*.

Findings of research studies indicate that women with type 1 diabetes are 2.4 times more likely to develop an eating disorder than women without diabetes *(35)*. In addition, type 1 diabetes is associated with higher rates of bulimia nervosa (binge eating followed by purging including vomiting and/or laxative use and self-evaluation unduly influenced by body shape and weight) *(36)*.

Patients' and providers' different views on how to manage body weight and blood glucose control is a major obstacle to the development of the treatment alliance. If a patient fears gaining weight, he or she will not or cannot collaborate on the goal of decreasing blood glucose levels and correctly managing insulin and food intake. Health care providers often feel frustrated in not being able to have their patients meet evidence-based blood glucose targets and may have difficulty forming a treatment partnership with patients whose goals for treatment include engaging in medically compromising behaviors.

In terms of building a working alliance, it is essential that treatment goals be discussed so that the building blocks for a patient–provider collaboration can be established. Goebel-Fabbri et al. *(33)* suggest that the treatment team must be willing to set attainable goals that patients are willing to try, and providers need to recognize that intensive glucose management is not a realistic treatment goal for patients who use insulin restriction for weight loss. Recognizing that this at-risk population requires flexibility in assessing treatment progress and may need more individualized treatment goals (e.g., prevention of DKA may serve as the most appropriate goal for which the health care provider and patient can collaborate) is important *(33)*. Table 1 provides a series of clinical questions to use when treating a female patient who presents with high A1c values.

Health care providers can become easily overwhelmed when their patients who restrict insulin for weight loss purposes require constant and vigilant medical and psychological treatment and have higher rates of hospitalization and

Table 1
Clinical Inquiry with Insulin Mismanagement Patients

1. Do you find yourself thinking too much about your weight and body shape?
2. How regular is your menstrual period?
3. Do you worry about your weight and blood glucose control? Please tell me about that.
4. Do you ever take less insulin that you need because of certain fears? What are these fears?
5. Do you ever adjust your insulin in order to lose weight? Please tell me about that.
6. Tell me about your experience with DKA.

emergency room visits, neuropathy and retinopathy, and higher A1C values than women who do not report restricting insulin (32,37,38). Treatment requires a multidisciplinary team with members who have experience working with diabetes and eating disorders, including an endocrinologist, nutritionist, nurse educator, psychologist/social worker for psychotherapy, and possibly a psychopharmocologist so that effective assessment and treatment can occur (33). Providers may begin to feel an extreme sense of ineffectiveness and helplessness that can interfere with the creation of a treatment alliance. Goebel-Fabbri and colleagues (33) recommend that health care providers take a "long-term view" and recognize that patients will make the most progress when they feel able to control their treatment at their own pace. It also is important that providers meet regularly as a treatment team to discuss the patient and their reactions to the treatment progress or lack of progress in order to avoid becoming too overwhelmed. In addition, seeking training and consultation through workshops, classes, and direct supervision is advised to aid in the treatment of this challenging population.

CHALLENGING PATIENTS AND CO-MORBID CONDITIONS

Diabetes, Depression, and Complications

Persons with type 1 and type 2 diabetes are reported to experience two to three times the rate of depression compared to persons in the general population (39). Ten to fifteen percent of patients with diabetes suffer from co-morbid major depression (39,40). In addition, depression is associated with diabetes complications such as retinopathy, neuropathy, nephropathy, hypertension, cardiac disease, and sexual dysfunction (41,42). In these situations, patients face multiple medical chronic illnesses and depression, itself a chronic condition, yet depression is under-recognized and underrated.

Patients with diabetes and co-morbid major depression in comparison to those with only diabetes are reported to have worse adherence to diet, exercise, and medication (40,43,44) and higher A1C levels (45). Interestingly, recent studies where patients with diabetes and depression have been effectively treated for their depression have not shown improvement in glycemic control (40,46,47). Furthermore, improvement in depressive symptomatology for persons with two or more diabetes complications also did not lead to improvement in glycemia (48). Therefore, an integrated biopsychosocial intervention program must focus both on depression and diabetes management in order to improve clinical outcomes in these co-morbid conditions (40).

Depression is sometimes unsuccessfully managed in primary care situations where multiple medical concerns present (49,50), and with both depression and diabetes complications, determining whether the depressive symptoms are secondary to the diabetes complications or exist on their own is difficult (48). De Groot and colleagues (41) consider that depression may be a secondary response to the onset of diabetes complications or may play a primary role in the development or exacerbation of diabetes complications. The temporal relationship remains unclear and further contributes to the complex nature of these challenging patient encounters.

Several studies report more dissatisfaction with health care encounters by patients with diabetes who are depressed (51–53). In addition, health care providers may view depressed and anxious patients with diabetes as "difficult" and less able to cope with their diabetes (54). Improved diagnosis and management of mental disorders in "difficult" patients may diminish the provider's experience of difficulty (55). Furthermore, when patients present with depression, diabetes, and diabetes complications the issue of competing clinical demands becomes more salient (48).

As health care providers, it is important to recognize depressed patients, to understand how depression may influence self-care behaviors and diabetes management, to acknowledge how these patients can make you feel as a health care provider, and to know how to respond to them. This is particularly true when patients with diabetes present not only with depression but also with diabetes complications. The following clinical vignette is given to illustrate a challenging patient encounter with a depressed patient who has diabetes and diabetes complications.

Clinical Vignette #3

Mary is a 58-year-old married woman who has had type 2 diabetes for 20 years. Her treatment includes NPH and Humalog insulins and oral medication. She reports experiencing episodes of depression for many years, including lack of interest in doing things she used to like to do and difficulty sleeping, concentrating, and managing her diabetes self-care in the last 6 months. She stated that she just forgets to take her insulin and that because of the neuropathy pain,

"I feel unsteady on my feet and cannot go shopping with my friends." Furthermore, she described that she was unhappy in her marriage and worried a great deal about her children. When asked if she had any goals for improving her diabetes self-care, she stated, "No, I don't think I can do anything different right now."

The following treatment suggestions are offered to diabetes educators in cases presenting similar to Mary. Encourage the patient to bring a family member (spouse, adult child) to the session in order to educate the family about the patient's depression and diabetes treatment, particularly daily insulin use, and to help the patient gain some support at home. Help the patient and family understand that depression is a medical problem that is not his/her fault and that diabetes is associated with a high rate of depression. Explain how symptoms of depression can negatively affect diabetes self-care and how sometimes people are ashamed to be depressed. Ask if the patient would mind taking a simple survey (such as Beck Depression Inventory (BDI) (56)) to assess the level of depression.

In order to form a working alliance with patients who have depression and neuropathy, diabetes educators should be aware that depression is most associated with patients' perceptions of diabetic peripheral neuropathy as "unpredictable" and as negatively affecting their social views of themselves (57). Ask patients about their concerns with neuropathy and, if unsteadiness is present, suggest mobility aids or a referral to a physiotherapist for gait training to improve confidence in walking. Arrange telephone follow-up within several days and outpatient follow-up within several weeks.

If the patient's mood continues to interfere with his/her diabetes self-care and daily functioning, then discuss a referral to a mental health clinician. Explain how certain forms of mental health treatment such as cognitive behavioral therapy are very effective in the treatment of depression (58) and that sometimes people with diabetes greatly benefit from anti-depressant medication (59,60). If the referral is refused, then discuss your talking with the endocrinologist or primary care doctor to let them know that the patient is depressed and to inform them of the treatment recommendations.

CREATING A WORKING ALLIANCE IN CHALLENGING PATIENT ENCOUNTERS

Increase Professional Self-Awareness

Diabetes health care providers often face challenging patient encounters. In these encounters, it is important to examine your own views of what motivates behavioral change in patients with diabetes and how these views shape the ways you inquire and interact with patients. If you have negative and doubting views that people can change, discuss this with colleagues and try to understand the effect this can have on your clinical diabetes work. In consultation with colleagues, discuss beliefs of how people with diabetes can change, what motivates positive change, how to instill hope for change, and brainstorm on ways to increase collaboration with patients.

Increase Understanding of Patients' Beliefs and Perceptions

Use inquiry as a means of gaining greater understanding of your patients' beliefs and perceptions of their world. Sincere curiosity allows patients to feel that you really want to know what they think and feel and that you are attempting to collaborate with them. Inquire about their knowledge of diabetes. Explore what is medically based knowledge and what is family folklore, i.e., stories told to them by other family members. Patients' views of diabetes may influence their sense of themselves as agents of change, i.e., their self-efficacy or the belief in their ability to organize and perform necessary behaviors to achieve their goals *(61)*. Inquire about the patient's perceptions of barriers to self-care behaviors as well as goals for treatment. What does the patient feel able to do or not to do and why? What interferes with his/her ability to improve self-care? How does the family and social environment either support or interfere with achieving improved self-care?

Create a Supportive Treatment Environment

Attempt to be non-judgmental and empathic and encourage the patient to make his/her own suggestions for overcoming barriers to change *(62,63)*. Discuss with the patient setting several attainable goals to try before meeting again. Encourage the patient to concentrate on only a few goals that are achievable in order to increase a sense of self-efficacy. Discourage patients' self-blame and viewing their blood glucose numbers as grades. Help patients silence their negative judgmental voices that evaluate blood sugars and behaviors as good or bad and contribute to a negative sense of self. Present the idea that blood sugars are information that allows patients to know something more about themselves in order to take appropriate actions. Use a multidisciplinary team for support and ideas in the discussion of clinical cases and with new approaches to treatment.

SUPPORT AN ACTIVE PROBLEM-SOLVING APPROACH

Type 1 and type 2 patients who described a more active problem-oriented coping style were found to have better HbA1c values *(64,65)*. Type 1 patients on the insulin pump who described themselves as more actively involved in their diabetes self-care had lower A1C values than type 1 insulin pump users who were more passive about these behaviors *(66)*. Feeling more in charge of one's diabetes management may help patients feel less frustrated by diabetes and therefore more able to engage in the working alliance. Active patients can begin to identify what needs to be done, act on their goals, and integrate successes into future goal-directed actions by viewing what is not yet accomplished as challenges to be met. Problem solving may be the important mediating variable between diabetes knowledge and effective self-management *(67)*.

CONCLUSION

Effective treatment for challenging patients with diabetes requires the building of a working alliance. This alliance begins with the establishment of a dialogue between patient and health care provider where the patient can begin to trust that the provider is really interested in what he/she thinks, feels, and wants. Both the provider and the patient need to be active members of the treatment team. They need to pay attention to their beliefs, motivations, moods, and interpersonal thoughts, feelings, and words. They particularly need to want to engage in a partnership where treatment and education occur in an environment of support and collaboration, and the goal is not just better glycemic control but the mutual development of coping strategies for living with diabetes.

REFERENCES

1. Rubin RR, M. P. Psychological issues and treatment for people with diabetes. J Clin Psychol 2001;57(4):457–78.
2. Peyrot M, Rubin RR, Lauritzen T, Snoek FJ, Matthews DR, Skovlund SE. Psychosocial problems and barriers to improved diabetes management: results of the Cross-National Diabetes Attitudes, Wishes and Needs (DAWN) Study. Diabet Med 2005;22(10):1379–85.
3. Kaplan SH, Greenfield S, Ware JE, Jr. Assessing the effects of physician-patient interactions on the outcomes of chronic disease. Med Care 1989;27(3 Suppl):S110–27.
4. Von Korff M, Gruman J, Schaefer J, Curry SJ, Wagner EH. Collaborative management of chronic illness. Ann Intern Med 1997;127(12):1097–102.
5. Bordin ES. The generalizability of the psychoanalytic concept of the working alliance. Psychotherapy: Theory, Res & Practice 1979;26(3):252–60.
6. Strauss GJ. Psychological factors in intensive management of insulin-dependent diabetes mellitus. Nurs clin North Am 1996;31(4):737–45.
7. Andersen RM. Revisiting the behavioral model and access to medical care: does it matter? J Health Soc Behav 1995;36(1):1–10.
8. Anderson RM, Funnell MM. Patient empowerment: reflections on the challenge of fostering the adoption of a new paradigm. Patient Educ Couns 2005;57(2):153–7.
9. Escudero-Carretero MJ, Prieto-Rodriguez MA, Fernandez-Fernandez I, March-Cerda JC. [Physician/patient relationship in diabetes mellitus type 1 treatment. A qualitative study]. Atencion primaria/Sociedad Espanola de Medicina de Familia y Comunitaria 2006;38(1):8–15.
10. Fuertes JN, Mislowack A, Bennett J, et al. The physician-patient working alliance. Patient Educ Couns 2007;66(1):29–36.

11. Gavin LA, Wamboldt MZ, Sorokin N, Levy SY, Wamboldt FS. Treatment alliance and its association with family functioning, adherence, and medical outcome in adolescents with severe, chronic asthma. J Pediatr Psychol 1999;24(4):355–65.
12. Strous RD, Ulman AM, Kotler M. The hateful patient revisited: Relevance for 21st century medicine. Eur J Intern Med 2006;17(6):387–93.
13. Ciechanowski PS, Katon WJ, Russo JE, Walker EA. The patient-provider relationship: attachment theory and adherence to treatment in diabetes. Am J Psychiatry 2001;158(1):29–35.
14. Wens J, Vermeire E, Royen PV, Sabbe B, Denekens J. GPs' perspectives of type 2 diabetes patients' adherence to treatment: A qualitative analysis of barriers and solutions. BMC Fam Pract 2005;6(1):20.
15. Cooper-Patrick L, Gallo JJ, Gonzales JJ, et al. Race, gender, and partnership in the patient-physician relationship. Jama 1999;282(6):583–9.
16. Koekkoek B, van Meijel B, Hutschemaekers G. "Difficult patients" in mental health care: a review. Psychiatr Serv 2006;57(6):795–802.
17. Robbins JM, Beck PR, Mueller DP, Mizener DA. Therapists' perceptions of difficult psychiatric patients. The Journal of nervous and mental disease 1988;176(8):490–7.
18. Macdonald M. Seeing the cage: stigma and its potential to inform the concept of the difficult patient. Clinical nurse specialist CNS 2003;17(6):305–10; quiz 11–2.
19. Peyrot M, Rubin RR. Levels and risks of depression and anxiety symptomatology among diabetic adults. Diabetes Care 1997;20(4):585–90.
20. Polonsky WH, Anderson BJ, Lohrer PA, et al. Assessment of diabetes-related distress. Diabetes Care 1995;18(6):754–60.
21. Welch GW, Jacobson AM, Polonsky WH. The Problem Areas in Diabetes Scale. An evaluation of its clinical utility. Diabetes Care 1997;20(5):760–6.
22. Ritholz MD, Jacobson AM. Living with hypoglycemia. J Gen Intern Med 1998;13(12):799–804.
23. Polonsky WH, Davis CL, Jacobson AM, Anderson BJ. Correlates of hypoglycemic fear in type I and type II diabetes mellitus. Health Psychol 1992;11(3):199–202.
24. Boyle S, Allan C, Millar K. Cognitive-behavioural interventions in a patient with an anxiety disorder related to diabetes. Behaviour research and therapy 2004;42(3):357–66.
25. Green L, Feher M, Catalan J. Fears and phobias in people with diabetes. Diabetes Metab Res Rev 2000;16(4):287–93.
26. Clark DM. Anxiety disorders: why they persist and how to treat them. Behaviour research and therapy 1999;37 Suppl 1:S5–27.
27. Cryer PE, Davis SN, Shamoon H. Hypoglycemia in diabetes. Diabetes Care 2003;26(6):1902–12.
28. Cox D, Gonder-Frederick L, Polonsky W, Schlundt D, Julian D, Clarke W. A multicenter evaluation of blood glucose awareness training-II. Diabetes Care 1995;18(4):523–8.
29. DCCT. Weight gain associated with intensive therapy in the diabetes control and complications trial. The DCCT Research Group. Diabetes Care 1988;11(7):567–73.
30. Hogel J, Grabert M, Sorgo W, Wudy S, Gaus W, Heinze E. Hemoglobin A1c and body mass index in children and adolescents with IDDM. An observational study from 1976–1995. Exp Clin Endocrinol Diabetes 2000;108(2):76–80.
31. Thompson CJ, Cummings JF, Chalmers J, Gould C, Newton RW. How have patients reacted to the implications of the DCCT? Diabetes Care 1996;19(8):876–9.
32. Polonsky WH, Anderson BJ, Lohrer PA, Aponte JE, Jacobson AM, Cole CF. Insulin omission in women with IDDM. Diabetes Care 1994;17(10):1178–85.
33. Goebel-Fabbri AE, Fikkan J, Connell A, Vangsness L, Anderson BJ. Identification and treatment of eating disorders in women with type 1 diabetes mellitus. Treat Endocrinol 2002;1(3):155–62.

34. Goebel-Fabbri AE, Fikkan J, Franko DL, Pearson K, Anderson BJ, Weinger K. Insulin restriction and associated morbidity and mortality in women with type 1 diabetes. Diabetes Care 2007;31(3):415–9.
35. Jones JM, Lawson ML, Daneman D, Olmsted MP, Rodin G. Eating disorders in adolescent females with and without type 1 diabetes: cross sectional study. BMJ 2000;320(7249): 1563–6.
36. Mannucci E, Rotella F, Ricca V, Moretti S, Placidi GF, Rotella CM. Eating disorders in patients with type 1 diabetes: a meta-analysis. J Endocrinol Invest 2005;28(5):417–9.
37. Affenito SG, Adams CH. Are eating disorders more prevalent in females with type 1 diabetes mellitus when the impact of insulin omission is considered? Nutr Rev 2001;59(6):179–82.
38. Biggs MM, Basco MR, Patterson G, Raskin P. Insulin withholding for weight control in women with diabetes. Diabetes Care 1994;17(10):1186–9.
39. Anderson RJ, Freedland KE, Clouse RE, Lustman PJ. The prevalence of comorbid depression in adults with diabetes: a meta-analysis. Diabetes Care 2001;24(6):1069–78.
40. Katon W, von Korff M, Ciechanowski P, et al. Behavioral and clinical factors associated with depression among individuals with diabetes. Diabetes Care 2004;27(4):914–20.
41. de Groot M, Anderson R, Freedland KE, Clouse RE, Lustman PJ. Association of depression and diabetes complications: a meta-analysis. Psychosom Med 2001;63(4):619–30.
42. Black SA, Markides KS, Ray LA. Depression predicts increased incidence of adverse health outcomes in older Mexican Americans with type 2 diabetes. Diabetes Care 2003;26(10): 2822–8.
43. Ciechanowski PS, Katon WJ, Russo JE, Hirsch IB. The relationship of depressive symptoms to symptom reporting, self-care and glucose control in diabetes. Gen Hosp Psychiatry 2003;25(4):246–52.
44. Ciechanowski PS, Katon WJ, Russo JE. Depression and diabetes: impact of depressive symptoms on adherence, function, and costs. Arch Intern Med 2000;160(21):3278–85.
45. Lustman PJ, Anderson RJ, Freedland KE, de Groot M, Carney RM, Clouse RE. Depression and poor glycemic control: a meta-analytic review of the literature. Diabetes Care 2000;23(7):934–42.
46. Georgiades A, Zucker N, Friedman KE, et al. Changes in depressive symptoms and glycemic control in diabetes mellitus. Psychosom Med 2007;69(3):235–41.
47. Lin EH, Katon W, Von Korff M, et al. Relationship of depression and diabetes self-care, medication adherence, and preventive care. Diabetes Care 2004;27(9):2154–60.
48. Kinder LS, Katon WJ, Ludman E, et al. Improving depression care in patients with diabetes and multiple complications. J Gen Intern Med 2006;21(10):1036–41.
49. Klinkman MS. Competing demands in psychosocial care. A model for the identification and treatment of depressive disorders in primary care. Gen Hosp Psychiatry 1997;19(2): 98–111.
50. Rost K, Nutting P, Smith J, Coyne JC, Cooper-Patrick L, Rubenstein L. The role of competing demands in the treatment provided primary care patients with major depression. Arch Fam Med 2000;9(2):150–4.
51. Katon WJ. Clinical and health services relationships between major depression, depressive symptoms, and general medical illness. Biol Psychiatry 2003;54(3):216–26.
52. Kroenke K, Jackson JL, Chamberlin J. Depressive and anxiety disorders in patients presenting with physical complaints: clinical predictors and outcome. Am J Med 1997;103(5): 339–47.
53. Wyshak G, Barsky A. Satisfaction with and effectiveness of medical care in relation to anxiety and depression. Patient and physician ratings compared. Gen Hosp Psychiatry 1995;17(2):108–14.
54. Jackson JL, Kroenke K. Difficult patient encounters in the ambulatory clinic: clinical predictors and outcomes. Arch Intern Med 1999;159(10):1069–75.

55. Hahn SR, Kroenke K, Spitzer RL, et al. The difficult patient: prevalence, psychopathology, and functional impairment. J Gen Intern Med 1996;11(1):1–8.
56. Beck AT, Ward CH, Mendelson M, Mock J, Erbaugh J. An inventory for measuring depression. Arch Gen Psychiatry 1961;4:561–71.
57. Vileikyte L, Leventhal H, Gonzalez JS, et al. Diabetic peripheral neuropathy and depressive symptoms: the association revisited. Diabetes Care 2005;28(10):2378–83.
58. Lustman PJ, Freedland KE, Griffith LS, Clouse RE. Predicting response to cognitive behavior therapy of depression in type 2 diabetes. Gen Hosp Psychiatry 1998;20(5):302–6.
59. Katon WJ, Von Korff M, Lin EH, et al. The Pathways Study: a randomized trial of collaborative care in patients with diabetes and depression. Arch Gen Psychiatry 2004;61(10):1042–9.
60. Lustman PJ, Freedland KE, Griffith LS, Clouse RE. Fluoxetine for depression in diabetes: a randomized double-blind placebo-controlled trial. Diabetes Care 2000;23(5):618–23.
61. Bandura A. Self-efficacy: toward a unifying theory of behavioral change. Psychol Rev 1977;84(2):191–215.
62. Miller WR, Rollnick S. Motivational Interviewing Preparing People for Change. New York: The Guilford Press; 2002.
63. Rollnick S, Mason P, Butler C. Health Behavior Change A Guide for Practitioners. Edinburgh: Churchill Livingstone; 1999.
64. Rose M, Fliege H, Hildebrandt M, Schirop T, Klapp BF. The network of psychological variables in patients with diabetes and their importance for quality of life and metabolic control. Diabetes Care 2002;25(1):35–42.
65. Kvam SH, Lyons JS. Assessment of coping strategies, social support, and general health status in individuals with diabetes mellitus. Psychol Rep 1991;68(2):623–32.
66. Ritholz MD, Smaldone A, Lee J, Castillo A, Wolpert H, Weinger K. Perceptions of psychosocial factors and the insulin pump. Diabetes Care 2007;30(3):549–54.
67. Norris SL, Engelgau MM, Narayan KM. Effectiveness of self-management training in type 2 diabetes: a systematic review of randomized controlled trials. Diabetes Care 2001;24(3): 561–87.

14 Diabetes and Sexual Health

Donna Rice, MBA, BSN, RN, CDE,
Janis Roszler, RD, CDE, LD/N,
and Jo Anne B. Farrell, BSN, RN, CDE

CONTENTS

> INTRODUCTION
> MEN'S SEXUAL HEALTH
> WOMEN'S SEXUAL HEALTH
> THE ROLE OF THE DIABETES EDUCATOR
> REFERENCES

ABSTRACT

Diabetes is a complex disease that affects both men and women, resulting in a myriad of physical and psychological conditions. Sexual dysfunction is a common, devastating complication of diabetes that significantly impacts quality of life, and as such must be addressed and treated. The most common complications in men with diabetes are erectile dysfunction, low testosterone, and premature ejaculation. Women with diabetes may suffer from decreased sexual arousal, reduced libido, and dyspareunia. In addition, because glucose levels fluctuate with female hormonal changes, glucose management is more difficult. The past 10 years have seen advances in awareness of sexual health in diabetes, tools for the assessment of sexual health, and treatment options. Despite these advances, sexual dysfunction is still the most under-recognized and undertreated complication of diabetes. The epidemic of this disease has created a need for diabetes educators to be proficient in all aspects of disease management, going well beyond blood glucose control.

From: *Contemporary Diabetes: Educating Your Patient with Diabetes*
Edited by: K. Weinger and C. A. Carver, DOI 10.1007/978-1-60327-208-7_14,
© Humana Press, a part of Springer Science+Business Media, LLC 2009

Key Words: Sexual health, Sexual dysfunction, Erectile dysfunction, Hypogonadism, Premature ejaculation, Vaginal dryness, Reduced libido, Dyspareunia.

INTRODUCTION

Diabetes is known to produce a myriad of physical and psychological conditions that affect quality of life. Sexual dysfunction is now recognized as a complication of diabetes among both men and women, and the past 10 years have brought significant advances in awareness, recognition, and treatment of this troubling problem. However, despite the mounting evidence in the literature that individuals with diabetes are at increased risk for sexual dysfunction, it remains one of the most under-recognized and undertreated complications of diabetes (1).

Complications in men with diabetes that affect sexual health are most often, erectile dysfunction, low testosterone, and premature ejaculation. In women with diabetes, sexual complications include vaginal dryness, decreased sexual arousal, reduced libido, and dyspareunia (painful intercourse).

The epidemic growth of diabetes and the association of erectile dysfunction in men with the disease in the past 10 years have led to a preponderance of research investigating this association. As a result of that research, a significant proportion of this chapter is devoted to erectile dysfunction. However, as awareness of diabetes-related erectile dysfunction has increased, more research has been focused on other complications to male sexual health and more recently to female sexual health in people suffering with diabetes. This chapter provides an overview of those complications, some of the risk factors that appear to be involved, treatment options, and the important role of the diabetes educator in addressing sexual health with patients.

MEN'S SEXUAL HEALTH

Erectile Dysfunction

Erectile dysfunction is the inability to obtain an erection rigid enough for vaginal penetration. Men with diabetes are at high risk for developing erectile dysfunction due to the co-morbid conditions associated with this disease (2). Men with diabetes are three times as likely to develop erectile dysfunction as non-diabetic males (3). Erectile dysfunction occurs in 32% of men with type 1 and 46% of men with type 2 diabetes (4). The Male Massachusetts Aging Study, a landmark study, predicted that by 2025, 300 million men worldwide will suffer from erectile dysfunction (5). Coupled with the epidemic of diabetes and obesity in the world, erectile dysfunction will emerge as a huge quality of life issue.

Male sexuality is a complex process that involves both physiological (organic) and psychological (psychogenic) interactions. Organic origins are most often the cause of erectile dysfunction, however, psychological involvement should always be a consideration when treating erectile dysfunction (6). Sexual adequacy and performance are intimately related to a man's self esteem, confidence, and overall well-being (7). For this reason, it is important to recognize and address this psychological component of organic erectile dysfunction. Counseling is an appropriate adjunct with any treatment option for optimal success.

Organic causes of erectile dysfunction are often categorized into vascular, endocrine, and neurological subsets. Vascular causes are the most common and involve endothelial deterioration (2). These complications are prevalent in type 2 diabetes. To better understand risk factors, onset, and treatments options of erectile dysfunction, a short overview of the anatomy and physiology of erectile dysfunction follows.

ERECTILE DYSFUNCTION ANATOMY AND PHYSIOLOGY

The penis is composed of three principle internal structures: the corpus spongiosum, two corpora cavernosa lateral and superior to the spongiosum, and a fairly inflexible sheath called the tunica albuginea (See Fig. 1). Within the corpora cavernosa are thousands of tiny vesicles called lacunae. They are made of endothelial cells and surrounded by smooth muscle. Blood flows through these lacunae via helcine arteries and emissary veins. Many of the emissary veins travel through the inner and outer layers of the tunica albuginea.

In the flaccid state, smooth muscle surrounding the lacunae is taut. An erection is initiated when nitrous oxide (NO) is released from nerve endings at the lacunae site. This release stimulates production of cyclic guanosine monophosphate (cGMP) which in turn will cause relaxation of the smooth muscle surrounding each lacunae. As this muscle relaxes, the lacunae swell as they accept blood from the helcine arteries. As they swell, pressure builds up against

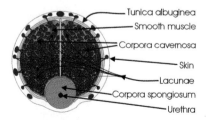

Fig. 1. Transection of penis with enlargement detailing blood supply to lacunae.
Reprinted from *Diabetes and Erectile Dysfunction* with permission from BellaVita Publications (22)

the inflexible sheath of the tunica albuginea causing constriction of emissary veins and further swelling (tumescence) of the penis. As pressure builds against the tunica albuginea, rigidity develops and an erection is obtained (8).

The erection will continue as long as these conditions persist. An erection is diminished normally when cGMP reacts with the enzyme, phosphodiesterase type 5 (PDE5). PDE5 breaks down cGMP, and, as the concentration of cGMP decreases, smooth muscle around the lacunae resumes its naturally taut state. Blood is forced out of the lacunae, pressure against the tunica is diminished, emissary veins are opened, and the naturally flaccid state is regained. Erectile dysfunction can ensue when damage to any one of these processes occur. There are numerous risk factors that increase chances for damage to occur.

ERECTILE DYSFUNCTION RISK FACTORS

Risk factors for erectile dysfunction are often categorized into three groups: organic, pharmacological, or lifestyle. Organic risk factors are most often disease states that predispose a person to erectile dysfunction. Diabetes, cardiovascular disease, hypertension, and hyperlipidemia are the principal organic risk factors. A 2004 study by Serfiel showed that among men with erectile dysfunction, 42% had hypertension, 42% had hyperlipidemia, and 20% had diabetes mellitus, while only 32% were free of these conditions (9). These risk factors are most commonly associated with vascular endothelial deterioration such as sclerosis of arterial walls and plaque formation (2). Endothelial deterioration of arteries and veins involved with erectile dysfunction occurs at the microvascular level, and for this reason erectile dysfunction may be an early warning sign for either of these risk factors. While endothelial deterioration is the principle cause of organic erectile dysfunction, autonomic neuropathies may also play a role. Autonomic neuropathies that affect the pelvic nerves are most commonly associated with erectile dysfunction "possibly through mechanisms of increased oxidative stress, nerve hypoxia, and raised protein kinase C production." (7).

Medication side effects also may be implicated. The prevalence of erectile dysfunction may range from 9% in patients receiving diuretics to 30% in patients receiving combinations of drugs (10). Some drugs believed to cause erectile dysfunction include antihypertensives, beta-blockers, thiazide diuretics, ACE inhibitors, vasodilators, and alpha-blockers. In addition, drugs affecting the central nervous system and endocrine system may also cause erectile dysfunction (10). An independent association between erectile dysfunction and pharmaceutical agents is the subject of some debate. In a multivariate analysis of drug classes, DeBardis found an independent link with erectile dysfunction and suggests that the drug association is "confounded" by the underlying medical condition (11). If a drug's effect on erectile function is questionable, it may be helpful to consider using an alternatively effective drug and compare sexual function.

Lifestyles that pose a significant risk of erectile dysfunction include smoking, obesity, and alcohol abuse (2,3,5). In the Male Massachusetts Aging Study, a group of men (n = 513) without co-morbid conditions were evaluated over a 10-year period (5). Men who were smokers at the beginning of the study had almost double the incidence of erectile dysfunction 10 years later. This statistic mirrors a similar study by Mirone, who reports that impairment of the endothelial smooth muscle relaxation and risk for coronary artery disease were amplified by cigarette smoking (12,13).

Obesity alone does not appear to be a risk factor for erectile dysfunction (3). However, obesity complicates diabetes management and predisposes a person to cardiovascular disease, hyperlipidemia, and hypertension, thereby increasing erectile dysfunction risk. A study by Chung comparing two groups of men above and below 120% of ideal body weight and without any vascular risk factors found no significant difference between the obese and the non-obese groups in the onset of erectile dysfunction (14).

Erectile dysfunction has been associated with alcohol abuse. Consumption of an excess of alcohol interferes with testosterone levels and can reduce libido. However research has more recently shown that moderate intake of alcohol and exercise may have a protective effect against the development of erectile dysfunction (15).

Some studies have ascribed a two-fold increase in erectile dysfunction in men suffering with depression (10,16). It should also be noted that there is a higher level of depression among men who have diabetes than in the general population and that depression is associated with numerous disease states and quality of life issues, including erectile dysfunction (11).

ERECTILE DYSFUNCTION TREATMENT OPTIONS

Erectile dysfunction involving endothelial damage does not appear to be reversible (17) and, as such, requires compensatory measures categorized as first, second, and third line therapies. These therapies, listed in Tables 1, 2, and 3, are tiered according to their level of invasiveness. It is important that educators emphasize that these treatment options compensate for a disease state that could easily worsen. The role of the educator is to present treatment options, but also, to emphasize lifestyle changes and disease management that will minimize further damage.

This wide variety of treatment options for erectile dysfunction gives men and their partners many choices to consider. Their ultimate decision will depend on personal preference, the extent and cause of the dysfunction, and the education and advice provided by knowledgeable healthcare professionals.

Table 1

First-Line Therapies for Treatment of Erectile Dysfunction in Men [Reprinted from *Diabetes and Erectile Dysfunction* with permission from Bella Vita Publications (22)]

Option	Device	Mode of action	Pros and cons	Teaching tips
Sex therapy Counseling		Guidance to help with acceptance of the condition and/or treatment option.	Effective, especially when partner is involved. Difficult to locate therapies in rural areas. Expensive if not covered by insurance.	Refer when individuals are having difficulty making decision.
Mechanical devices Non-invasive devices-variety of sizes/styles-Available at retail stores or by prescription Relatively easy to use-effective	Construction rings	Ring placed at the base of the penis constricts blood flow out of penis. Rings often remediate venous leakage.	Inexpensive and simple Placing elastic rings on or off may be painful Penis is wobbly at the base and may seem cool.	Ring should not be left on more than 30 minutes.
	Vacuum devices	Cylinder is placed over the penis and vacuum is applied which forces blood into the penis. A constriction ring is placed at the base of the erect penis.	One time cost. Manual and battery operated devices available. May be part of foreplay. May be clumsy or difficult for some men. Ring concerns apply.	Education practice is essential for success (partner should be included). Ring concerns apply.

Penile sleeve	Plastic sleeve slips over the flaccid penis and fastens under the testes. Sleeve is covered with a condom that is open at the head of the penis. Often used with premature ejaculation problems. Dispose of after single use.	May be difficult or clumsy to use for some men. The partner may feel some discomfort.	Education/practice is essential to improve comfort level.
Oral medications PDE5 inhibitors Effective in 50–60% of men with diabetes.	Viagra® Sildenafil)*	Inhibit the action of PDE5, thereby maintaining high levels of cGMP. High levels of cGMP induce an erection. Stimulation/arousal remains necessary to release cGMP.	Take on an empty stomach. Fats interfere with uptake. Take 30 minutes prior to sex. May be effective up to 4h.	Do not take with any forms of nitroglycerin. Mild flushing, headache, dizziness may occur. Vision problems may occur and must be addressed.
	Levitra® (Vardenafil HCl)[†]		Take 10–15 minutes prior to sex. May be effective up to 12h.
	Cialis® (Tadalafil)[‡]		Take 15 minutes prior to sex. May be effective up to 36h.

*Viagra is a registered trademark of Pfizer Inc.
[†]Levitra is a registered trademark of Baker Inc.
[‡]Cialis is a registered trademark of Eli Lilly Corp.

Table 2
Second-Line Therapies for Treatment of Erectile Dysfunction in Men

Option	Device	Mode of action	Pros and Cons	Teaching tips
Intra-urethral suppository	Alprostadil (Muse®*)	Relaxes smooth muscle and dilates blood vessels to allow blood to flow into the penis.	30–50% effective (18). Easy to use. Lasts $^{1}/_{2}$–1 h. Urethral burning, pain in testicles and irritation may occur. Needs to be refrigerated.	Education and counseling needed for proper insertion. Use of condoms if partner is pregnant.
Penile injection therapy	Alprostadil (Caverject®† or Edex®‡)	Relaxes smooth muscle and dilates blood vessels allowing blood flow into the penis.	70–90% effective (19). Lasts 0.5–1 h. Strong erections are reported. Men are reluctant to inject their penis. Pain, scarring, priapism may occur. Only inject 3× per week. Refrigerate.	Education and counseling needed to teach injection procedure. Follows specific physician instructions on dosage.

*Muse is a registered trademark of Vivus, Inc.
†Caverject is a registered trademark of Pfizer, Inc.
‡Edex is a registered trademark of Schwarz Pharma.
Reprinted from *Diabetes and Erectile Dysfunction* with permission from BellaVita Publications (22)

Table 3
Third-Line Therapies for Treatment of Erectile Dysfunction in Men

Option	Device	Mode of action	Pros and Cons	Teaching tips
Penile implants Surgically implanted prosthetic device Usually a last resort procedure Permanently affects structure of the penis Involves standard complications of surgery	Semi-rigid devices	Surgical implant of semi-rigid cylinders. Constant pressure inside the penis may cause injury in some men. Questionable implant for men with diabetes.	Penis remains semi-rigid and may be difficult to conceal. Overall positive satisfaction rating of patient and partner.	Counseling and education prior to surgery is essential. Diabetes must be controlled prior to surgery.
	2-Piece inflatable device.	Surgical implant of inflatable cylinders in the penis and a pump/reservoir in the scrotum. Manual manipulation of pump inflates/deflates penis.	Mechanical failures are possible though < 1% bulky pump/reservoir may be uncomfortable. Very-high satisfaction rate (20).	Pre/post-op care important to prevent infection. Infection almost always involve surgery and replacement.
	3-Piece inflatable device	Surgical implant of inflatable cylinders in the penis, pump in the scrotum and reservoir in the abdominal wall.	95% patient and partner satisfaction rate. Low mechanical failures (< 1%) (21). No restrictions on frequency of use allows for increased spontaneity.	Penis tip remains soft.

Reprinted from *Diabetes and Erectile Dysfunction* with permission from BellaVita Publications (22)

Testosterone Deficiency in Men

A recent U.S. epidemiological survey estimated the prevalence of testosterone deficiency in males, 45 years of age and older, to be at 13.8 million in primary care settings *(23)*. Certain conditions exist that may contribute to the high prevalence of low testosterone. These include sellar mass (of which pituitary adenomas are the most common), medications that affect testosterone production or metabolism, HIV-associated weight loss, end-stage renal disease, COPD, infertility, osteoporosis or low trauma fracture, and type 2 diabetes *(24)*.

Emerging evidence has shown that low testosterone may predispose men to insulin resistance and type 2 diabetes *(25,26)*. Endocrine Society and the American Association of Clinical Endocrinologists recommend that a diagnosis of testosterone deficiency include a low testosterone level ($<$ 300 ng/dl), along with consistent signs and symptoms of the disorder *(24,27)*. A serum total testosterone level needs to be measured in the morning with a repeat measurement to confirm diagnosis *(24)*. The usual normal serum T level range is 300–1,000 ng/dl in adult men *(28)*.

Recognizing the signs and symptoms of testosterone deficiency may be vague and difficult for the man with type 2 diabetes to describe. The use of an assessment tool will be helpful in identifying these symptoms, which include a progressive decrease in muscle mass, loss of libido, erectile dysfunction, hot flashes, poor ability to concentrate, and an increased risk of osteoporosis *(24,27)*. When the patient is diagnosed with testosterone deficiency, his healthcare practitioner will prescribe replacement therapy. Available delivery formulations include pellet implants, intramuscular injectables, transdermal patches, transdermal gels, and buccal tablets (Table 4) *(24)*. The goal of therapy is to restore serum testosterone levels to a mid-normal range. It is important for the patient to understand the benefits as well as the risks of therapy. Testosterone therapy is contraindicated in men with known prostate or breast cancer. In addition, older men may be at risk for the development for enlarged prostate and prostate cancer. Monitoring is essential while the patient is on replacement therapy. Healthcare practitioners should be periodically checking testosterone levels, hemoglobin and hematocrit, cholesterol, liver function, breast discomfort, prostate, and symptom relief.

In conclusion, there is a higher prevalence of testosterone deficiency in men with type 2 diabetes. Low testosterone is often unrecognized, and therefore may be under-treated. In symptomatic patients with confirmed low serum testosterone levels, replacement therapy should restore testosterone levels to the normal to mid-normal range, and these patients can experience relief of their low testosterone symptoms. Patients need to be fully informed of the benefits and risks of therapy, and be properly monitored as recommended by the Endocrine Society. Diabetes Educators have a unique opportunity and responsibility to initiate discussion and education to guide their patients with low

Table 4
Testosterone Replacement Therapies Available in United States

Formulation	Brand name	Delivery route	Dosing	Pros	Cons
Testosterone buccal system	Striant®	Bio-adhesive buccal tablet	30 mg bid	Testosterone levels with physiologic range.	Possible taste alteration, gum irritation, bid dosing.
Testosterone gel	AndroGel® Testim®	Topical gel	5–10 g/day	Testosterone levels within physiologic range, steady state concentrations.	Potential transfer to partner.
Testosterone injectables – Testosterone enanthate – Testosterone cypionate	Delatestryl® Depo-Testosterone®	Intramuscular	50–400 mg every 2–4 weeks or 100 mg/week or 200 mg every 2 weeks 50–100 mg every 2–4 weeks or 100 mg/week or 200 mg every 2 weeks	Corrects symptoms of androgen deficiency, inexpensive if self-administered.	Peaks and valleys in serum testosterone levels, mood fluctuations, requires an injection.

(Continued)

Table 4 (*Continued*)

Formulation	Brand name	Delivery route	Dosing	Pros	Cons
Testosterone patch	Androderm®	Skin patch	5 mg/day	Mimics circadian rhythm.	Skin irritation.
Testosterone pellets	Testopel®	Pellets	Four to six 400 mg pellets injected sc	Corrects symptoms of androgen deficiency.	Requires surgical incision for pellet insertion, pellets may extrude spontaneously.

Adapted from Nature Clinical Practice Urology.2006; 3; 5:260–267
Androderm® trademark of Watson Pharma, Corona, CA. 2005.
AndroGel® trademark of Solvay Pharmaceuticals, Inc, Marietta, GA. 2007.
Delatestryl® trademark of SAB-Pharma, Inc. Boucherville, QC, Canada. 2005.
Depo-Testosterone® trademark of Pharmacia/Pfizer. Kalamazoo, MI. 2002.
Testim® trademark of Auxillium Pharmaceuticals, Inc, Norristown, PA. 2003.
Boehringer. Comparison of testosterone replacement products. The Pharmacist's Letter. 2003:19.
Striant™ trademark of Columbia Laboratories Inc., Livingston, NJ. 2003.
Testopel® trademark of Bartor Pharmacal Co., Rye, NJ. 1992.

testosterone in order to achieve a better understanding of the disorder, treatment options, proper monitoring, and required follow-up.

Premature Ejaculation

Men with diabetes have a higher-than-normal incidence of premature ejaculation (PE). Until recently, premature ejaculation was considered a psychological etiology requiring psychological counseling *(29)*. Premature ejaculation is now known to have a neurobiological component, and diagnosis and management has come to the forefront. PE is defined as an "ejaculation that occurs sooner than desired either before or shortly after penetration, causing distress to either one or both partners" *(30)*. The American Urological Association Guidelines on the Pharmacologic Management of Premature Ejaculation suggest that 5–30% of men suffer from premature ejaculation. *(30)*.

DIAGNOSIS AND MANAGEMENT OF PREMATURE EJACULATION

Most studies agree that the diagnosis of premature ejaculation should be based principally on self-reported sexual history *(30,31)*. There is no known physiological test at present that can characterize premature ejaculation. Factors to consider when recording the sexual history of premature ejaculation are frequency and duration, whether it is partner specific, the degree of stimulation prior to the episode, the emotional and psychological impact on the individual and/or his partner, the impact of on sexual activity and quality of life, and the presence of premature ejaculation *(29)*.

Treatment options include topical anesthetics, selective serotonin reuptake inhibitors (SSRIs), the penile sleeve discussed in Table 2, and behavioral and psychological therapies. At present there are no FDA-approved drugs. Antidepressant agents that have been shown to be effective in treating premature ejaculation include the SSRIs fluoxetine, paroxetine, and sertraline, and the tricyclic antidepressant clomipramine *(30)*. These treatments have not been approved by the FDA, and as such, the contraindications and adverse reactions regarding the physiology of premature ejaculation are not understood.

At present there are two significant documents that deal with diagnosis and treatment of premature ejaculation as a neurobiological syndrome. One is from the American Urological Association *(30)* and the other reports on the Second International Consultation on Sexual Medicine: Sexual Dysfunction in Men and Women *(31)*.

WOMEN'S SEXUAL HEALTH

Comprehensive studies investigating sexual health as it relates to women with diabetes are extremely limited in number. Considering that complications to sexual health occur in almost 50% of all women with diabetes *(32)*, investigative research and awareness will hopefully continue to improve in the coming years.

Common Female Sexual Problems

The most common sexual problems reported in women with diabetes are slowed or inadequate lubrication and decreased sexual arousal *(32)*. Other complaints include reduced libido, difficulty achieving orgasm, dyspareunia (painful intercourse), and frequent vaginal infections that interfere with the ability to participate in sexual relations. The underlying causes in women appear to be a combination of psychological and physical issues that interfere with a woman's ability to become sexually aroused *(33)*. Neuropathy, vascular impairment, and psychological complaints were initially believed to be the primary causes of sexual dysfunction in the female diabetic population, but early studies that credited these factors were found to have methodological flaws. They lacked properly segmented control groups, used inadequate sample sizes, neglected to characterize the subjects' diabetes type, neglected to note the presence or number of diabetic complications (including depression), and disregarded the subjects' psychological adjustment to having diabetes *(32)*. More recent studies show a poor correlation between sexual difficulties and age, body mass index, duration of diabetes, glycemic control, hormonal therapy, diabetic complications, and menopausal status *(7)*. The results from five controlled prevalence studies *(32,34–37)* on sexual dysfunction in women with diabetes are shown in Table 5.

The Mind–Body Connection

A woman's mood sets the process of sexual enjoyment into motion *(33)*. Her psychological desire is followed by physical responses that include the secretion of lubricating moisture in the vaginal area, relaxation of pelvic floor muscles, and engorgement of the labia and clitoris *(33)*. The initial sexual interest that initiates this process is affected by a number of emotional factors.

A significant barrier to this process in women is depression *(7)*. Depression is twice as common in individuals with diabetes, and women with diabetes have 1.6 times the risk of depression compared with their male counterparts *(38)*. Selective serotonin reuptake inhibitor (SSRI) medications, frequently used to treat depression, can also negatively affect a woman's libido *(39)*.

Other emotional factors known to interfere with the female sexual experience include marital discord, stress, fatigue, hormonal status, distractions in the immediate environment, fear of pregnancy, and the fear of contracting a sexually transmitted disease *(37,38)*. If a woman attempts to engage in intercourse without being adequately aroused, physical trauma may take place and impede

Table 5
Sexual Dysfunction in Women with Diabetes: Results from Five Controlled Studies

Study instrument	Mean age in years (range)	Diabetes type (n)	Low desire	Low arousal	Reduced lubrication	Orgasm difficulties	Pain	Dissatisfaction	Predictors of female sexual dysfunction
Premenopausal Women‖									
IFSF (33)	39 (25–47)	Type 2 (72)	78%	Not studied	38%	49%	42%	42%	No association with HbA1C, BMI, duration, or nephropathy
		Controls (60)	20%	Not studied	20%	0%	20%	7%	
IFSF (34)	43 (39–50)	Type 1 (7)		Not studied	*	*	*	*	No correlation with sensory loss
		Type 2 (23)							
		Controls (20)							
Premenopausal and postmenopausal women‖									
BSFI,DSIF (35)	40 (20–76)	Type 1 (36)	NS	NS	40%	38%‡	31%	NS	Fear of dependence correlated with retinopathy and nephropathy
		Type 2 (24)	NS	NS	47%	31%‡	42%	NS	
		Controls (67)			34%	33%‡	26%		
UKU (31) (adapted)	37 (20–72)	Type 1 (120)	17%	NS	14%	14%	12%		Depression
		Controls (180)	9%		6%	10%	6%		No association with postmenopausal estrogen treatment

(Continued)

227

Table 5 (*Continued*)

Study instrument	Mean age in years (range)	Diabetes type (n)	Low desire	Low arousal	Reduced lubrication	Orgasm difficulties	Pain	Dissatisfaction	Predictors of female sexual dysfunction
FSFI (36)	41 (21–64)	Type 1 (21)	85%	76%*	57%*	66%*	61%	52%	No risk factors identified§
		Type 2 (50)	82%	68%*	38%*	38%*	46%	50%	No association with menopausal status
		Controls (56)	66%	41%	28%	39%	39%	37%	

IFSF, Index of Female Sexual Function; *BSFI*, Brief Sexual Function Inventory Questionnaire; *DISF*, Derogates Interview for Sexual Functioning; *UKU*, "Udvalg for Kliniske Undersoegelser" (Questionnaire for clinical studies); *FSFI*, Female Sexual Function Index; *NS*, not significant.
*Significant difference between diabetes patients and controls (p < 0.05).
†On the basis of IFSI score ≤ 30.
‡Orgasm difficulties with intercourse but only 8–13% had difficulties with self-stimulation
§Diabetic complications not studied
¶Postmenopausal status=Basson et al.: T1=19%, T2=44.4%; Enzlin et al.: T1=15%; Erol et al.: did not record; Doruk et al.: T1 and T2=31%
Reprinted from *The Lancet* 2007 with permission from Elsevier (7).

the physical response *(33)*. If pain occurs during intimate activity, a woman may become apprehensive about engaging in subsequent experiences *(40)*. If her fear becomes a significant problem, sexual counseling may be needed *(41)*.

Hormones Fluctuations, Glucose Control, and Sexual Health

Sexual hormones play a key role in blood glucose metabolism and insulin resistance *(42)*. They may also play a lesser known role in the ability for a woman to enjoy a satisfactory sexual experience. Salonia et al. *(34)* links sexual problems occurring in women with type 1 diabetes to their menstrual cycle. During the luteal phase, these women may experience greater problems with arousal, lubrication, and orgasm and have increased discomfort or pain during sexual penetration *(34)*. Puberty, menarche, and menopause affect diabetes control due to hormone excursions and the insulin resistance associated with changing levels of hormones *(43)*. There is evidence to suggest that the use of hormone therapy may play a role in reducing the risk of type 2 diabetes in postmenopausal women *(44)*. If this evidence bears scrutiny, there may be a preventative role for estrogen therapy. Estrogen was also noted as a possible way to reduce insulin sensitivity after menopause *(45)*. Care needs to be taken to further assess the use of oral contraception and hormone replacement on a case-by-case basis weighing the benefits against the risks in every individual.

Other Issues

Women with type 2 diabetes may develop hypertension, hyperlipidemia, and coronary artery disease, which can interfere with the blood flow and engorgement needed for sexual satisfaction. Medicines used to treat these conditions may also impair sexual function in many women in both well controlled and uncontrolled type 2 diabetes *(46)*. Polycystic ovarian disease, a marker for insulin resistance that often identifies women at risk for the development of type 2 diabetes *(47)* is not generally associated with sexual issues, but the potential infertility issues that it may cause can create a myriad of psychological issues that bring stress to an intimate relationship.

Treatments

Good glycemic control should always be the first consideration when attempting to manage the complications of sexual health in diabetes. Educators and healthcare providers should help patients understand the relationship between hormones levels and blood glucose control. Emphasis should be placed on management as a means to avoid or delay the development of diabetic complications and vaginal infections. Vaginal dryness can be treated with vaginal and estrogen lubricants *(48)* and physical manipulation, which can encourage a physical response if psychological arousal does not occur *(33)*. Sildenafil may be used in certain women to improve clitoral blood flow *(49)*. Stress can be reduced with the use of reliable birth control and relaxation techniques. Consideration should be given to the longer arousal periods required for women for sexual intimacy.

Relationship building and couples counseling to increase awareness of the "romantic needs" of women should be emphasized. Romantic dates, long walks, cuddling, bonding conversations, are all contributing factors that "set the mood" and should be encouraged to enhance an intimate relationship *(50)*. A woman's inability to achieve an orgasm may be caused by physical and emotional factors as well as her lack of knowledge of her own body. Self-stimulation can help her understand the steps that the body takes as it reaches and achieves sexual satisfaction. Couple's sexual counseling can help a woman achieve an orgasm during intimate sexual activity with a partner. All the suggestions listed above that help a woman experience improved vaginal lubrication, libido, and arousal should help lead her to a satisfactory sexual climax.

Many women with diabetes experience sexual dysfunction. Intimacy and intimate relationships are an essential part of a full and rewarding life. When diabetes interferes in this personal arena, it can undermine the emotional and physical support needed for a patient to successfully complete diabetes self-care tasks and enjoy life to its fullest.

THE ROLE OF THE DIABETES EDUCATOR

Diabetes educators must play an instrumental role to initiate dialogue, instruct on different treatment options, make referrals for appropriate care, and most importantly, provide follow up that monitors the level of success for a chosen treatment option. Today, sexuality is rarely assessed and barely addressed in the classroom setting or during individual consultations. Time rarely permits healthcare providers to broach the subject, and individuals are often shy or embarrassed to discuss intimate and personal details. Furthermore, cultural or religious beliefs may also inhibit forthright discussion on any issues related to sexuality. Other barriers such as reimbursement issues, lack of training in sexual medicine, and insufficient resources exist for diabetes educators that further segregate sexuality from the scope of diabetes care. As a result, sexuality takes a back seat to the many other and more easily discussed issues. There is no easy answer or training for clinicians to learn how to overcome these barriers. A solution to the problem begins with openness, understanding, and tools and resources to assist diabetes educators in assessment, education, and treatment. The development of an internal process within the diabetes education program or clinic can assist diabetes educators to begin the conversation and assess for these sexuality issues. A simple four-step approach can be the answer that will open the doors to restoring sexual health.

1. Use an assessment tool to begin the dialogue around the relationship of diabetes and sexual health. Appropriate assessment tools for sexual health in men and women can be found in the literature *(51,52)*. These provide an excellent means to assess sexual health and its relationship to diabetes. Moreover, these tools provide an excellent opportunity to discuss the value of blood glucose control and its effect on sexuality.

2. Incorporate sexuality issues and treatment options in an educational context. Sexual health is often compromised in people with diabetes, and should be readily discussed, just as neuropathies and heart disease would be. Developing educational content around treatment options is often a best way to begin to develop a comfort level for discussing sexual health. Education also develops an atmosphere of hope to individuals who suffer from sexual issues and are too embarrassed to openly discuss the topic. Knowing that there are treatment options is often the ice breaker that encourages discussion.

3. Provide appropriate referrals to the right provider. Educators must build their referral base to provide optimal care for individuals. That list should include urologists, sex therapists, psychologists, social workers, and marriage counselors, in addition to the team members for routine diabetes care. Each member plays a unique supportive role.

4. Follow up on treatment choices and success. Diabetes educators must continue to follow up over time in order to obtain both clinical and behavioral outcomes. Success around a chosen treatment option should be questioned and discussed at follow-up visits. Just as there is a need to change a diabetes treatment plan, a change in strategy or therapy may be warranted with sexual complications as well.

Diabetes educators are emerging as the "change agents" – the professionals who educate, coach, and counsel on the necessary steps to create positive and effective health habits, which in turn, lead to improved health outcomes. The epidemic of diabetes has created the need for diabetes educators to be proficient in diabetes care that goes well beyond blood glucose management. Sexual health is emerging as a new subspecialty, and educators need to be prepared to address all types of quality of life issues. Sexual health is too important to ignore, and diabetes educators are the key providers to greatly impact total care in all individuals suffering with diabetes. Our patients deserve it.

REFERENCES

1. DeBerardis G, Franciosi M, Belfiglio M, et al. Erectile dysfunction and quality of life in type 2 diabetic patients. Diabetes Care 2002;25:1807–1811.
2. Muneer A, Borley N, Ralph DJ. Erectile dysfunction. In: European Endocrine Disease. London: Business Briefings, 2007; 93–96.
3. Cirino G, Fusco F, Imbimbo C, Mirone V. Pharmacology of erectile dysfunction in man. Pharm Thera 2006; 111:400–423.

4. Vickers MA, Wright EA. Erectile dysfunction in the patient with diabetes mellitus. Am J Man Care 2004;10 (suppl):S3–S11.
5. Feldman HA, Goldstein I, Hatzichristou DG, Krane RJ, McKinlay JB. Impotence and its medical and psychosocial correlates: results of the Massachusetts Male Aging Study. J Urol 1994; 151:54–61.
6. Giommi R, Corona G, Maggi M. The therapeutic dilemma: how to use psychotherapy. Int J Androl 2005;28(suppl 2):81–85.
7. Bhasin S, Enzlin P, Basson R. Sexual dysfunction in men and women with endocrine disorders. Lancet 2007;369:597–611.
8. Krane RJ, Goldstein I. Impotence period. N Engl J Med. 1989;321:1648–1659.
9. Serftel AD, Sun P, Swindle R. The prevalence of hypertension, hyperlipidemia, diabetes mellitus and depression among men with erectile dysfunction. J Urol 2004;171:2341–2345.
10. Vinik A, Richardson D. Erectile dysfunction in diabetes. Diabetes Rev 1998;6:16–33.
11. DeBerardis G, Pellegrini F, Franciosi M, et al. Identifying patients with type 2 diabetes with a higher likelihood of erectile dysfunction: the role of the interaction between clinical and psychological factors. J Urol 2003;169:1422–1428.
12. Mirone V, Imbimbo C, Bortolotti A, et al. Cigarette smoking as a risk factor for erectile dysfunction: results from an Italian epidemiological study. Eur Urol 2002;41:294–297.
13. Jeunemann KP, Lue TF, Luo JA, Benowitz NL, Abozeid M, Tanagho EA. The effect of cigarette smoking on penile erection. J Urol 1987;138:438–441.
14. Chung WS, Sohn JH, Park YY. Is obesity an underlying factor in erectile dysfunction? Eur J Urol 1999;36:68–70.
15. Kalter-Leibovici, Wainstein J, Ziv A, et al. Clinical, socioeconomic, and lifestyle parameters associated with erectile dysfunction among diabetic men. Diabetes Care 2005;28:1739–1744.
16. Montorsi F, Padma-Nathan H, Glina S. Erectile function and assessments of erection hardness correlate positively with measures of emotional well-being, sexual satisfaction, and treatment satisfaction in men with erectile dysfunction treated with sildenafil citrate (Viagra). Urology 2006;68(suppl):26–37.
17. Yaman O, Akand M, Gursoy A, Erdogan MF, Anafarta K. The effect of diabetes mellitus treatment and good glycemic control on the erectile function in men with diabetes mellitus-induced erectile dysfunction: a pilot study. J Sex Med 2006;3:344–348.
18. Linet OI, Neff LL. Intracavernous prostaglandin Ei and erectile dysfunction. Clin Investig 1994;72:139–149.
19. Brant WO, Bella AJ, Lue TF. Treatment options for erectile dysfunction. Endocrinol Metab Clin N Am 2007;36:465–479.
20. Moore DR, Wang R. Pathophysiology and treatment of diabetic erectile dysfunction. Asian J Androl 2006;8:675–684.
21. Lux M, Reyes-Vallejo L, Morgentaler A, Levine LA. J Urol 2007;177:262–266.
22. Rice D, Rice B. Diabetes and Erectile Dysfunction: A Quick 'n' Easy Handbook For The Diabetes Educator. Brighton, MI: Bella Vita Publications, 2006: Appendix 3.
23. Mulligan T, Frick MF, Zuraw QC, et al. Prevalence of hypogonadism in males aged at least 45 years: the HIM study. Int J Clin Pract 2006;60:762–769.
24. Bhasin S, Cunningham GR, Hayes F, et al. Testosterone therapy in adult men with androgen deficiency syndromes: an Endocrine Society clinical practice guideline. J Clin Endocrinol Metab 2006; 91:1995–2010.
25. Kapoor D. Goodwin E. Channer KS, et al. Testosterone replacement therapy improves insulin resistance, glycemic control, visceral adiposity and hypercholesterolaemia in hypogonadal men with type 2 diabetes. European J Endo 2006; 154:899–906.
26. Pitteloud N, Hardin M, Dwyer A, et al. Increasing insulin resistance is associated with a decrease in Leydig cell testosterone secretion in men. J Clin Endocrinol Metab 2005; 91: 2636–2641.

27. Petak SM, Nankin HR, Spark RF, et al. American Association of Clinical Endocrinologists medical guidelines for clinical practice for the evaluation and treatment of hypogonadism in adult male patients—2002 update. Endoc Pract 2002;8:440–456.
28. Winters SJ, Clark BJ. Testosterone synthesis, transport, and metabolism. In: Bagatell C, Bremner W, eds. Androgens in Health and Disease. Totowa, NJ: Humana Press, 2003:3–22.
29. Sharlip ID. Guidelines for the diagnosis and management of premature ejaculation. J Sex Med 2006;3(suppl 4):309–317.
30. Montague DK, Barada JH, Belker AM, et al. Clinical guidelines panel on erectile dysfunction: summary report on the treatment of organic erectile dysfunction. J Urol 1996;156:2007–2011.
31. Lue TF, Basson R, Rosen R, et al, eds. Second international consultation on sexual medicine: sexual dysfunction in men and women. Paris: Health Publications, 2004.
32. Enzlin P, Mathieu, Van den Bruel A, et al. Sexual dysfunction in women with type 1 diabetes. Diabetes Care 2002;25:672–677.
33. Jovanovic L. Finally it is our turn! Diabetes Care 2002;25:787–788.
34. Salonia A, Lanzi R, Scavini M, et al. Sexual function and endocrine profile in fertile women with type 1 diabetes. Diabetes Care 2006;29:312–316.
35. Erol B, Tefekli A, Sanli O, et al. Sexual dysfunction in type II diabetic females: a comparative study. J Sex Marital Ther 2002; 28 (suppl 1): 55–62.
36. Erol B, Tefekli A, Sanli O, et al. Does sexual dysfunction correlate with deterioration of somatic sensory system in diabetic women?. Int J Impot Res 2003; 15: 198–202.
37. Basson RJ, Rucker BM, Laird PG, et al. Sexuality of women with diabetes. J Sex Reprod Med 2001;1:11–20.
38. Ruggiero L, Wagner J, de Groot M. Understanding the individual: emotional and psychological challenges. In: American Association of Diabetes Educators' The Art and Science of Diabetes Self-Management Education. Chicago: AADE, 2006:59–89.
39. Kanaly KA, Berman JR. Sexual side effects of SSRI medications: potential treatment strategies for SSRI-induced female sexual dysfunction. Curr Womens Health Rep 2002; 6:409–16.
40. Payne KA, Binik YM, Amsel R, et al. When sex hurts, anxiety and fear orient attention towards pain. European J Pain 2005; 4:427–36.
41. Muniyappa R, Norton M, Dunn ME, et al. Diabetes and female sexual dysfunction: moving beyond "benign neglect". Curr Diabetes Report 2005; 3:230–6
42. Costrini NV, Kalkhoff, RK. Relative effects of pregnancy, estradiol, and progesterone on plasma insulin and pancreatic islet insulin secretion. J Clin Invest 1971; 5:992–9.
43. Goran MI, Gower BA. Longitudinal study on pubertal insulin resistance. Diabetes Care 2001; 24:1144–1150.
44. Rossi R, Origlianni G, Modena M. Transdermal 17 β-Estradiol and risk of developing type 2 diabetes in a population of healthy, nonobese postmenopausal women. Diabetes Care 2004; 27:645–9.
45. Sites CK, L'Hommedieu GD, Toth MJ, et al. The effect of hormone replacement therapy on body composition, body fat distribution, and insulin sensitivity in menopausal women. J Clin Endo Metab. 2005; 5:2701–7.
46. Clayton AH. Female sexual dysfunction related to depresión and antidepressant medications. Curr Womens Health Rep 2002; 3:182–7.
47. Ehrmann DA, Barnes RB, Rosenfield RL, et al. Prevalence of impaired glucose tolerance and diabetes in women with polysystic ovary síndrome. Diabetes Care. 1999; 1:141–6.
48. Doruk EH, Akabay E, Cayan S, et al. Effect of diabetes mellitus on female sexual function and risk factors. Arch Androl 2005; 51:1–6
49. Caruso S, Rugolo S. Mirabella D, et al. Changes in clitoral blood flow in premenopausal women affected by type 1 diabetes after single 100-mg administration of sildenafil. Urology 2006;68:161–165.

50. Roszler J, Rice D. For her. In: Sex and Diabetes. Alexandria: American Diabetes Association, 2007:71–87.
51. Rice D, Jack L. Use of an assessment tool to enhance the diabetes educator's ability to identify erectile dysfunction. Diabetes Educ. 2006;32:373–380.
52. Roszler J, Rice D. Chapter 1. In: Sex and Diabetes. Alexandria: American Diabetes Association, 2007:10–11.

15 Diabetes in Pregnancy

Elizabeth S. Halprin, MD

CONTENTS

INTRODUCTION
METABOLIC CHANGES DURING PREGNANCY
WOMEN WITH PRE-EXISTING DIABETES MELLITUS
GESTATIONAL DIABETES
BREASTFEEDING FOR WOMEN WITH PRE-EXISTING
    DIABETES MELLITUS OR GESTATIONAL DIABETES
CONTINUING CARE
REFERENCES

ABSTRACT

A review of present practices in the assessment and treatment of diabetes during pregnancy is presented, including preconception counseling, insulin therapy, nutrition and exercise therapy of patients with pre-existing diabetes, care of patients with gestational diabetes, and post-partum care for infants and mothers of both conditions.

Key Words: diabetes, pregnancy, gestational diabetes, preconception counseling, glucose management

INTRODUCTION

Women with diabetes were told in the past that they could not have babies. This is no longer the case, but this cannot be achieved without significant work on the part of the family and the provider. Similarly, for women in whom

From: *Contemporary Diabetes: Educating Your Patient with Diabetes*
Edited by: K. Weinger and C. A. Carver, DOI 10.1007/978-1-60327-208-7_15,
© Humana Press, a part of Springer Science+Business Media, LLC 2009

diabetes develops during pregnancy, proper attention and treatment ensures a healthy outcome.

METABOLIC CHANGES DURING PREGNANCY

Many hormonal and metabolic changes occur during pregnancy. Placental hormones cause an increase in insulin resistance for women with and without diabetes. In the case of no pre-existing diabetes, if insulin production cannot keep pace with growing insulin resistance, relative carbohydrate intolerance develops with resulting elevated blood glucose levels. This presents toward the end of the second trimester or beginning of the third trimester and is referred to as gestational diabetes (GDM) *(1)*. This glucose intolerance may present earlier in the pregnancy and may be an indicator of predisposition for development or continuation of diabetes post partum *(2)*. For insulin-dependent women with pre-existing diabetes, insulin requirements increase dramatically at this time.

WOMEN WITH PRE-EXISTING DIABETES MELLITUS

The best service we can offer our patients is to stress that they should plan for pregnancy, as opposed to aiming for rapid glycemic improvement once already pregnant.

Preconception Counseling

Addressing diabetes control well before conception decreases risk of poor pregnancy outcome *(3)*. Despite the fact that many women of childbearing age do not intend to get pregnant in the immediate future, it is common that they have no plan in place for contraception. Every visit for a woman with diabetes of childbearing age must address this issue – a direct question about contraception methods. Intentions to begin a family are often impetus enough for a woman who previously did not keep her glucose in target range to begin doing so. All too often, this motivation begins only once pregnancy develops *(4)*.

Preconception achievement of tight glucose control results in remarkable outcome improvement *(5)*. However, two-third of pregnancies today are unplanned. Although preconception care has improved in the type 1 population, it has decreased in the type 2 population of childbearing years, which is growing *(6)*. The populations at particular risk require a proactive approach to preconception care. Women with diabetes who do *not* seek preconception care are poorer, more likely to belong to an ethnic or racial minority, more likely to be uninsured, have less family support, and less substantive relations with their medical providers than those that do seek preconception care *(7)*. Consequently, they require more focused attention. *All women with diabetes of childbearing age should use effective contraception and be counseled on the risks of pregnancy and poor metabolic control* (Table 1).

The pioneer physician in attention to women with diabetes was Joslin Clinic's Priscilla White. By recognizing the different factors of diabetes that negatively influenced pregnancy, she stratified her patients. The specific factors she identified were age, duration of diabetes, presence or lack of complications (particularly retinopathy, nephropathy, and cardiac disease), and presence or lack of hypertension *(8)*. The White classification system, while not always strictly applied to each patient today, is a warning flag that particular attention is required for all women with diabetes. All women, except for those with diet-controlled GDM or diet-controlled type 2 diabetes, should be treated with insulin *(9)*.

Fetal Risks

MALFORMATION

Research shows women with diabetes who presented for care prior to conception bore infants with a 2–3% risk of malformation, while women who presented for care post-conception had infants with 6–10% risk of malformation *(10)*. Studies also suggest a relationship between maternal hyperglycemia and congenital malformation. In one study, patients with an A1C <8.5% bore infants with malformations 3.4% of the time, while patients with an A1C >8.5% bore infants with malformations 22.4% of the time *(11)*. Common malformations (neural tube, renal, and cardiac) occur before the 7th week after conception and are more severe if they occur during blastogenesis (1st 4 weeks post conception) than during organogenesis (weeks 4–5 post conception) *(12)*. All malformations can increase the risk of spontaneous abortion *(13)*.

MACROSOMIA

Macrosomia (a fetus with > 90th percentile weight for gestational age) has been shown to be more closely related to postprandial hyperglycemia than with fasting hyperglycemia *(14)*. Therefore, while strict A1C targets are crucial, they are not sufficient on their own to encompass treatment. Maintaining postprandial blood glucose levels within the goal of <130 at 1 h postprandial is key in preventing macrosomia. Macrosomic infants show increased risk of birth trauma, neonatal hypoglycemia, hyperbilirubinemia, respiratory distress, erythrocytosis, and hypertrophic cardiomyopathy *(15)*.

INTRAUTERINE GROWTH RESTRICTION (IUGR)

IUGR is typically seen in women with type 1 diabetes with poor placental perfusion related to microvascular disease *(16)*.

Table 1

Preconception Evaluation and Counseling

Counseling	Medical evaluation	Laboratory	Skills/parameters
• Glucose and A1c goals • Risks to mother and fetus outlined • Contraception until goals reached • Exercise and nutrition assessment • Prenatal vitamins • Recommendation for high-risk obstetrician • Smoking cessation • Alcohol cessation	• Diabetes history • Complications • Previous pregnancies • Past medical history • Referrals to ophthalmology, cardiac evaluation, renal as needed • Medications – changing from oral agents to appropriate insulin regimen, stopping medications contraindicated in pregnancy (ACE, ARB, Statins, etc) • Blood pressure evaluation, treatment with pregnancy appropriate medications	• Hgb A1c • Microalbumin • Lipids • Renal function • Thyroid function • Cardiac testing as indicated	• Assessment of techniques • Self-management • Sick-day rules • Exercise adjustments

Maternal Risks

HYPOGLYCEMIA

Given the risk of hyperglycemia and the need for tight control to avoid fetal malformation, hypoglycemia will likely increase as blood glucose trends within target range. The maternal risks are clear – loss of consciousness, seizures, accidents, etc. Less is known about risk to the fetus. Studies have shown that women at risk for severe hypoglycemia have a history of severe hypoglycemia in the 4 months prior to gestation, have had diabetes for >10 years, are on a daily insulin dose of >0.1 unit/kg or have an A1C <6.5%. Pregnancy itself can predispose to severe hypoglycemia due to nausea and vomiting. In addition, it is possible that pregnancy decreases the counter-regulatory responses for hypoglycemia (17).

DIABETIC KETOACIDOSIS (DKA)

Ketonuria is common in pregnancy but can be avoided by using more frequent meals and snacks. However, due to accelerated metabolism during pregnancy, DKA may occur more rapidly (18). Treatment for DKA is similar to that for non-pregnant patients, but if the patient is unable to tolerate any glucose orally, it is of utmost importance to supply 100–150 grams of intravenous glucose to meet the increased demands of pregnancy. The risk of fetal mortality in DKA is very high, but decreases dramatically once the patient is hospitalized and treated (19).

RETINOPATHY

Retinopathy can be directly affected by pregnancy. Mild to moderate non-proliferative retinopathy can worsen during pregnancy and generally returns to prepregnancy state after the baby is born. Severe non-proliferative retinopathy, however, may require laser intervention prior to pregnancy and even during pregnancy in some cases (20). If proliferative retinopathy is present prior to conception, disease is likely to progress more rapidly after conception. Patients with higher A1Cs prior to pregnancy are at higher risk for worsening retinal disease during pregnancy, which argues in favor of achieving excellent glucose control slowly and steadily prior to conception (21). Each patient should have a dilated eye exam prior to conception to assess the degree of retinopathy and the safety of proceeding with pregnancy (22). Most patients are seen by an ophthalmologist at least once during each trimester, and then again post partum.

Renal Function

In non-diabetic pregnancies, there is an increase in glomerular filtration rate and protein excretion, both of which return to normal post partum (23). However, if there is pre-existing advanced renal disease, the added stress of pregnancy may cause these changes to be permanent. Increased protein excretion is more marked during the last weeks of pregnancy and peaks one week post partum. By six weeks post partum, protein excretion should return to normal; hypertension may exacerbate this progression. Women with frank proteinuria are at increased risk of chronic hypertension and preeclampsia (24). Fetal complications are also increased in this group of women, with an increase in intrauterine growth retardation, preterm delivery, and neonatal respiratory distress syndrome in 15–25% (13). As ACE inhibitors are contraindicated for use in all pregnancies, they should not be used in women even considering pregnancy (due to the risk of congenital malformations) (25). If creatinine is greater than 1.5 mg/dl or creatinine clearance is <50 ml/min, then consider delaying pregnancy until renal function is improved and stable. Methyldopa, calcium channel blockers, and labetolol can be used to treat hypertension in pregnant women. ACE inhibitors should be stopped prior to conception but can be restarted post partum even if the patient plans on breastfeeding.

HYPERTENSIVE DISORDERS

Hypertension during pregnancy is classified as (26):

- chronic hypertension, which is blood pressure >140/90 mmHg noted before pregnancy or up to the 20th week of gestation
- preeclampsia-eclampsia, after 20 weeks gestation, with proteinuria of >0.3 g per 24 hour specimen
- preeclampsia-eclampsia superimposed on chronic hypertension, associated with a sudden increase in blood pressure, associated with new proteinuria, HELLP syndrome (hemolytic anemia, elevated liver enzymes, low platelet counts)
- gestational hypertension, diagnosed after 20 weeks gestation, without signs of preeclampsia
- transient hypertension

Treatment includes sodium restriction, increased exercise, and medications listed above (27).

GLUCOSE MANAGEMENT

Glucose goals during pregnancy are very strict but are still tailored to prevent hypoglycemia. Prior to conception, approach the goals that will be required when pregnant and aim for an A1C of <6.5% (28). See Table 2 for blood glucose goals for women with type 1 or type 2 diabetes.

The goals for a patient with type 2 diabetes should be achieved on the regimen she will need to be on during pregnancy. It is not sufficient or optimal to have an A1C of <6.5% on her oral agent regimen, or on insulins not used in pregnancy, only to change to a different regimen once she has conceived.

Table 2
Target Goals for Women with Type 1 or Type 2 Diabetes

Target Goals – glucose	Preconception	During Pregnancy
Fasting	80–110	60–99
1 h post prandial	Not monitored	< 130
2 h post-prandial	100–155	<120

Insulin should be changed to at least 2 doses of NPH and premeal fast acting, either lispro or aspart. As many as 4 smaller doses of NPH may be used, which confers a more peakless basal insulin level. The patient should be assessed for the ability to count carbohydrates and adjust premeal insulin based on carbohydrate content of the meal, including a correction for elevated blood glucose. The insulin pump is another treatment option, even for type 2 patients planning pregnancy. Tight control can be reached more easily on the pump when it is used in the right population. However, there is a higher risk of DKA due to pump failure and the prevention of this should be reviewed thoroughly (29). Human regular insulin may be used in some women with gastroparesis, but otherwise does not address the issue of peak postprandial blood glucose and increases the risk of hypoglycemia. Glargine insulin is not approved in pregnancy at this time, as there is little information on safety. Increased IGF-1 receptor affinity and mitogenic potency compared with human insulin have made this a hypothetical risk for teratogenicity (30).

Medical Assessment

Medical assessment should include a review of other past medical history. Functional cardiac evaluation should be undertaken if the woman is over 35, has had 20 or more years of diabetes and one or more additional cardiac risks (hypertension, tobacco use, family history, high lipids, microalbumin, nephropathy) (31). Hypertension needs to be strictly controlled and cholesterol should be checked. Triglycerides increase during pregnancy; omega 3 fatty acids can be used to treat this prior to and during gestation. Any other lipid-lowering agents should be discontinued (32). Thyroid status should be evaluated. Thyroid replacement dose usually requires adjustment upward by 4–6 weeks and can be by as much as 30–50%. A monthly thyroid stimulating hormone (TSH) should be measured and adjustments made in thyroid hormone replacement (33). If the patient is on any psychiatric medications, she should meet with her prescribing provider to help adjust pregnancy-safe psychiatric medications. The gynecologic and obstetric history should also be reviewed.

MEDICATIONS

Oral agents are discontinued and supplanted with insulin, ideally prior to conception (34). Metformin is the possible exception, if used in the treatment of polycystic ovary disease prior to conception. It can be continued through the first trimester and should be discontinued with simultaneous increases in insulin (35). The insulin regimen may be initiated or changed at the first preconception visit.

Management During Pregnancy

The work involved on the part of the patient to maintain glucose levels within goal is significant and time-consuming and must be both acknowledged and appreciated. All benefits and decreased risk associated with tight control must be continually stressed to the patient. Blood glucose should be monitored daily premeal, one hour post meal, at bedtime and occasionally overnight according to prescribed goals.

Nutrition

Nutrition counseling should begin before conception, and all pregnant women should see a registered dietitian. Daily records of diet are encouraged, at least initially. Women should be instructed in either basic or advanced carbohydrate counting skills for consistent carbohydrates or individualized insulin to carbohydrate ratios (36). A meal plan that is successful addresses not only the researched issues listed in Table 3, but also takes into account the individual characteristics that make up each woman, such as cultural, religious, psychosocial, work and family schedules, and finances.

Exercise

Exercise has both positive and detrimental effects on glucose control during pregnancy. While it lowers glucose levels acutely and chronically, it must be taken into account when planning an individual diabetes program. Exercise in the first trimester may increase the risk of spontaneous abortion; exercise also increases insulin sensitivity and enhances insulin action in extramuscular tissue (38), which can cause hypoglycemia. If the exercise program makes it harder for a woman with type 1 diabetes to maintain blood glucose control, then it becomes a risk for early spontaneous abortion (39). Absolute contraindications to exercise during pregnancy in diabetes are the same as for women without diabetes and can be found in corresponding texts.

Table 3
Nutritional Recommendations for Pre-existing diabetes mellitus in pregnancy (*37*)

Calories (distributed over 6–8 small meals and snacks)	BMI (Institute of Medicine)	Kcal/kg prepregnancy weight	Recommended weight gain (lbs)
	Underweight (<19.8)	36–40	28–40
	Normal (1.8–26)	30	25–35
	Overweight (26.1–29)	24	15–25
	Obese (>29)	Not <1800 kcal total daily	> 15
	Twins/Triplets	?	35–55
Carbohydrates	45–55% of total calories (Ex. 30/15/45/15/60/15). Minimum of 175 g carb/day Fiber 25–35 g/day		
Protein Fat	0.8 g/kg DBW plus and additional 25 g/day (20–25% of total calories) 30–35% total calories with <10% from saturated fat		
Nutritive and non-nutritive sweeteners	Although not proven to be detrimental in fetal health, women who consume "calorie-free" soft drinks and candies are likely missing more nutritious foods and drinks. • Sugar alcohols are safe, but may be laxative • Non- nutritive – aspartame, acesulfame potassium, sucralose = safe • No saccharin		

Ketones

Urine ketones should be checked every morning on the first urine of the day. These serve as an indicator of the body's use of fat for fuel during times of relative "starvation," or when food intake is spaced out. Many women, trying to keep insulin doses down, will drastically limit their carbohydrate ingestion and induce ketone production, particularly in the morning after an overnight without food. There is some suggestion, albeit not firm, that ketone production in the mother is associated with lower IQ in the baby *(40,41)*. As ketones are monitored, the meal plan should be adjusted to try to decrease them. In some cases, ensuring frequent small meals and a good bedtime snack will eliminate ketone production.

Delivery

The timing and method of delivery for women with diabetes mellitus is influenced by the specifics of diabetes and its complications in addition to the usual obstetric guidelines. If active retinopathy is present, then cesarean section is recommended to avoid the increased pressure of active labor. Cesareans are also recommended based on estimated baby weight at delivery (42,43).

Euglycemia is the goal during delivery. If the delivery is planned, then the usual nighttime NPH insulin is given the night before and approximately 1/2 of the morning NPH. While still eating, women can use their usual bolus dose of fast acting insulin. Once in active labor, or during cesarean section, an IV insulin infusion should be initiated together with a 10% dextrose drip to maintain the glucose level between 80 and 110 mg/dl. If the patient has been on an insulin pump, it can be continued during delivery, but should be replaced with an IV insulin infusion if blood glucose levels cannot be maintained between 80 and 110 mg/dl. Elevated glucose levels in the mother during delivery increase the risk of neonatal hypoglycemia within the first hours of delivery (44).

Postpartum Management

Insulin requirements for the mother decrease markedly immediately postpartum. At this point, blood glucose goals should be liberated, although many women will have become fixated on the very tight control they obtained during pregnancy. One-half to one-third of the *preconception* insulin dose should be used in the immediate postpartum visit. These requirements will increase slowly over the coming weeks (13). Breastfeeding adds to the risk of hypoglycemia for the mother, and it is common for a woman to need to feed herself as she feeds her baby. A postpartum visit at 2 weeks is an appropriate time to assess insulin regimen as glucose levels will be somewhat stabilized. At the 6-week postpartum visit laboratory assessment of urine microalbumin, renal function, thyroid function should be done. ACE inhibitors are considered safe for breastfeeding and can be restarted or initiated at this time if indicated (45). A postpartum dilated eye exam should be scheduled. Thyroid replacement should be returned to the preconception dose immediately post partum (46). Once again, the issue of contraception should be addressed and the importance of planning for future pregnancies stressed (47).

GESTATIONAL DIABETES

Definition and Significance

Gestational diabetes (GDM) is a carbohydrate intolerance that presents or is first recognized during pregnancy (2). It is important to identify gestational diabetes both to maintain a closer eye on the fetus during pregnancy and to identify women at risk for development of type 2 diabetes. There are varying degrees of GDM prevalence, depending on the population (44). Intensive management of GDM has decreased intrauterine fetal demise to a level not much higher than in the general population. Morbidity, however, still is elevated in this population. This is related to excessive fetal growth, which is directly related to maternal hyperglycemia, increased glucose delivery to the fetus, and a subsequent increase in fetal insulin levels. Increased fetal size, in turn, can result in birth trauma, maternal trauma, possible long-lasting glucose intolerance and obesity in the offspring, as well as increase in rate of cesarean section *(48)*. Preeclampsia is also more common in GDM pregnancy. Complications that are more prevalent in the infants of GDM pregnancies include hypoglycemia, hyperbilirubinemia, hypocalcemia, and poor feeding *(49)*. Details on screening and diagnosis of GDM can be found in multiple other sources.

Management of Gestation Diabetes

All women with GDM should be instructed in self-monitoring and provided with a glucose meter in order to check glucose both fasting and 1 hour after every meal. Target goals are similar to those for women with pre-existing diabetes (see Table 2). Initial evaluation will include assessment of the woman's body mass index, level of physical activity, and present diet. Nutritional changes may be sufficient to control the fasting and postprandial glucose levels, but in at least 50% of women with GDM, insulin treatment is required *(36)*. Basics for nutritional treatment of GDM fulfill nutrient requirements for pregnancy without inducing weight loss, ketone production, or excessive weight gain. A registered dietitian should be part of the medical team to work with the patient to create a meal plan that is individualized and culturally appropriate *(50)*. Calorie restriction can improve blood glucose levels, but excessive restriction will limit weight gain during pregnancy and induce undesirable ketone production. Weight gain recommendations for women with GDM are similar to those for women with pre-existing diabetes mellitus in Table 3. Women with GDM have often surpassed these recommendations by the time they are diagnosed. Studies have shown that restricting calories to <1500 calories per day (50%), increases ketonuria and ketonemia, while a more modest restriction of 1600–1800 calories (33%) controls weight gain without ketone production *(51)*. To control postprandial glucose levels, we adjust the carbohydrate content of each meal, as outlined in Table 3.

EXERCISE

Exercise is very important in decreasing the insulin resistance of GDM. Women should not initiate a strenuous exercise program if they were previously sedentary, but a walking program can be very useful in decreasing postprandial glucose peaks *(52)*.

ORAL MEDICATIONS

If blood glucose remains elevated with the changes mentioned above in nutrition and exercise, medication is required. Oral medications are not indicated in pregnancy, although this is an area of great debate. Of all the oral agents, the sulfonylurea glyburide seems to have the least placental transfer, therefore inducing less insulin production in the fetus (53). It is rarely used in mild GDM cases of women who are not morbidly obese. We do not generally use any oral agents in GDM.

INSULIN

GDM insulin is initiated based on fasting and 1 hour postprandial blood glucose levels. As insulin resistance increases with the progression of the pregnancy, doses will need to be added and/or increased on a regular basis. The insulin regimen must be individualized, and adjusted regularly. Patients should check in via faxed or emailed logbooks at least weekly. There is some discussion regarding the use of abdominal circumference to determine the need for insulin and the blood glucose goals for each woman, but there is no clear consensus on this practice (54).

Obstetric Considerations

MATERNAL SURVEILLANCE

Prematurity increases in untreated or poorly controlled GDM. The use of corticosteroids is not contraindicated, despite the likely increase in glucose levels. Insulin needs to be adjusted during the 48 hours of steroid treatments (44). The risk of hypertension increases in association with GDM – therefore, blood pressure and urinary protein should be measured at each prenatal visit.

DELIVERY

If the mother did not require insulin during the pregnancy then insulin will likely not be required during delivery. However, the same glucose goals of 80–110 mg/dl apply, with insulin drip only if necessary (55).

POSTPARTUM

Mother – Once the baby and placenta have been delivered, the insulin resistance that was caused by the conceptus resolves rapidly and blood glucose levels return to normal. In the hospital, blood glucose levels are checked at fasting and 2 hours postprandially for 24 hours. If glucose levels are high enough that medications are required and breastfeeding is planned, insulin must be continued. There are no specific recommendations for the prevention of future type 2 diabetes, the risk of which is approximately 50% in the following 20 years (56). A 2 hours 75 grams oral glucose tolerance test is performed from 6 to 12 weeks post partum and random glucose levels should be measured annually. Some studies indicate that a 5–7% loss of prepregnancy weight will markedly decrease the risk of developing type 2 diabetes *(57)*. Additionally there is an increased risk of GDM in future pregnancies and testing should be undertaken earlier in the future pregnancies than for women of lower risk.

Infant – In the immediate postpartum period, there is an increased risk of neonatal hypoglycemia, stemming from the fetus' own insulin production in response to glucose levels of the mother *(58)*. Once the baby is delivered, that glucose source no longer exists, but insulin levels may remain elevated for a short period. Assessment of the baby's glucose level should be done in the first hour of life.

Childhood obesity may be related to the level of hyperglycemia in the mother during pregnancy. Therefore, it is even more important to screen for and treat gestational diabetes in hopes of further prevention of obesity in an increasingly younger population *(59)*.

BREASTFEEDING FOR WOMEN WITH PRE-EXISTING DIABETES MELLITUS OR GESTATIONAL DIABETES

It is well established that breastfeeding is beneficial to both woman and child. This is also true for diabetic pregnancy, as there is evidence for decreased risk of future type 2 diabetes in the mother, as well as protection against breast and ovarian cancer *(60)*. For the baby, breastfeeding provides protection against over- and under-nutrition in early childhood. It may also decrease risk in the offspring of obesity, hypertension, cardiovascular disease, and diabetes. Breastfeeding seems to improve glucose tolerance in the baby's early postpartum period, but whether it confers a decrease in risk of developing type 2 diabetes is less clear *(61)*.

CONTINUING CARE

Although the post partum visits are often overlooked by both practitioner and patient, they are an invaluable opportunity to encourage all women to continue taking as good care of themselves as they did during their pregnancy. This opportunity to educate women who have withstood a pregnancy complicated by pre-existing or gestational diabetes mellitus is integral in the prevention of future type 2 diabetes for both mother and child. Continuing a healthy diet, exercising regularly, and maintaining a healthy weight for the rest of their lives will be key in this process for all women that have successfully navigated pregnancy with diabetes mellitus. For women with pre-existing diabetes, their glucose control may never have been so excellent. Although their lives with a new baby are certainly not going to be any easier, staying healthy for their family's sake may be inspiration enough for them to continue excellent diabetes control.

REFERENCES

1. Catalano PM, Tyzbir ED, Wolfe RR, et al. Carbohydrate metabolism during pregnancy in control subjects and women with gestational diabetes. *Am J Physiol* 1993; 264; E60–E6.
2. Buchanan T, Xiang A, et al. What is gestational diabetes?. *Diabetes Care* 2007; 30 (2): S105.
3. KitzmillerJL, Buchanan TA, Kjos S, Combs CA, Ratner RE. Pre-conception care of diabetes, congenital malformations, and spontaneous abortions. *Diabetes Care* 1996; 19:514–541.
4. Steel JM, Johnstone FD, Hepburn DA, Smith AF. Can prepregnancy care of diabetic women reduce the risk of abnormal babies?. *BMJ* 1990; 301: 1070–1074.
5. Temple R, et al. Prepregnancy care and pregnancy outcomes in women with type 1 diabetes. *Diabetes Care* 2006; 29: 1744–1749.
6. Willhoite MB, Bennert HW, Palomake GE, Zaremba MM, Herman WH, Williams JR, Spear NH. The Impact of preconception counseling pregnancy outcomes: the experience of the Maine diabetes in pregnancy program. *Diabetes Care* 1993 16:450–455.
7. Holing EV, Beyer CS, Brown ZA, Connell FA. Why don't women with diabetes plan their pregnancies?. *Diabetes Care* 1998 21: 889–895.
8. White P. Pregnancy complicating diabetes. *Am J Med* 1949; 7:609–616.
9. Hare J, White P. Gestational diabetes and the white classification. *Diabetes Care* 1980;3:394.
10. Miller E, Hare JW, Cloherty JP, et al. Elevated maternal hemoglobin A1c in early pregnancy and major congenital anomalies in infants of diabetic mothers. *N Engl J Med* 1981; 304: 1331–1334.
11. Greene M, Hare JW, Cloherty JP, et al. First trimester hemoglobin A1 and risk for major malformations. *Teratology* 1989; 39:225–331.
12. Mills JL, Baker L, Goldman AS. Malformations in infants of diabetic mothers occur before the seventh gestational week. Implications for treatment. *Diabetes* 1979; 28:292–293.
13. Brown, F, Goldfine A. Diabetes and pregnancy. In: Joslin's Diabetes Mellitus, 14th Eds. Lippincott Williams & Wilkins, 2005: 1035–1048.
14. Jovanovic-Peterson L, Peterson CM, Reed GF, Metzger BE, Mills JL, Knopp RH, Aarons JH. Maternal postprandial glucose levels and infant birth weight: the diabetes in early pregnancy study. *Am J Obstet Gynecol* 1991; 164:103–111.
15. Yang J, Cummings EA, O'Connell C, Jangaard K. Fetal and neonatal outcomes of diabetic pregnancies. *Obstet Gynecol* 2006; 108:644–650.
16. Farrell T, Neale L, Cundy T. Congenital anomalies in the offspring of women with type 1, type 2, and gestational diabetes. *Diabet Med* 2002; 19:322–326.
17. Inge M, Evers, et al. Risk Indicators predictive for severe hypoglycemia during the first trimester of Type 1 diabetic pregnancy. Diabetes Care; 2002; 24:554–559.
18. Barbour L, Friedman J. Management of diabetes in pregnancy in EndoText.com 2003
19. Cullen MT, Reece EA, Homko CJ et al. The changing presentations of diabetic ketoacidosis during pregnancy. *Am J Pernat* 1996; 13(7):449–51.
20. Chew, EY, et al. Metabolic control and progression retinopathy. The diabetes in early pregnancy study. National Institute for Child Health and Human Development Diabetes in Early Pregnancy Study. *Diabetes Care* 1995; 18: 631–637.
21. Diabetes Control and Complications Trial Research Group. Effect of pregnancy on microvascular complications in the diabetes control and complications trial. *Diabetes Care* 2000; 23:1084–91.
22. Lauszus F, Klebe JG, Bek T. Diabetic retinopathy in pregnancy during tight metabolic control. *Acta Obstet Gynecol Scand* 2000; 79(5):367–70.
23. Biesenbach G, Zazgornik J. Incidence of transient nephrotic syndrome during pregnany in diabetic women with and without pre-existing microalbuminuria. *BMJ* 1989;299:366–7.
24. Rossing K, Jacobsen P, Hommel E, Mathiesen E, Svenningsen A, Rossing P, Parving HH. Pregnancy and progression of diabetic nephropathy.*Diabetologia* 2002; 45(1):36–41.

25. Cooper, William, et al. Major congenital malformations after first-trimester exposure to ACE inhibitors. NEJM 2006; 354:2443–2451.
26. Roberts, JM. et al. Summary of the NHLBI working group on research on hypertension during pregnancy. *Hypertension* 2003;41: 437–445.
27. Leguzamon G, Reece EA. Effect of medical therapy on progressive nephropathy: influence of pregnancy, diabetes, and hypertension. *J Mat-Fet Med* 2000; 9(1):70–78.
28. Casson IF, Clarke CA, Howard CV, McKendrick O, Pennycook S, Pharoah POD, et al. Outcomes of pregnancy in insulin dependent diabetic women: results of a five year population cohort study. *Br Med J* 1997; 315:275–78.
29. Gabbe SG, Holing E, Temple P, Brown ZA. Benefits, risks, costs, and patient satisfaction associated with insulin pump therapy for the pregnancy complicated by type 1 diabetes mellitus. *Am J Obstet Gynecol* 2000; 182:1283–91.
30. Hofmann T, Horstmann G, Stammberger I. Evaluation of the reproductive toxicity and embryotoxicity of insulin glargine (LANTUS) in rats and rabbits. *Int J Tox* 2002; 21(3): 181–9.
31. Barbour LA, Laiffer SA. Preconception counseling. In Lee RV, Rosene-Montella K, Barbour LA, Garner PR, Keely E (eds). Medical care of the pregnant patient, Philadelphia, American College of Physicians 2000:1–18.
32. Hsia SH, Connelly PW, Hegele RA. Successful outcome in severe pregnancy-associated hyperlipemia: a case report and literature review. *Am J Med Sci* 1995; 309:213–218.
33. Abalovich M, et al. Management of thyroid dysfunction during pregnancy and postpartum: an endocrine society clinical practice guideline. *The Journal of Clinical Endocrinology & Metabolism* 2007; 92: S1–S47.
34. Hellmuth E, Damm P, Molsted-Pedersen L. Oral hypoglycaemic agents in 118 diabetic pregnancies. *Diabetic Med* 2000;17(7):507–11.
35. Jakubowicz DJ, Iuorno MJ, Jakubowicz S, Roberts KA, Nestler JE. Effects of metformin on early pregnancy loss in the polycystic ovary syndrome. *J Clinical Endo Metab* 2002;89(2):524–9.
36. Reader D. Medical nutrition therapy and lifestyle interventions. *Diabetes Care* 2007; 30:S188–S193
37. Position of the American Dietetic Association. *J Am Diet Assoc* 2002; 102:1470–1490.
38. Harris GD, White RD. Diabetes management and exercise in pregnant patients with diabetes. *Clin Diabetes* 2005; 23: 165–168.
39. Jovanovic L, et al. In: Guide to Physical Activity, American Association of Clinical Endocrinologists Physical Activity for Pregnant Women with Diabetes, 2006; 55–63.
40. Churchill JA, Berendes HW, Nemore J. Neuropsychological deficits in children of diabetic mothers: a report from the Collaborative Study of Cerebral Palsy. *Am J Obstet Gynecol* 1969; 105: 257–268.
41. Gin H, Vambergue A, Vasseur C. Blood ketone monitoring: a comparison between gestational diabetes and non-diabetic pregnant women. *Diabetes & Metabolism* 2006,32, 6: 592–597.
42. Mazouni C, Rouzier R, Collette E, Menard JP, Magnin G, Gamerre M, Deter R. Development and validation of a nomogram to predict the risk of cesarean delivery in macrosomi. *Acta Obstet Gynecol Scand* 2008;87(5):518–23. 43, (43)
43. Hod M, Bar J, Peled Y, et al. Antepartum management protocol. Timing and mode of delivery in gestational diabetes. *Diabetes Care* 1998;21 Suppl 2:B113–B117.
44. Metzger, Boyd E et al. Summary and recommendations of the fifth international workshop-conference on gestational diabetes mellitus. *Diabetes Care* 2007; 30: S251–260.
45. Briggs GC, Freeman RK, Yaffee SJ. Drugs in pregnancy and lactation, 6th edition. Baltimore: Williams and Wilkins 2001.
46. Abalovich AUM, Gutierrez S, Alcaraz G, Maccallini G, Garcia A. Overt and subclinical hypothyroidism complicating pregnancy. *Thyroid* 2002 Jan;12(1):63–8.

47. Kjos SL. Postpartum care of the woman with diabetes. *Clinical Obstet Gynecol* 2000; 43: 75–90.
48. Kuhl C. Etiology and pathogenesis of gestational diabetes. *Diabetes Care* 21:B19–26, 1998.
49. Uvena-Celebrezze J, Catalano P. The Infant of the woman with gestational diabetes mellitus. *Clinical Ob Gyn* 2000; 43(1):127–139.
50. ADA. Nutrition Recommendation and Interventions for diabetes. *Diabetes Care* 2007; 30: S48–S65.
51. Knopp RH, Magee MS, Raisys V, Benetti T. Metabolic effects of hypocaloric diets in management of gestational diabetes. *Diabetes* 1991; 40(Suppl 2):165–171.
52. Carpenter MW. The role of exercise in pregnant women with diabetes mellitus. *Clinical Obstet Gynecol* 2000; 43(1):56–64.
53. Langer O, Conway DL, Berkus MD, Xenakis EM-J, Gonzales O. A comparison of glyburide and insulin in women with gestational diabetes. *N Engl J Med* 343:1134–8, 2000.
54. Buchanan TA, Kjos SI, Montoro MN et al. Use of fetal ultrasound to select metabolic therapy for pregnancies complicated by mild gestational diabetes. *Diabetes Care* 1994; 17(4); 275–83.
55. Conway DL. Obstetric management in gestational diabetes. *Diabetes Care* 2007; 30: S175–S179.
56. Diabetes Prevention Program Research Group. Reduction in the incidence of type 2 diabetes with lifestyle intervention or metformin. *N Engl J Med* 2002; 346:393–403.
57. Ratner R. Prevention of type 2 diabetes in women with previous gestational diabetes. *Diabetes Care* 2007; 30:S242–245.
58. Silverman BL, Landsberg L, Metzger BE. Fetal hyperinsulinism in the offspring of diabetic mothers. Association with the subsequent development of childhood obesity. *Ann N Y Acad Sci* 1993; 699:36–45.
59. Silverman BL, Metzger BE, Cho NH, et al. Impaired glucose tolerance in adolescent offspring of diabetic mothers. Relationship to fetal hyperinsulinism. *Diabetes Care* 1995; 18:611–617.
60. Gunderson, E. Breastfeeding after gestational diabetes pregnancy. *Diabetes Care* 2007; 30:S161–168.
61. Martorell R, Stein AD, Schroeder DG. Early nutrition and later adiposity. *J Nutrition* 2001; 131(3):874S–80S

16 Pediatric Diabetes Education: A Family Affair

Arlene Smaldone, DNSc, CPNP, CDE
and Margaret T. Lawlor, MS, CDE

Contents

INTRODUCTION
DEVELOPMENT: THE FRAMEWORK
    OF DIABETES EDUCATION
ESSENTIALS OF DIABETES EDUCATION
PREPARATION FOR TRANSITIONS
SUMMARY
REFERENCES

ABSTRACT

Implementation of findings of the Diabetes Control and Complications Trial (DCCT) has dramatically changed diabetes care for pediatric patients. The purpose of this chapter, within the broader scope of this book, is to examine unique issues in caring for children and adolescents with diabetes and provide a synopsis of current clinical practice and research findings relevant to care of this population. Normative aspects of growth and development provide background to the need for tailoring diabetes education and self-care expectations according to a child's age and developmental stage. The role of the diabetes educator working with children and families during specific transition points through childhood is examined: school issues, camping diabetes style, adolescence, and transition to young adulthood.

Key Words: Diabetes, Children, Adolescents, Family, School, Camp, Depression, Eating disorders.

From: *Contemporary Diabetes: Educating Your Patient with Diabetes*
Edited by: K. Weinger and C. A. Carver, DOI 10.1007/978-1-60327-208-7_16,
© Humana Press, a part of Springer Science+Business Media, LLC 2009

INTRODUCTION

The purpose of this chapter is to examine unique issues in caring for children and adolescents with diabetes and provide a synopsis of current clinical practice and research findings relevant to care of this population. It begins with a review of the epidemiology and statistics for children with types 1 and 2 diabetes and changes in pediatric diabetes care since the Diabetes Control and Complication Trial (DCCT) *(1,2)*. This is followed by a brief discussion of the normative aspects of growth and development as rationale for tailoring diabetes education according to a child's age and developmental stage. The role of the diabetes educator is specifically examined during transition points through childhood: school issues, camping diabetes style, adolescence, and the post high school years. Throughout, the importance of a team approach and the role of parents and family in the management of diabetes are emphasized. Children and adolescents with diabetes can accomplish anything. However, living a normal life, in spite of diabetes, means that everyone must work diligently for it takes support, planning, and state-of-the-science diabetes care to accomplish this goal.

Diabetes is the second most common chronic disease in childhood. In 2001, the largest standardized registry of childhood diabetes in the United States was compiled as part of the Search for Diabetes in Youth Study *(3)* and provides current epidemiological estimates of incidence and prevalence for both type 1 and type 2 diabetes in youth. Findings of this study demonstrate that the incidence of type 1 diabetes in youth is higher than reported previously and varies by age, race, and ethnic background. Collectively, types 1 and 2 diabetes affect approximately 1.8 per 1,000 children in the United States. This translates to 154,369 children less than 20 years of age living with diabetes *(4)*. The incidence of pediatric type 1 diabetes is also rising worldwide *(5)*. Although children are most often diagnosed during the time of puberty, the highest age-specific increase has occurred in young children *(6)* with approximately 20% of new cases diagnosed in children ≤5 years *(7)*. Although type 1 diabetes remains the most prevalent form of diabetes in childhood, type 2 diabetes among youth *(8)* and the pediatric obesity epidemic have emerged as national public health concerns. Although still relatively infrequent in American youth compared to type 1 diabetes, the highest rates of type 2 diabetes are observed among older adolescents of all racial/ethnic minority groups *(3)*.

The DCCT *(1,2)* clearly demonstrated the importance of glycemic control in preventing or forestalling long-term complications of diabetes. The Epidemiology of Diabetes Interventions and Complications (EDIC) Study *(9,10)* continues to prospectively monitor DCCT participants and provides ongoing evidence that the improved metabolic control achieved for those in the intensively treated group remains protective against the long-term complications of diabetes. It is important to remember that, although more than 1,400 research subjects participated in the DCCT, fewer than 200 were adolescents; children

<13 years did not meet inclusion criteria for DCCT participation. During the DCCT, severe hypoglycemia was three times more frequent in adolescents compared to adults (2). Therefore, clinicians were initially cautious of the application of DCCT findings to pediatric patients because of risk of hypoglycemia (2) and safety of intensive insulin regimens when young children were away from parental supervision. However, recent reports (11–16) provide evidence that intensive insulin regimens are both safe and efficacious even when used in young children.

Advancements in technology have allowed incorporation of DCCT findings into routine care of children with diabetes in all settings and are not merely limited to care provided at major pediatric diabetes centers. Intensive management is now as much a part of diabetes treatment for children as it is for adults. Current American Diabetes Association standards of care for children with type 1 diabetes (17) reflect both lower glycemic targets and intensive insulin regimens using multiple daily injections or insulin pump therapy as the means to achieve them.

DEVELOPMENT: THE FRAMEWORK OF DIABETES EDUCATION

Combine diabetes with its chronic nature and management complexities with the normal tasks of childhood or adolescence and it is easy to understand why glycemic control presents special challenges to children and adolescents with diabetes and their families. Several multi-center pediatric studies have demonstrated that only a minority of patients achieve an A1C <8.0% (18–20). Optimal glycemic control requires a high level of daily commitment to diabetes management tasks. Parental involvement is key to effective pediatric diabetes self-management (17,21,22).

Physical, cognitive, and psychosocial growth and development patterns of children and adolescents with diabetes should mimic peers without diabetes. However, these domains both impact and are impacted by diabetes. For example, psychosocial factors such as positive family involvement (21,22) are prerequisites to optimal glycemic control in children and adolescents whereas other factors such as diabetes-specific family conflict (23–25) and diabetes burnout are detrimental. Therefore, recognizing and anticipating how diabetes and its management may influence normative growth and development patterns is important.

Development occurs over a continuum throughout the life cycle. Attainment of each new stage requires mastery of the preceding one. Children and adolescents with diabetes travel this continuum in the same sequence as those who do not have diabetes. Use of developmental frameworks enables us to understand normative cognitive and psychosocial development in children and adolescents.

Further, it provides both the practitioner and the family with a foundation for understanding the child or adolescent with diabetes because it may be difficult to differentiate whether a particular behavior reflects normative development or a response to diabetes or its daily management tasks. This background provides an ongoing opportunity for the diabetes health care team, in particular the diabetes educator, to revisit developmentally appropriate realistic expectations, problem solving techniques, and anticipatory guidance to the child or adolescent with diabetes and his/her family (17) at each new developmental stage.

The works of Jean Piaget (26) and Erik Erikson (27) lend insight into understanding the normal stages of childhood and adolescence and help us to identify how diabetes and its management influence those stages. These theories of how the child or adolescent develops in the cognitive and psychosocial domains provide an understanding of how the child or adolescent conceptualizes diabetes. Knowledge of developmental norms allows families and providers to realize that certain tasks are not appropriate at a certain stage and can only be managed at a later stage. With repeated interactions with the tasks of diabetes – insulin administration, meal planning, physical exercise, blood glucose monitoring, and taking action for hypo and hyperglycemia, the child or adolescent learns to associate actions with outcomes (missed insulin dose leads to a high blood glucose level) and begins to gain insight and knowledge of the consequences of an action for future decision-making. Since Piaget's and Erikson's stages are hierarchical in nature and somewhat age specific, they provide broad individual guidelines for when it is appropriate to assume shared responsibility with diabetes tasks. Guidelines for the care and education of children/adolescents with diabetes and their families stress the importance of diabetes care and education to be individualized, developmentally relevant, culturally sensitive, and appropriately paced (17).

The goal for the child or adolescent with diabetes is to achieve or even exceed normative developmental expectations while managing the demands of a chronic health condition. Child and adolescent growth and development are daunting tasks onto themselves; add diabetes to the mix and the child/adolescent with diabetes and his/her family are at risk of becoming overwhelmed. The diabetes health care team needs to work with the entire family and other support personnel to ensure optimal glycemic control as well as successful attainment of normative milestones.

ESSENTIALS OF DIABETES EDUCATION

Pediatric diabetes education is a family affair (28–30). Children and adolescents need adults in a variety of settings to assume or share the responsibility of diabetes management. Diabetes self-management may mean self-care by the child/adolescent with diabetes or be better understood as "parent management" or "family management." Recent pediatric-specific guidelines published by the American Diabetes Association provide recommendations for the management, treatment, and support of children with type 1 *(17)* and type 2 *(31–33)* diabetes by a pediatric diabetes health care team.

Despite the fact that some parents, health care professionals, and school personnel would find age-specific guidelines for when the child/adolescent should assume responsibility for diabetes self-care tasks useful, rigid guidelines are rarely successful. In addition to age, child/adolescent temperament, cognitive abilities, motor skills, as well as diabetes duration and family support must all be considered throughout the transition from dependence to independence *(17,34)*. Assuming responsibility of these diabetes tasks occurs over a continuum of time. Some aspects of diabetes self-management such as insulin management, problem solving, and scheduling medical and education appointments are always best if shared, with interdependence being the goal.

Pediatric diabetes education includes two specific stages: survival education and ongoing education *(35,36)*. Survival education occurs at time of diagnosis and may be effectively provided in either a hospital or outpatient setting *(37,38)*. This initial education is generally individual based due to immediate need and provides an introduction to essential skills: injection technique, drawing up insulin, blood glucose monitoring, and introduction to meal planning. During the ongoing or continuing stage, education incrementally builds upon knowledge, skills, and support to the child/adolescent and family. Content is revisited at each developmental stage to reflect age-appropriate diabetes management issues, psychosocial concerns, and expectations for the growing and developing child/adolescent with diabetes *(29,34)*. Some ongoing education may be provided individually whereas some may be more beneficial when provided in group settings *(39,40)*. Diabetes education should provide the knowledge, skills, and tools to reach age-specific blood glucose (BG) and A1C goals. Table 1 lists current treatment goals for children/adolescents with type 1 diabetes *(17,41)*. Because young children are more vulnerable to hypoglycemia, target glucose ranges are more generous in this age group. By adolescence recommended targets for blood glucose values and A1C approximate those of adults.

Although diabetes management has made dramatic strides, one must remember that a diagnosis of diabetes is a major event in the life of a child and his family. Diabetes educators and other health team members often hear parents refer to life events "before" and "after" their child's diagnosis of diabetes. Though a "new normal" is usually realized by these families, diabetes has a major impact on family life due to its serious nature, chronicity, and complexity of treatment. The following provides a brief synopsis of current recommendations regarding medications, medical nutrition therapy, physical activity,and blood glucose monitoring for children and adolescents.

Table 1
Plasma blood glucose and A1C goals for type 1 diabetes by age group (*17,41*)

Values by age	Plasma blood glucose goal range (mg/dl)			A1C	Rationale
	Before meals	Bedtime/overnight			
Toddlers and preschoolers (<6 years)	100–180	110–200		<8.5 (but >7.5) %	• High risk and vulnerability to hypoglycemia
School age (6–12 years)	90–180	100–180		<8%	• Risks of hypoglycemia and relatively low risk of complications prior to puberty
Adolescents and young adults (13–19 years)	90–130	90–150		<7.5%*	• Risk of hypoglycemia • Developmental and psychological issues

Key concepts in setting glycemic goals:
- Goals should be individualized and lower goals may be reasonable based on benefit–risk assessment
- Blood glucose goals should be higher than those listed above in children with frequent hypoglycemia or hypoglycemia unawareness
- Postprandial blood glucose values should be measured when there is a disparity between preprandial blood glucose values and A1C levels

*A lower goal (<7.0%) is reasonable if it can be achieved without excessive hypoglycemia. Reprinted with permission from the American Diabetes Association.

Medication

All children/adolescents with type 1 diabetes require insulin as part of their treatment. Intensive insulin regimens achieved through either multiple (three or more) daily injections (MDI) of long- and short-acting insulin analogues or insulin pump therapy are currently widely used in the management of children with type 1 diabetes *(42)*. These "basal/bolus" regimens supply insulin in a more physiologic way. Onset, peak, and duration of the particular insulin used and the specific regimen dictate the insulin protocol developed for the child/adolescent. It is important to remind families of the importance of administering insulin, by either injection or insulin pump bolus, prior to meals. Though there may be occasional exceptions, such as toddlers with unpredictable eating habits, after-meal insulin dosing should be the exception rather than the rule.

Clinically we have observed that when children/adolescents plan an after-meal insulin dose, blood glucose levels far exceed the pre meal reading by the time the dose is administered. It is also common for the insulin dose to be forgotten when given regularly after meals *(43)*. Education regarding site rotation for both injections and infusion set insertion is important. It is not uncommon for certain sites to be overused due to habit and/or increasing physical comfort for the child/adolescent at sites that have hypertrophy. However, hypertrophy is in fact tissue damage and results in insufficient absorption of insulin.

Children and adolescents with type 2 diabetes may be treated with a variety of medications. Currently, metformin and insulin are the only medications approved by the Food and Drug Administration for use in this population *(32,33)*. However, recent advances in different classes of medications for adults with type 2 diabetes have led to "off label" use in children with type 2 diabetes, and it is important that educators are well versed with the medications used in their particular setting. In addition, medication may also be prescribed to control hypertension and hyperlipidemia, two frequent comorbidities in type 2 diabetes in youth. Children and families should receive oral and written instruction for each prescribed medication including purpose, dose, frequency, and potential side effects. Furthermore, medication adherence should be assessed at each patient encounter with particular emphasis during adolescence.

Medical Nutrition Therapy

Medical Nutrition Therapy (MNT) is best achieved by working with a registered dietitian, preferably with experience in both diabetes and pediatric populations. The meal plan should be individualized and realistic with consideration to the child's developmental stage, food preferences, and cultural background. Calorie recommendations should be sufficient for growth, reduced in the case of overweight or obese children, provide optimal nutrition, provide satiety, and match medication and exercise/physical activity *(44–46)*.

Physical Activity

Physical activity is important to the health of all children and should be encouraged. However, for children/adolescents with type 1 diabetes, hypoglycemia is a risk *(47–49)*. The timing, intensity, and duration of physical activity, peaking of insulin, or inadequate carbohydrate intake may cause hypoglycemia. Because of the spontaneous nature of physical activity in youth, it is important to make efforts to prevent hypoglycemia with blood glucose monitoring; intake of carbohydrate before, during, and/or after exercise based on blood glucose values; and speedy treatment in the event of hypoglycemia.

Physical activity has multiple benefits for the child or adolescent with type 2 diabetes. In addition to lowering blood glucose levels, activity helps to burn fat, increase insulin sensitivity, increase energy expenditure, and has beneficial effects on blood pressure and lipid levels. Hypoglycemia is rare for children with type 2 diabetes who are not taking insulin or oral secretogogues *(41)*. Because of their more sedentary lifestyle pattern, children/adolescents with type 2 diabetes may need ongoing encouragement to initiate an exercise program and should be counseled to start slowly, gradually increase intensity, and build physical activity into lifetime habits.

Blood Glucose Monitoring

Blood glucose monitoring provides the child/adolescent and their families, as well as the diabetes team, vital information to make short- or long-term changes in diabetes management. Interpreting a blood glucose level as "high," "low," or "in-range" versus "good" or "bad" uses the blood glucose reading as information, thereby removing an emotional response from the assessment. Using the term "blood sugar check" versus "blood sugar test" removes the concept of pass/fail from the monitoring process. Home blood glucose monitoring provides up-to-the-minute information, whereas the A1C provides a larger retrospective picture of average blood glucose control over the past few months.

Currently two continuous glucose monitors (CGM) are approved by the Food and Drug Administration for use in pediatric patients (http://www.childrenwithdiabetes.com/continuous.htm). Both systems require placement of a catheter in subcutaneous tissue and use a sensor, transmitter, and receiver to measure and report both interstitial glucose levels and directional trending graphs every few minutes. Alarms warn of low and high blood glucose levels using individually determined preset blood glucose ranges. As insurance reimbursement becomes routine and next-generation products become available, more children and adolescents will use these devices, bringing this new technology, as well as its potential challenges, to pediatric diabetes care *(50,51)*.

Children and Adolescents with Type 2 Diabetes

Lacking the strong evidence base of pediatric type 1 diabetes, treatment of type 2 diabetes in youth is in its infancy. The Today Study is a multi-center randomized controlled trial to identify the best "Treatment Options for Type 2 Diabetes in Adolescents and Youth" (http://www.todaystudy.org/index.cgi). The study compares the effectiveness of treatment using metformin (currently the only oral diabetes agent approved for use in children) versus two alternative treatment approaches: metformin plus rosiglitazone and metformin plus an intensive lifestyle intervention *(33)*.

Though the trial continues, evidence supports the benefits of healthy eating both in terms of nutritional value and portion size as well as physical activity *(41)*. The National Diabetes Education Program offers specific educational materials regarding type 2 diabetes in youth. The emphasis of care for children and adolescents with type 2 diabetes is behavior change therapy *(52,53)*. Though it may appear to many as not as much of a challenge, both research *(33,52)* and common sense support the notion that behavior change is difficult for virtually everyone.

PREPARATION FOR TRANSITIONS

Transitions are exciting adventures and denote moving from one developmental stage to the next or embarking on new and different experiences. However, for many children and families, transitions may be marked by feelings of uncertainty regarding the unknown. This is certainly true when a child has diabetes because of concern regarding who will assist with diabetes management and how this will be accomplished in new and unfamiliar settings. Diabetes educators, as part of the pediatric diabetes team, are important to successful transitions of children with diabetes, be it the first day of kindergarten or a child's first sleep-away camp experience. We specifically address the role of the diabetes educator during four transition periods: school, attendance at diabetes camp, adolescence, and the young adult post high school.

Diabetes Care at School

Children and adolescents spend many hours at school. The first priority for students with diabetes is a medically safe school environment. For many students, diabetes care in the post DCCT era involves more intensive management and greater use of technology. Therefore, to keep children and adolescents with diabetes healthy and safe, it is necessary that the health needs of the student with diabetes be accommodated during the school day and at school-sponsored activities. The family, diabetes health care team, and school personnel must partner to ensure optimal diabetes management in a safe learning environment. Further, schools must provide students with diabetes equal access to all school activities available to similar-age peers.

The pediatric obesity epidemic and its risk of type 2 diabetes have highlighted the need for primary prevention efforts at schools. Since 2003, many states have implemented legislation directed at school lunch programs, vending machine choices available to children, and promotion of physical activity (54). The increasing incidence of both type 1 and type 2 diabetes, occurrence of type 1 diabetes in younger children, and more intensive diabetes management strategies mandate that a well-educated school staff be available to provide care and to assist children in diabetes care management tasks.

Traditionally, the school nurse has been the professional entrusted with the responsibility for administering care, assistance, and health care supervision to children with diabetes in the school setting. Although diabetes professionals advocate that a nurse trained in all aspects of diabetes management should be assigned to each school, this is not a reality in many communities. The National Association of School Nurses recommends that the school nurse to student ratio be 1:750 for optimal care during the school day (55). However, the current ratio is 1 school nurse for every 1,350 children and differs widely by state with less than half of the schools meeting the recommended school nurse to student ratio (56). Research has demonstrated that presence of a school nurse is associated with receipt of services by children with diabetes (57). Currently only 16 states have policies regarding school nurse staffing ratios and these range from 1 nurse per school to 1 nurse per 5,000 students (58).

Two studies (59,60) have examined in-school care and support for children with diabetes including teacher training and diabetes-specific policies and procedures regarding care provided at school. Findings in both studies were similar in that a significant minority of schools lacked teachers or school staff who had received diabetes education and training and/or a school diabetes policy. The American Diabetes Association takes the position that, in the absence of a school nurse, non-medical school personnel should be educated and trained to provide safe and effective care and assistance to children with diabetes (61). Though this offers a reasonable solution, state laws and regulations as well as philosophy may prohibit non-medical school personnel from performing tasks, in particular the administration of insulin and glucagon (62). Hellems and Clarke (63) surveyed a large group of parents to examine diabetes management support provided by non-nurse school personnel. Approximately one-third of parents reported that their child's school lacked a full-time school nurse; in these cases, diabetes care and assistance was provided by part-time nurses and supplemented by teachers, administrators, coaches, and cafeteria workers with no adverse consequences.

Diabetes management plans vary widely depending on age, duration of diabetes, and intensity of therapy and must be clearly communicated to school personnel for effective partnership and diabetes care delivery during the school day. Pediatric diabetes educators need to be aware of school policies within their locality and assist parents in knowing how to advocate for their child within the school setting. In addition, diabetes educators may be called upon by parents or schools to facilitate training of school personnel. *Helping the Student Succeed: A Guide for School Personnel* (http://ndep.nih.gov/resources/school.htm), developed by the National Diabetes Education Program (NDEP), provides comprehensive information about diabetes care in the school setting. This publication may be ordered or downloaded free of charge. In addition, the American Diabetes Association (ADA) position statement *Diabetes Care in the School and Day Care Setting* (http://care.diabetesjournals.org/cgi/reprint/30/suppl_1/S66) outlines general guidelines for diabetes care, responsibilities of the various partners in care, background of several federal laws, as well as a template for the diabetes medical management plan (DMMP).

Each year the pediatric diabetes team, in conjunction with the family, should develop a written diabetes treatment plan for the school reflecting the child's unique needs. In addition, modifications to the plan should be communicated whenever significant changes, such as initiation of insulin pump therapy, occur. There are four types of written diabetes management plans:

- Diabetes medical management plan (DMMP)
- Individual health care plan (IHP) or nursing care plan
- "504" plan
- Individual education program (IEP)

Two of these plans, the 504 plan and IEP, are legal documents developed under provisions of the Rehabilitation Act of 1973 and the Individuals with Disabilities Education Act, respectively. Both plans are signed agreements between the child's parents/guardians and representatives of the school; the school is legally bound to implement the recommendations incorporated in the plan.

The question often arises as to which type of plan is best for a particular student. Unfortunately the answer is not simple. Some parents and/or school systems feel most comfortable with either a 504 Plan or an IEP since they are legally binding documents. However, others feel that the DMMP or IHP is sufficient. The decision must be individualized according to the specific needs of the child or adolescent. Sample DMMPs and 504 plans are available at http://www.diabetes.org/advocacy-and-legalresources/discrimination/school/504plan.jsp#dmmp.

Routine school activities such as participation in field trips, class parties, and school lunch programs generally require extra planning for the student with diabetes. Other more diabetes-specific activities such as what to do with an insulin

pump when playing sports, insulin injections, pump boluses, designated loca-
tions for blood glucose monitoring, and identification of school personnel to
provide diabetes-specific assistance are often stumbling blocks for provision of
optimal diabetes care at school. The best way to avert stumbling blocks is to
be proactive in their prevention. The DMMP, IHP, 504 plan, and/or IEP facilitate communication among the family, school, and diabetes care team. Whether
the student has type 1 or type 2 diabetes, school presents special challenges for
diabetes management. All students with diabetes need a written plan so that the
student can be a student first and a student with diabetes second!

Camping Diabetes Style

For more than 80 years, children and adolescents have benefited from sharing
a commonality of living with diabetes at diabetes camps. Camp attendance provides the atypical opportunity of being "the norm" through living in a situation
where the majority of campers and staff alike have diabetes. This experience
enables children/adolescents with diabetes to build a support system unlike any
other. They learn that they are not alone as well as how to live better with
diabetes through diabetes education and exposure to new tools for managing
diabetes. Parents get a much needed respite from the daily tasks of diabetes care.
Diabetes camps are empowering, and many former campers return to camp as
counselors.

Although the vast majority of camps are for children and adolescents
with type 1 diabetes, several camps offer programs for children and families with type 2 diabetes. Up-to-date information regarding specific diabetes
camps and their programs may be found on the following websites: Diabetes Education and Camping Association at http://www.diabetescamps.org/,
American Diabetes Association at http://diabetes.org/communityprograms-and-
localevents/diabetescamps.jsp, and Children With Diabetes at http://www.
childrenwithdiabetes.com/camps/

Diabetes educators play many roles in the diabetes camping experience. They
are often resources who inform families about diabetes camping and assist
parents with navigating through the application process for both camp enroll-
ment and "camperships" (scholarship support for camp attendance). Diabetes
educators are often a part of the health care team at diabetes camps. Living
with campers and staff who have diabetes provides a "real-life" immersion
in diabetes self-management. Diabetes educators may also act as resources to
camp staff via e-mail and telephone communication; educators may not be
able to get away from the office or clinic but can bring their experience and
knowledge of individual campers to on-site camp staff. The American Diabetes
Association position statement, *Diabetes Care at Diabetes Camp*, provides

recommendations regarding management of the child/adolescent at a diabetes camp *(64)*.

Adolescence

During adolescence profound cognitive, psychosocial, and physical changes occur. Despite maturation in their cognitive ability, adolescents with chronic illness, similar to their peers without diabetes, are primarily concerned with the present *(25)* and are less influenced by long-term health risks *(65)*. From a psychosocial perspective, the adolescent/parent relationship changes as the adolescent becomes increasingly independent. Adolescents with diabetes begin to assume increasing responsibility for self-management tasks, a process that often creates tension and conflict within the family *(23,25)*. Finally, hormonal changes during puberty lead to significant insulin resistance *(66)*, resulting in higher insulin requirements and need for frequent insulin adjustment during this time *(67)*. The interplay of these factors place adolescents with diabetes at high risk for deterioration in metabolic control.

Ongoing parent involvement in diabetes care *(21,22,68)* during the assumption of appropriate levels of self-management autonomy by the adolescent is critical during this period. Decreased parental involvement in diabetes care during adolescence is associated with decreased performance of self-care tasks *(21,23)*. Adolescents with greater responsibility for diabetes self-management make more self-care mistakes, demonstrate less treatment adherence, and have poorer metabolic control compared to children with parental involvement.

Poor diabetes control during adolescence often extends into young adulthood *(69)*, suggesting that adolescence is a critical time period for embedding positive or negative lifetime diabetes self-management habits. Diabetes educators can play an important role in providing anticipatory guidance to both the adolescent and the family regarding appropriate levels of responsibility during transition to self-care autonomy and monitoring its ongoing progress. Diabetes education during this period is directed toward diabetes problem solving, decision-making, and reinforcing positive behaviors with the goal of achieving gradual self-care autonomy by the end of high school. Parent(s) and the entire diabetes health care team need to be attentive in terms of recognition and early intervention for problems for which adolescents are at particular risk: engagement in risky behaviors, depression, and eating disorders.

Adolescence is a time of discovery and experimentation. Studies have examined tobacco, alcohol, and illicit drug use and sexual behavior among high school students with and without diabetes. Compared to peers without diabetes, students with diabetes use tobacco, alcohol, and drugs less frequently during early high school years; however, by the end of high school substance use is similar to peers without diabetes *(70)*. Similarly, sexual behaviors including age at first intercourse, frequency of sexual activity, or pregnancy history are similar for girls with diabetes compared to peers *(71)*. One study *(72)* demonstrated that teens with diabetes lack information regarding preventing unplanned pregnancies. These findings support the need for reproductive health education, ongoing prevention and/or cessation efforts regarding tobacco and illicit drug use, and education regarding responsible use of alcohol and effect of alcohol on blood glucose levels for all adolescents with diabetes.

Children with chronic illness are at higher risk to develop depression compared to healthy peers *(73–75)*. The combination of diabetes with a comorbid psychiatric condition places a child at further risk for poor medical outcomes *(73,76–78)*. Despite the fact that children with chronic illness have greater exposure to health care professionals, depression often remains unrecognized; therefore, adolescents with chronic conditions are no more likely to receive mental health services compared to healthy peers *(79)*.

Kovacs et al. *(80)* studied a group of Pittsburgh children from the time of diagnosis and reported that by the tenth year following diagnosis of diabetes, approximately half developed psychiatric comorbidity, with the highest incidence rates occurring within the first year of diabetes diagnosis. In two more recent cross-sectional studies *(75,81)*, 15–23% of youth with diabetes reported depressive symptoms. Adolescents with depression are more frequently re-hospitalized for diabetic ketoacidosis *(77,82)* and have more hospital and emergency room visits *(78,81)*. These findings highlight the importance of routine screening for depression in children and adolescents with diabetes, maintaining a high index of suspicion of depression in adolescents with "frequent flyer" DKA hospitalizations, and prompt initiation of treatment when depression is identified.

Eating disorders are among the most lethal psychiatric disorders that exist. Eating disorders encompass a wide spectrum of behaviors that involve insufficient or excessive food intake. Diabetes provides a unique opportunity to control calorie utilization and weight gain through deliberate insulin reduction or omission. Insulin omission behaviors meet the criteria of the Diagnostic and Statistical Manual of Psychiatric Disorders, 4th version (DSM-IV) as "eating disorder not otherwise specified" *(83)*. For those with type 2 diabetes, unhealthy eating behaviors may precede a diagnosis of diabetes and be further compounded by calorie limitation as part of the diabetes treatment plan.

Eating disorders occur more frequently in adolescent girls with type 1 diabetes compared to both similar-age girls without diabetes *(84)* and boys with diabetes *(85)*. In one survey of adolescents with diabetes, although both girls and boys (38% and 16%, respectively) reported efforts to control their weight, girls were more likely to report unhealthy behaviors such as severely restricting food intake or skipping meals and/or deliberate skipping or decreasing insulin dose *(85)*. Although less frequent, competitive sports such as wrestling may place undue emphasis on weight and should be considered when students with diabetes participate in these activities. The consequences of eating disorders are serious: poor glycemic control (84–86) and long-term complications of diabetes (87–89).

Weight loss in a child or adolescent with diabetes should always be investigated and examined in conjunction with A1C values. When weight loss and poor glycemic control coexist, a high index of suspicion should be given to insulin omission as a possible cause. Similar to depression, screening for the presence of eating disorders should be routinely incorporated into clinical practice. For adolescents who wear insulin pumps, downloading pump information at each office visit provides a good means to screen for routine insulin omission.

Psychological functioning is essential for positive adaptation to a diagnosis of diabetes (90) and long-term metabolic control (69,77,91,92). Diabetes educators need to be aware that both depression and eating disorders may be unrecognized factors in adolescents with deterioration in glycemic control, school performance, or family/peer relationships. Broad screening questions may elicit problems in these areas warranting more targeted screening and/or referral for mental health services.

Young Adulthood

Older adolescents require special attention from the pediatric team to enable a successful transition to the role of young adult with diabetes. Senior year of high school is filled with decisions regarding college, vocational school, or employment; residential living or commuting to school; college lifestyle; establishing new friendships; and establishing a new level of independence. These changes and their resulting demands on the young adult with diabetes may be overwhelming and may become a distraction from effective diabetes self-management (93). Although the literature has focused on the needs and concerns of college students with diabetes (94–96), the issues identified apply generally to the age group at large.

Preparation and education regarding the transition to college is important to receipt of optimal health services during the college years (96). Students and parents need to know options for their ongoing relationship with the pediatric diabetes team during the college years. In addition, parents and students should be encouraged to initiate a relationship with the college health facility to understand the level of services available and develop a plan if care is needed on an emergent basis. How diabetes supplies will be ordered and stored, meal options, receipt of influenza vaccine, sick day management, and disclosure of diabetes to a roommate and others are topics that benefit from early planning and discussion. The current insulin regimen should be re-examined for its utility in preparation for irregular eating schedules that go hand in hand with college life.

Finally, safe use of alcohol and sexual health including contraception options, prevention of sexually transmitted infections, and the importance of preconception planning for women with diabetes should be addressed regardless of whether the student currently engages in these practices.

SUMMARY

Whether it be a child or adolescent with type 1 or type 2 diabetes, effective diabetes self-management requires a high level of ongoing commitment by the child and family. Pediatric diabetes educators, as part of a pediatric diabetes team, are essential to promote positive adaptation of the child/adolescent and his family to the demands of diabetes, provide a developmentally appropriate foundation for caring for and supporting the child/adolescent with diabetes, and serve as an ongoing resource for development of diabetes knowledge, skills, and lifelong learning through the period of childhood to young adulthood. The five phrases that best summarize the essence of pediatric diabetes self-management are team approach, family based, pediatric specific, culturally sensitive, and kid friendly.

REFERENCES

1. The effect of intensive treatment of diabetes on the development and progression of long-term complications in insulin-dependent diabetes mellitus. The Diabetes Control and Complications Trial Research Group. N Engl J Med 1993;329(14):977–86.
2. Effect of intensive diabetes treatment on the development and progression of long-term complications in adolescents with insulin-dependent diabetes mellitus: Diabetes Control and Complications Trial. Diabetes Control and Complications Trial Research Group. J Pediatr 1994;125(2):177–88.
3. Dabelea D, Bell RA, D'Agostino RB, Jr., et al. Incidence of diabetes in youth in the United States. JAMA 2007;297(24):2716–24.
4. Liese AD, D'Agostino RB, Jr., Hamman RF, et al. The burden of diabetes mellitus among US youth: prevalence estimates from the SEARCH for Diabetes in Youth Study. Pediatrics 2006;118(4):1510–8.
5. Incidence and trends of childhood Type 1 diabetes worldwide 1990–1999. Diabetes Med 2006;23(8):857–66.
6. Green A, Patterson CC. Trends in the incidence of childhood-onset diabetes in Europe 1989–1998. Diabetologia 2001;44 Suppl 3:B3–8.
7. Roche EF, Menon A, Gill D, Hoey H. Clinical presentation of type 1 diabetes. Pediatr Diabetes 2005;6(2):75–8.
8. Dabelea D, Pettitt DJ, Jones KL, Arslanian SA. Type 2 diabetes mellitus in minority children and adolescents. An emerging problem. Endocrinol Metab Clin North Am 1999;28(4):709–29, viii.
9. Effect of intensive therapy on the microvascular complications of type 1 diabetes mellitus. JAMA 2002;287(19):2563–9.
10. White NH, Cleary PA, Dahms W, Goldstein D, Malone J, Tamborlane WV. Beneficial effects of intensive therapy of diabetes during adolescence: outcomes after the conclusion of the Diabetes Control and Complications Trial (DCCT). J Pediatr 2001;139(6):804–12.

11. Litton J, Rice A, Friedman N, Oden J, Lee MM, Freemark M. Insulin pump therapy in toddlers and preschool children with type 1 diabetes mellitus. J Pediatr 2002;141(4):490–5.

12. DiMeglio LA, Pottorff TM, Boyd SR, France L, Fineberg N, Eugster EA. A randomized, controlled study of insulin pump therapy in diabetic preschoolers. J Pediatr 2004;145(3): 380–4.

13. Fox LA, Buckloh LM, Smith SD, Wysocki T, Mauras N. A randomized controlled trial of insulin pump therapy in young children with type 1 diabetes. Diabetes Care 2005;28(6): 1277–81.

14. Wilson DM, Buckingham BA, Kunselman EL, Sullivan MM, Paguntalan HU, Gitelman SE. A two-center randomized controlled feasibility trial of insulin pump therapy in young children with diabetes. Diabetes Care 2005;28(1):15–9.

15. Mack-Fogg JE, Orlowski CC, Jospe N. Continuous subcutaneous insulin infusion in toddlers and children with type 1 diabetes mellitus is safe and effective. Pediatr Diabetes 2005;6(1): 17–21.

16. Jeha GS, Karaviti LP, Anderson B, et al. Insulin pump therapy in preschool children with type 1 diabetes mellitus improves glycemic control and decreases glucose excursions and the risk of hypoglycemia. Diabetes Technol Ther 2005;7(6):876–84.

17. Silverstein J, Klingensmith G, Copeland K, et al. Care of children and adolescents with type 1 diabetes: a statement of the American Diabetes Association. Diabetes Care 2005;28(1): 186–212.

18. Mortensen HB, Hougaard P. Comparison of metabolic control in a cross-sectional study of 2,873 children and adolescents with IDDM from 18 countries. The Hvidore Study Group on Childhood Diabetes. Diabetes Care 1997;20(5):714–20.

19. Danne T, Mortensen HB, Hougaard P, et al. Persistent differences among centers over 3 years in glycemic control and hypoglycemia in a study of 3,805 children and adolescents with type 1 diabetes from the Hvidore Study Group. Diabetes Care 2001;24(8):1342–7.

20. Rosilio M, Cotton JB, Wieliczko MC, et al. Factors associated with glycemic control. A cross-sectional nationwide study in 2,579 French children with type 1 diabetes. The French Pediatric Diabetes Group. Diabetes Care 1998;21(7):1146–53.

21. Anderson B, Ho J, Brackett J, Finkelstein D, Laffel L. Parental involvement in diabetes management tasks: relationships to blood glucose monitoring adherence and metabolic control in young adolescents with insulin-dependent diabetes mellitus. J Pediatr 1997;130(2): 257–65.

22. Laffel LM, Vangsness L, Connell A, Goebel-Fabbri A, Butler D, Anderson BJ. Impact of ambulatory, family-focused teamwork intervention on glycemic control in youth with type 1 diabetes. J Pediatr 2003;142(4):409–16.

23. Anderson BJ, Vangsness L, Connell A, Butler D, Goebel-Fabbri A, Laffel LM. Family conflict, adherence, and glycaemic control in youth with short duration Type 1 diabetes. Diabetes Med 2002;19(8):635–42.

24. Laffel LM, Connell A, Vangsness L, Goebel-Fabbri A, Mansfield A, Anderson BJ. General quality of life in youth with type 1 diabetes: relationship to patient management and diabetes-specific family conflict. Diabetes Care 2003;26(11):3067–73.

25. Weinger K, O'Donnell KA, Ritholz MD. Adolescent views of diabetes-related parent conflict and support: a focus group analysis. J Adolesc Health 2001;29(5):330–6.

26. Piaget J. Piaget's theory. In: Mussen P, ed. Carmichael's manual of child psychology. New York: John Wiley & Sons; 1970.

27. Erikson E. Identity, youth and crisis. New York: W.W. Norton & Co., Inc.; 1968.

28. La Greca AM. It's "all in the family": responsibility for diabetes care. J Pediatr Endocrinol Metab 1998;11 Suppl 2:379–85.

29. Butler D, Lawlor MT. It takes a village: Helping families live with diabetes. Diabetes Spectr 2004;17(1):26–31.

30. Wiebe DJ, Berg CA, Korbel C, et al. Children's appraisals of maternal involvement in coping with diabetes: enhancing our understanding of adherence, metabolic control, and quality of life across adolescence. J Pediatr Psychol 2005;30(2):167–78.
31. Type 2 diabetes in children and adolescents. American Diabetes Association. Diabetes Care 2000;23(3):381–9.
32. Atkinson A, Radjenovic D. Meeting quality standards for self-management education in pediatric type 2 diabetes. Diabetes Spectr 2007;20(1):40–6.
33. Zeitler P, Epstein L, Grey M, et al. Treatment options for type 2 diabetes in adolescents and youth: a study of the comparative efficacy of metformin alone or in combination with rosiglitazone or lifestyle intervention in adolescents with type 2 diabetes. Pediatr Diabetes 2007;8(2):74–87.
34. Halvorsen M, Yasuda P, Carpenter S, Kaiserman K. Unique challenges for pediatric patients with diabetes. Diabetes Spectr 2005;18(3):167–73.
35. Mensing C, Boucher J, Cypress M, et al. National standards for diabetes self-management education. Diabetes Care 2007;30 Suppl 1:S96–S103.
36. Swift PG. Diabetes education. ISPAD clinical practice consensus guidelines 2006–2007. Pediatr Diabetes 2007;8(2):103–9.
37. Gage H, Hampson S, Skinner TC, et al. Educational and psychosocial programmes for adolescents with diabetes: approaches, outcomes and cost-effectiveness. Patient Educ Couns 2004;53(3):333–46.
38. Clar C, Waugh N, Thomas S. Routine hospital admission versus out-patient or home care in children at diagnosis of type 1 diabetes mellitus. Cochrane Database Syst Rev 2007(2):CD004099.
39. Grey M, Boland EA, Davidson M, Li J, Tamborlane WV. Coping skills training for youth with diabetes mellitus has long-lasting effects on metabolic control and quality of life. J Pediatr 2000;137(1):107–13.
40. Anderson BJ, Wolf FM, Burkhart MT, Cornell RG, Bacon GE. Effects of peer-group intervention on metabolic control of adolescents with IDDM. Randomized outpatient study. Diabetes Care 1989;12(3):179–83.
41. Standards of medical care in diabetes – 2007. Diabetes Care 2007;30 Suppl 1:S4–S41.
42. Weintrob N, Benzaquen H, Galatzer A, et al. Comparison of continuous subcutaneous insulin infusion and multiple daily injection regimens in children with type 1 diabetes: a randomized open crossover trial. Pediatrics 2003;112(3 Pt 1):559–64.
43. Burdick J, Chase HP, Slover RH, et al. Missed insulin meal boluses and elevated hemoglobin A1c levels in children receiving insulin pump therapy. Pediatrics 2004;113(3 Pt 1):e221–4.
44. Nutrition recommendations and principles for people with diabetes mellitus. American Diabetes Association. Tenn Med 2000;93(11):430–3.
45. Franz MJ. Evidence-based medical nutrition therapy for diabetes. Nutr Clin Pract 2004;19(2):137–44.
46. Evert A. Nutrition management tools and techniques for working with students with diabetes. School Nurse News 2005;22(1):12–6.
47. Toni S, Reali MF, Barni F, Lenzi L, Festini F. Managing insulin therapy during exercise in type 1 diabetes mellitus. Acta Biomed 2006;77 Suppl 1:34–40.
48. Admon G, Weinstein Y, Falk B, et al. Exercise with and without an insulin pump among children and adolescents with type 1 diabetes mellitus. Pediatrics 2005;116(3): e348–55.
49. Kollipara S, Warren-Boulton E. Diabetes and physical activity in school. School Nurse News 2004;21(3):12–6.
50. Wilson DM, Beck RW, Tamborlane WV, et al. The accuracy of the FreeStyle Navigator continuous glucose monitoring system in children with type 1 diabetes. Diabetes Care 2007;30(1):59–64.

51. Buckingham B, Beck RW, Tamborlane WV, et al. Continuous glucose monitoring in children with type 1 diabetes. J Pediatr 2007;151(4):388–93, 93 e1–2.
52. Kaufman FR, Schantz S. Current clinical research on type 2 diabetes and its prevention in youth. School Nurse News 2007;24(3):13–6.
53. Burnet D, Plaut A, Courtney R, Chin MH. A practical model for preventing type 2 diabetes in minority youth. Diabetes Educ 2002;28(5):779–95.
54. Boehmer TK, Brownson RC, Haire-Joshu D, Dreisinger ML. Patterns of childhood obesity prevention legislation in the United States. Prev Chronic Dis 2007;4(3):A56.
55. Vail K. The medicated child. Am Sch Board J 2004,191(12):26–8.
56. Brener ND, Wheeler L, Wolfe LC, Vernon-Smiley M, Caldart-Olson L. Health services: results from the School Health Policies and Programs Study 2006. J Sch Health 2007;77(8): 464–85.
57. Guttu M, Engelke MK, Swanson M. Does the school nurse-to-student ratio make a difference? J Sch Health 2004;74(1):6–9.
58. Healthy schools: State-level school health policies. 2007. (Accessed November 26, 2007, at http://www.nasbe.org/HealthySchools/States/Topics.asp?Category=B&Topic=4.)
59. Melton D, Henderson J. Do public schools provide optimal support for children with diabetes? Prev Chronic Dis 2007;4(3):A78.
60. Lewis DW, Powers PA, Goodenough MF, Poth MA. Inadequacy of in-school support for diabetic children. Diabetes Technol Ther 2003;5(1):45–56.
61. Diabetes care in the school and day care setting. Diabetes Care 2007;30 Suppl 1:S66–73.
62. Healthy schools: State level school health policies: State-by-state administration of medications. National Association of State Boards of Education. (Accessed January 7, 2008, at http://www.nasbe.org/HealthySchools/States/Topics.asp?Category=D&Topic=2.)
63. Hellems MA, Clarke WL. Safe at school: a Virginia experience. Diabetes Care 2007;30(6):1396–8.
64. Diabetes care at diabetes camps. Diabetes Care 2007;30 Suppl 1:S74–6.
65. Sawyer SM, Aroni RA. Self-management in adolescents with chronic illness. What does it mean and how can it be achieved? Med J Aust 2005;183(8):405–9.
66. Amiel SA, Sherwin RS, Simonson DC, Lauritano AA, Tamborlane WV. Impaired insulin action in puberty. A contributing factor to poor glycemic control in adolescents with diabetes. N Engl J Med 1986;315(4):215–9.
67. Laffel L, Pasquarello C, Lawlor MT. Treatment of the child and adolescent with diabetes. In: Kahn CR, Weir GC, King GL, Jacobsen AM, Moses AC, Smith RJ, eds. Joslin's diabetes mellitus. 14th ed. ed. Philadelphia: Lippincott Williams & Wilkins; 2005:711–36.
68. Wysocki T, Taylor A, Hough BS, Linscheid TR, Yeates KO, Naglieri JA. Deviation from developmentally appropriate self-care autonomy. Association with diabetes outcomes. Diabetes Care 1996;19(2):119–25.
69. Bryden KS, Peveler RC, Stein A, Neil A, Mayou RA, Dunger DB. Clinical and psychological course of diabetes from adolescence to young adulthood: a longitudinal cohort study. Diabetes Care 2001;24(9):1536–40.
70. Martinez-Aguayo A, Araneda JC, Fernandez D, Gleisner A, Perez V, Codner E. Tobacco, alcohol, and illicit drug use in adolescents with diabetes mellitus. Pediatr Diabetes 2007;8(5): 265–71.
71. Suris JC, Resnick MD, Cassuto N, Blum RW. Sexual behavior of adolescents with chronic disease and disability. J Adolesc Health 1996;19(2):124–31.
72. Charron-Prochownik D, Sereika SM, Falsetti D, et al. Knowledge, attitudes and behaviors related to sexuality and family planning in adolescent women with and without diabetes. Pediatr Diabetes 2006;7(5):267–73.
73. Grey M, Whittemore R, Tamborlane W. Depression in type 1 diabetes in children: natural history and correlates. J Psychosom Res 2002;53(4):907–11.

74. Bennett DS. Depression among children with chronic medical problems: a meta-analysis. J Pediatr Psychol 1994;19(2):149–69.
75. Hood KK, Huestis S, Maher A, Butler D, Volkening L, Laffel LM. Depressive symptoms in children and adolescents with type 1 diabetes: association with diabetes-specific characteristics. Diabetes Care 2006;29(6):1389–91.
76. Dantzer C, Swendsen J, Maurice-Tison S, Salamon R. Anxiety and depression in juvenile diabetes: a critical review. Clin Psychol Rev 2003;23(6):787–800.
77. Stewart SM, Rao U, Emslie GJ, Klein D, White PC. Depressive symptoms predict hospitalization for adolescents with type 1 diabetes mellitus. Pediatrics 2005;115(5):1315–9.
78. Garrison MM, Katon WJ, Richardson LP. The impact of psychiatric comorbidities on readmissions for diabetes in youth. Diabetes Care 2005;28(9):2150–4.
79. Suris JC, Parera N, Puig C. Chronic illness and emotional distress in adolescence. J Adolesc Health 1996;19(2):153–6.
80. Kovacs M, Goldston D, Obrosky DS, Bonar LK. Psychiatric disorders in youths with IDDM: rates and risk factors. Diabetes Care 1997;20(1):36–44.
81. Lawrence JM, Standiford DA, Loots B, et al. Prevalence and correlates of depressed mood among youth with diabetes: the SEARCH for Diabetes in Youth study. Pediatrics 2006;117(4):1348–58.
82. Liss DS, Waller DA, Kennard BD, McIntire D, Capra P, Stephens J. Psychiatric illness and family support in children and adolescents with diabetic ketoacidosis: a controlled study. J Am Acad Child Adolesc Psychiatry 1998;37(5):536–44.
83. Crow SJ, Keel PK, Kendall D. Eating disorders and insulin-dependent diabetes mellitus. Psychosomatics 1998;39(3):233–43.
84. Jones JM, Lawson ML, Daneman D, Olmsted MP, Rodin G. Eating disorders in adolescent females with and without type 1 diabetes: cross sectional study. Bmj 2000;320(7249):1563–6.
85. Neumark-Sztainer D, Patterson J, Mellin A, et al. Weight control practices and disordered eating behaviors among adolescent females and males with type 1 diabetes: associations with sociodemographics, weight concerns, familial factors, and metabolic outcomes. Diabetes Care 2002;25(8):1289–96.
86. Meltzer LJ, Johnson SB, Prine JM, Banks RA, Desrosiers PM, Silverstein JH. Disordered eating, body mass, and glycemic control in adolescents with type 1 diabetes. Diabetes Care 2001;24(4):678–82.
87. Rydall AC, Rodin GM, Olmsted MP, Devenyi RG, Daneman D. Disordered eating behavior and microvascular complications in young women with insulin-dependent diabetes mellitus. N Engl J Med 1997;336(26):1849–54.
88. Nielsen S. Eating disorders in females with type 1 diabetes: An update of a meta-analysis. Eur Eat Disord Rev 2002;10(4):241–54.
89. Steel JM, Young RJ, Lloyd GG, Clarke BF. Clinically apparent eating disorders in young diabetic women: associations with painful neuropathy and other complications. Br Med J (Clin Res Ed) 1987;294(6576):859–62.
90. Lernmark B, Persson B, Fisher L, Rydelius PA. Symptoms of depression are important to psychological adaptation and metabolic control in children with diabetes mellitus. Diabet Med 1999;16(1):14–22.
91. Whittemore R, Kanner S, Singleton S, Hamrin V, Chiu J, Grey M. Correlates of depressive symptoms in adolescents with type 1 diabetes. Pediatr Diabetes 2002;3(3):135–43.
92. Nakazato M, Kodama K, Miyamoto S, Sato M, Sato T. Psychiatric disorders in juvenile patients with insulin-dependent diabetes mellitus. Diabetes Res Clin Pract 2000;48(3):177–83.
93. Anderson BJ, Wolpert HA. A developmental perspective on the challenges of diabetes education and care during the young adult period. Patient Educ Couns 2004;53(3):347–52.

94. Ramchandani N, Cantey-Kiser JM, Alter CA, et al. Self-reported factors that affect glycemic control in college students with type 1 diabetes. Diabetes Educ 2000;26(4):656–66.
95. Wdowik MJ, Kendall PA, Harris MA. College students with diabetes: using focus groups and interviews to determine psychosocial issues and barriers to control. Diabetes Educ 1997;23(5):558–62.
96. Mellinger DC. Preparing students with diabetes for life at college. Diabetes Care 2003;26(9):2675–8.

17 The Challenge of Weight and Diabetes Management in Clinical Practice

Ann E. Goebel-Fabbri, PhD,
Gillian Grant Arathuzik, RD, LDN, CDE,
and Jacqueline I. Shahar, M.Ed., RCEP, CDE

CONTENTS

RATES, RISKS, AND RISK REDUCTION
LIFESTYLE INTERVENTIONS
    FOR OBESITY AND DIABETES
BEHAVIORAL STRATEGIES FOR
    WEIGHT AND DIABETES MANAGEMENT
NUTRITION RECOMMENDATIONS FOR
    WEIGHT AND DIABETES MANAGEMENT
EXERCISE RECOMMENDATIONS FOR
    WEIGHT AND DIABETES MANAGEMENT
TYPES OF EXERCISE
EXERCISE INTENSITY
EXERCISE DURATION AND FREQUENCY
EXERCISE SAFETY – INJURY PREVENTION
    AND BLOOD GLUCOSE MANAGEMENT
CONCLUSION – LIFESTYLE
    APPROACHES IN CLINICAL PRACTICE
REFERENCES

From: *Contemporary Diabetes: Educating Your Patient with Diabetes*
Edited by: K. Weinger and C. A. Carver, DOI 10.1007/978-1-60327-208-7_17,
© Humana Press, a part of Springer Science+Business Media, LLC 2009

ABSTRACT

Behavioral approaches to weight loss and diabetes management have been studied for decades. Effective lifestyle programs successfully combine three primary interventions – dietary changes, increased physical activity, and behavioral weight loss strategies. The goal of such a multi-pronged approach is to teach patients the skills they need to maintain a balanced meal plan, a long-term exercise program, and integrate these new habits with cognitive and behavioral principles tailored to their unique potential triggers for relapse. The treatment ideal would consist of a comprehensive and multi-disciplinary diabetes team. Without access to such a team, these interventions require clinicians to be familiar with behavioral weight loss techniques, nutrition recommendations, and exercise goals for weight and diabetes management. The principles outlined here are intended to provide practical, empirically supported techniques for improving diabetes and weight-related wellness in this burgeoning patient population.

Key Words: Lifestyle approach, Behavioral weight loss, Exercise, Obesity, Nutrition.

RATES, RISKS, AND RISK REDUCTION

Type 2 diabetes and obesity are both recognized as important American and global public health problems. From 1990 to 1998, as the prevalence of obesity in the United States rose by 49%, the prevalence of type 2 diabetes also rose by 33% (from 4.6% in 1990 to 6.5% in 1998) *(1–3)*. Diabetes affects an estimated 21 million people and is currently the sixth leading cause of death by disease in the United States *(4)*.

The majority of patients with type 2 diabetes (an estimated 60–90%) are overweight or obese *(5,6)*. Obesity is closely associated with insulin resistance, which not only promotes hyperglycemia in diabetes but also is a major risk factor for hypertension, hyperlipidemia, and other markers of cardiovascular disease *(7)*. Indeed, cardiovascular disease is the primary cause of death in diabetes *(8)*.

The United Kingdom Prospective Diabetes Study (UKPDS), the largest and longest prospective study of type 2 diabetes to date, found that for every one point reduction in hemoglobin A1c there was a corresponding 35% reduction in risk of the development of diabetes complications *(9–11)*. As such, treatment for type 2 diabetes is aimed at lowering and stabilizing average daily blood glucose levels through dietary changes, exercise, home blood glucose monitoring, and oral medication and/or insulin treatment. Approximately 28% of adults with diabetes are treated with insulin *(4)*.

The American Diabetes Association recommends that overweight patients with diabetes lose 5–7% of their body weight in order to improve insulin sensitivity and glycemic control *(12)*. However, a common side effect of pharmacotherapy for type 2 diabetes – many oral agents and insulin therapy – is weight gain *(7)*. UKPDS results indicated that patients treated with insulin gained an average of 5 kg *(11)*. Several reasons have been postulated as underlying causes for this weight gain, such as improvements in glycosuria, direct fat and muscle building effects of insulin, increasing calorie intake to prevent hypoglycemia, and proposed central nervous system effects of insulin that could influence appetite and eating behavior *(7)*.

Weight gain is an undesirable result of diabetes management because added weight in turn increases insulin resistance and has been linked to increased cardiovascular risks *(7)*. Additionally, the motivational challenge presented by added weight must be understood as a particular burden to patients who have been struggling with long-standing weight problems and who have likely been counseled to try to lose weight for some time. Metformin is currently the most widely prescribed oral diabetes agent and is known to be weight neutral or to promote modest weight loss. For this reason, it is often recommended as a first-line or combination treatment in type 2 diabetes. Two newer injected agents, pramlintide and exenatide, may also be helpful in managing weight in patients with type 2 diabetes because both have been shown to promote modest weight loss while improving glycemic control. Sitagliptin (Januvia, Merck, Whitehouse Station, NJ) is a newer oral agent with early evidence of weight neutrality.

LIFESTYLE INTERVENTIONS FOR OBESITY AND DIABETES

Behavioral approaches to weight loss have been studied for decades. Most research evidence supports the effectiveness of combining moderate dietary changes and increased physical activity – an approach referred to as a lifestyle intervention – for achieving modest weight loss and maintaining weight improvements over time. Long-term evidence supports the power of lifestyle interventions to prevent the onset of type 2 diabetes in high-risk populations *(13,14)*; however, early research indicated that patients already diagnosed with diabetes had a harder time achieving and maintaining weight loss than patients without diabetes *(8)*.

More recent evidence from the LookAHEAD trial (Action for Health in Diabetes), a large-scale, multi-center clinical trial investigating the impact of lifestyle intervention on cardiac outcomes in over 5,000 patients with type 2 diabetes, supports the successful impact of lifestyle interventions in achieving weight loss and improved glycemic control in type 2 diabetes patients. Participants in the lifestyle arm lost an average of 8.6% of their initial weight and experienced a mean decrease in A1c from 7.3 to 6.6% during their first year of LookAHEAD. Additionally, lifestyle participants showed improvements in blood pressure, cholesterol and triglycerides, and urine albumine-to-creatinine ratios *(15)*. Ultimately, LookAHEAD will track participant outcomes for 5 or more years to determine not only the sustainability of their weight loss but its impact on cardiac health *(16)*. However, current results already support the use of lifestyle interventions by clinicians aiming to help patients with diabetes improve their overall health and wellness. These interventions require clinicians to be familiar with behavioral weight loss techniques, nutrition recommendations, and exercise goals for weight and diabetes management.

BEHAVIORAL STRATEGIES FOR WEIGHT AND DIABETES MANAGEMENT

Provider Stance and Approach

Surveys of overweight and obese people reveal that they are frequently the targets of weight-based stigmatization from family members, co-workers, and even healthcare providers *(17)*. Indeed, negative attitudes toward obese people have been reported in studies of healthcare professionals including medical students, dietitians, nurses, and physicians. A recent study of weight management and obesity experts reported somewhat lower levels of bias but concluded that direct care for obese patients did not eliminate anti-fat bias in these professionals *(18)*. For this reason, clinicians should keep their patient's history of stigmatization in mind and examine their own internalized biases about overweight and obese patients to ensure their delivery of sensitive, patient-centered care. Providers should strive to establish a collaborative rapport by conveying a sense of acceptance, warmth, and appreciation of their patient's unique motivations to change. Motivational interviewing is an example of one such client-centered counseling approach that has been suggested as an adjunct treatment in behavioral weight loss *(19)*.

Realistic Goal Setting

A recent meta-analysis of lifestyle approaches to weight management reports that these interventions typically achieve modest weight losses with an average weight loss of 7 pounds *(20)*. Large-scale trials in diabetes have found that 7–10% reductions in weight are both achievable and sustainable over time *(13,15,16)*. Such a modest weight loss goal may appear to be trivial and disappointing to patients because it leaves them unlikely to achieve their ideal weight. However the health benefits of modest weight loss are proven. Patients should be encouraged to establish realistic goals for themselves in order to achieve an overall goal of sustainable improvements in their quality of health and quality of life.

Self-Monitoring and Stimulus Control

A fundamental technique for weight and diabetes management involves daily monitoring of food intake (calorie and macronutrient breakdown), blood glucose fluctuations, exercise, and weight. By tracking patterns of successful behavior change and slips into old behavior patterns, patients increase their awareness of their own unique behavior patterns. Developing new problem-solving strategies and specific targets for behavior change is a natural outgrowth of reviewing self-monitoring records in collaboration with a health professional.

Cognitive Restructuring

As patients identify behavior patterns through self-monitoring, they can also begin to identify automatic thought patterns that serve to reinforce unhealthy weight and diabetes self-management behaviors. Health professionals should work with patients to identify these thoughts and work on changing them in order to promote active problem-solving and positive health behaviors.

Stress Management and Alternative Coping

Teaching patients how to reduce their reactions to stress will be especially helpful for those patients who have turned to overeating as a stress management strategy in the past. Establishing an exercise routine is a fundamental part of lifestyle interventions for weight and diabetes management, and many patients learn to use exercise as a means of coping rather than turning to food for comfort.

Relapse Prevention

Long-term weight loss maintenance remains an ongoing problem for clinicians and researchers alike. One year after losing weight, the majority of patients regain up to 30% of their lost weight *(8)*. Studies with longer follow-up show a return to baseline weight by about 50% of people at the 5 year mark *(21)*. These data again underscore the importance of helping patients to establish realistic goals for themselves at the beginning of a weight loss attempt. They also reinforce the importance of teaching relapse prevention strategies to help patients anticipate difficulties in their future and establish coping strategies ahead of time.

NUTRITION RECOMMENDATIONS FOR WEIGHT AND DIABETES MANAGEMENT

When it comes to recommending a meal-planning approach for both diabetes and weight management, dietitians and diabetes educators have a broad range of options from which to choose. Caloric intake must be reduced to initiate weight loss, but whether or not macronutrient distribution makes a difference in weight loss and glycemic control has been debated. A limited number of studies have evaluated the long-term effectiveness of different weight loss plans. One such study compared the effectiveness and sustainability of four popular weight loss diets, each recommending a different macronutrient composition: Atkins (low carbohydrate diet), Zone (macronutrient-balanced diet), Weight Watchers (daily calorie-restricted diet), or Ornish (low-fat diet). While the Atkins diet group lost more weight in the first 6 months of study participation, by 1 year, study results found that all four diets led to equivalent weight reductions and improvements in cardiovascular risk factors (22). More long-term research is needed to evaluate the effectiveness of weight loss meal plans designed with varying macronutrient distribution.

After a comprehensive review of the literature on diabetes and weight management, the clinical oversight committee at Joslin Diabetes Center developed clinical nutrition guidelines for overweight and obese adults with type 2 diabetes (23). The goal was to provide a structured meal-planning approach to induce weight loss and improve blood glucose targets in patients with diabetes. These guidelines recommend a caloric distribution consisting of 40% calories from carbohydrate, 20–30% calories from protein, and 30–35% calories from fat. Minimum carbohydrate intake per day is 130 g. Carbohydrate sources should be low in glycemic index/glycemic load and fiber intake should be at least 20–35 g per day. Both protein and fat sources should be low in saturated and trans fats.

Registered dietitians and diabetes educators can use equations such as Harris–Benedict or Mifflin–St. Jeor (see Table 1) to estimate basal metabolic rate (BMR) and determine a daily calorie goal. First, the total daily calories for weight maintenance are estimated by multiplying the BMR by an activity factor. Equations are referenced in the table below. Next, the Joslin guidelines recommend decreasing the daily maintenance caloric intake by 250–500 calories to establish an initial daily calorie goal for weight loss. To promote optimal health and gradual weight loss, the recommended calorie levels range from 1,000 to 1,800 calories per day. Daily caloric intake for women should be no less than 1,000 calories per day and for men no less than 1,200 calories per day. Patients with renal disease should consult a nephrologist before starting a higher protein meal plan, even though with caloric reduction the total protein intake will be less than what is typically consumed and therefore should not aggravate renal function.

As patients lose weight, insulin sensitivity improves and diabetes medications can be reduced or even discontinued. It is critical for patients with diabetes undergoing any weight loss attempt to be closely monitored by their diabetes team so that medication changes can occur, as patterns of hypoglycemia become an issue. If patients experience frequent hypoglycemia and medications are not reduced, they will need to consume additional calories to treat the hypoglycemia

Table 1
Daily Calorie Consumption Formulas

Harris–Benedict formula
Men: BMR $= 66.5 + (13.75 \times$ weight in kg$) + (5.003 \times$ height in cm$) - (6.775 \times$ age$)$
Women: BMR $= 655.1 + (9.563 \times$ weight in kg$) + (1.850 \times$ height in cm$) - (4.676 \times$ age$)$

Mifflin–St. Jeor equations
Men: BMR $= 10 \times$ weight in kg $+ 6.25 \times$ height in cm $- 5 \times$ age $+ 5$
Women: BMR $= 10 \times$ weight in kg $+ 6.25 \times$ height in cm $- 5 \times$ age $- 161$
  1. Sedentary people (little or no exercise): Calorie $-$ Calculation $=$ BMR $\times 1.2$
  2. Lightly active people (light exercise/sports 1–3 days/week):
     Calorie calculation $=$ BMR $\times 1.375$
  3. Moderately active people (moderate exercise/sports 3–5 days/week):
     Calorie calculation $=$ BMR $\times 1.55$
  4. Very active people (hard exercise/sports 6–7 days a week):
     Calorie calculation $=$ BMR $\times 1.725$
  5. Extra active people (very hard exercise/sports & physical job):
     Calorie calculation $=$ BMR $\times 1.9$

and weight loss may plateau. This can leave patients feeling frustrated and at risk for returning to old eating patterns.

As patients learn how to implement the nutrition guidelines into everyday eating patterns, they will need help understanding which foods fall into specific nutrient categories and also how to determine their appropriate portion sizes. As with any meal-planning approach, it must be tailored to meet the patient's educational background, level of motivation, and complexity of treatment regimen. For example, some patients may benefit most from a simplified meal planning like "the plate method." Patients are taught that one third of the plate will be designated for the carbohydrates, one third for the proteins/fats, and one third for the vegetables. Other patients are interested in learning to do more sophisticated calculations of the calories provided by each food in a particular meal. This allows them to better determine portion sizes that fit their desired macronutrient distribution. Patients taking multiple daily insulin injections or using an insulin pump will benefit from advanced carbohydrate counting principles and algorithms for making adjustments to their insulin to carbohydrate ratios and correction factors as their weight loss progresses and insulin sensitivity improves.

Use of meal replacements is supported by the guidelines as a viable option to assist in weight loss and glycemic improvements. The benefits of meal replacements include clearly defined portion control and limiting food choice, both of which can improve adherence to a structured meal plan *(21)*. Research supports safely using meal replacements for up to 4 years *(24)*. However, for long-term weight loss maintenance, patients should be encouraged to practice other methods of designing their own portion controlled, nutrient-balanced meals.

Diabetes professionals face a difficult task in helping patients with diabetes lose weight, improve glycemic profiles, and maintain these achievements long term. Portion control, especially when eating outside the home, is a challenging hurdle. Average restaurant portions have grown over time along with larger plates, glasses, and silverware, leaving many patients unaware of the added calories they are regularly consuming. Brian Wansink and colleagues *(25)* studied this issue by comparing the calories consumed by a group served soup from a standard soup bowl with another group served from a soup bowl that was surreptitiously being refilled. Participants who ate from the refilling bowls ate 73% more soup but reported feeling no more satiated than the comparison group. This study clearly demonstrates the idea that people perceive the serving size they are given as the appropriate portion size and will eat accordingly.

Obesity researchers, like Kelly Brownell, have referred to the growing problem of portions size and cheap high-calorie foods in the United States as "a toxic food environment." However, patients can be taught to make healthier choices *(26)*. Patients need concrete strategies especially when dining out. For example, patients can be encouraged to measure foods at home and compare appropriate portion sizes to reference items such as a compact disc, deck of cards, or the palm of their hand in order to use these visual reminders to guide their portion decisions. It is critical for patients to learn to identify menu items that are higher in calories because of ingredients or food preparation, like adding cream sauces or frying foods. This awareness will assist patients to either avoid these choices or learn how to request lower calorie alternatives. When patients have favorite restaurants that they frequent, they can be encouraged to look up that restaurant's nutrition information on their website or request more detailed information from the restaurant's management. This again can help patients by giving them familiarity with healthier menu choices ahead of time.

EXERCISE RECOMMENDATIONS FOR WEIGHT AND DIABETES MANAGEMENT

Exercise and increased physical activity is key to weight loss. Exercise has been shown to reduce adipose tissue and insulin resistance, and improve glycemic control *(29)*. Obesity and sedentary lifestyle lead to insulin resistance, which causes the inhibition of GLUT 4, a protein carrier that transports glucose into the cells. Therefore, glucose is not transported and metabolized as efficiently in adipose and muscle tissue *(27–29)*. Muscle contractions during exercise increases glucose uptake by muscles, and as frequency and duration of exercise increases, the amount of GLUT 4 available for glucose transport increases *(30)*.

Metabolic demand increases in a single bout of exercise through the following process. Initially, muscles utilize glycogen stores, but within approximately 5–10 min of exercise, the liver becomes the main energy source for the active muscles by releasing stored glycogen to the blood stream. Insulin secretion is reduced, and epinephrine is released to signal the release of glucose by the liver. As activity continues, the muscles use free fatty acids (stored fat) as energy in addition to glucose. During low-to-moderate intensity exercise the role of epinephrine (adrenaline) is minor and blood glucose typically drops, however with vigorous exercise, the release the counter-regulatory hormones including epinephrine (adrenaline) triggers the liver to produce glucose causing blood glucose levels to rise (31). Post-exercise session, glucose uptake from the blood stream continues for about 24 h or more since muscles need to replenish themselves with energy (32). Individuals taking insulin injections and some oral medications are at greater risk for hypoglycemia during and after exercise and may require medication adjustments to prevent this problem (see blood glucose management section below).

Designing an Individualized Exercise Plan

Exercise recommendations for patients with diabetes are similar to individuals without diabetes with respect to the mode, frequency, duration and intensity of exercise. The exercise prescription should be individualized in accordance to the patient's current exercise capacity, medical status, age, weight, duration of diabetes, and personal goals. Sedentary people often have specific barriers related to increasing their physical activity. The Centers for Disease Control developed a questionnaire, the Barriers to Being Active Quiz, as an efficient tool to help identify barriers, such as lack of time, skill, resources, energy, willpower, fear of injury, and social support, as part of a comprehensive exercise assessment (33).

A careful assessment helps prevent exacerbation of diabetes complications and orthopedic issues. Before starting an exercise program, individuals with diabetes should undergo a complete physical examination to identify neurological, microvascular, or macrovascular complications, which may require exercise modifications (34). Depending on the individual's age and diabetes duration, a graded exercise test should be performed. Blood pressure should be controlled. If systolic blood pressure is above 200 mmHg or diastolic blood pressure is above 110 mmHg, exercise should be avoided. A dilated eye exam should also be performed 2–3 months prior to the start of an exercise plan. Individuals who develop foot injuries or infections should avoid water-based exercise and limit themselves to upper body exercise only, as feet should stay dry and protected until they have healed.

With nephropathy, exercise intensity should be low to moderate and blood pressure controlled. Autonomic neuropathy causes orthostatic hypotension and changes in heart rate. Using the Rate of Perceived Exertion scale rather than a target heart rate is preferred (see intensity of exercise section below). With peripheral neuropathy, exercise should combine weight-bearing and non-weight-bearing activities at short duration, and their exercise recommendations should be designed to reduce the risk of losing balance *(35)*. Exercise accommodations must also be tailored to the severity of retinopathy. For example, in moderate-to-severe non-proliferative diabetic retinopathy, heavy weight lifting and breath holding should be avoided. With proliferative diabetic retinopathy or macular edema, high impact aerobic, running, racquet sports, weight lifting, exercises with the head down, or any other activities that increase blood pressure should be avoided *(35)*.

TYPES OF EXERCISE

An exercise prescription for the individual with diabetes should include cardiovascular (aerobic), resistance (strength training), and flexibility (stretching) exercises. These modes of exercise will help develop and maintain cardiovascular fitness, muscular strength, and range of motion in joints. The components of any exercise session should include a warm-up and cooldown. Warm-up refers to the first 5–10 min of the exercise session, which helps the body adjust from rest to exercise. It increases body temperature and blood flow, and as a result avoids musculoskeletal injury. Cooldown refers to the last 5–10 min of the exercise session, which provides recovery for the working muscles.

A combination of resistance training and aerobic exercise has been shown to improve glycemic control, improve muscle strength and lean body mass, and reduce waist circumference and systolic blood pressure *(36–38)*. Evidence suggests that a combination of aerobic and resistance exercises increases exercise adherence as compared to either type of exercise alone *(38)*.

Aerobic exercise refers to activities that use major muscles groups over a long period of time. Aerobic exercise improves cardio-respiratory fitness, reduces the cardiac risk factors, decreases blood pressure, and improves lipids and triglycerides. Aerobic exercise includes walking, cycling, dancing, swimming, and the use of aerobic exercise machines.

It is important to identify a suitable mode of exercise that can be performed safely while maximizing energy expenditure. Weight-bearing activities, such as walking, jogging, running, or hiking, can be performed by many patients. However, individuals with peripheral neuropathy, vascular disease, foot problems, or other orthopedic issues may require modified non-weight-bearing or low-impact activities. These activities include water aerobics, swimming, and aerobic machines such as the recumbent bicycle, Nu Step, or Airdyne. If an individual cannot perform exercises using their legs because of injury or complications, an Arm bike is another safe alternative *(34)*.

Resistance exercise is also called weight or strength training and involves use of resistance in the form of free weights, stretching bands, or machines to increase muscle strength or endurance. Muscle tissue decreases while fat tissue increases with age, and as a result energy metabolism is reduced. Resistance training increases muscle mass and metabolism which promotes weight loss; increases muscle tone, muscle strength, and bone density, reducing the risk of injury from falls. Resistance training also reduces intra-abdominal and subcutaneous fat, hemoglobin A1c, LDL, triglycerides, and total cholesterol *(36)*.

Resistance machines such as Cybex or Nautilus are easy to learn to use. With free weights, more muscles and motor units are required to maintain proper form. Stretching/tubing bands are elastic bands with handles where the resistance level of a band corresponds to a different color or thickness. They require little storage space and are lightweight enough for use during travel. Bands are especially useful for deconditioned people because they allow the individual to perform many exercises in a seated position *(39)*.

Flexibility exercise or stretching involves loosening the muscles to prevent them from cramping after exercise. Muscles tighten up following exercise and this can cause pain or reduce the range of motion in joints. Therefore, stretching exercise should be performed when muscles are warm or at the end of an exercise session.

EXERCISE INTENSITY

A number of tools can be used to measure exercise intensity. An individual can follow the Heart Rate (HR) Reserve formula: (Heart rate = {50–85% intensity × (HR max − HR rest)} + HR rest). Max HR can be calculated using the following equation: 220–age. For a person age 40: max HR is 180 bpm, resting HR 70 bpm. (Heart rate = {50–85% intensity × (180–70)} + 70). In this example, the target HR would be: 90–153 bpm. The Rate of Perceived Exertion (RPE) scale is another tool which correlates well with heart rate and workload and is recommended for patients with autonomic neuropathy, those who have difficulty measuring their own heart rate, or those taking medication that affect their heart rate. When using the RPE, an individual is asked to rate their exertion on a scale ranging from 0 to 10, where a "0" estimates exertion as "nothing at all" and "10" as "extremely strong." The range between 3 and 5 indicates moderate exercise intensity *(34)*.

"The Talk Test" is the simplest guide and refers to attempting a conversation during exercise. An individual, who can have a conversation, but cannot whistle during exercise, is most likely exercising at a moderate intensity. If the individual is short of breath, exercise intensity is vigorous and slowing the pace or reducing the resistance should be recommended. If the individual can whistle or sing while exercising, the intensity is low and the pace or resistance should be increased. If at any point the individual experiences joint or muscle pain or chest discomfort, they should be encouraged to stop exercising *(40)*.

EXERCISE DURATION AND FREQUENCY

The American College of Sports Medicine (ACSM) suggests that aerobic exercise should be done for a minimum of 30 min at moderate intensity; however, exercise bouts of 10 min or more added together throughout the day also achieve this goal. For weight loss and weight loss maintenance, 60–90 min of exercise at a moderate level of intensity is recommended *(41)*. The ACSM suggests that individuals should perform aerobic exercise 5 or more days per week for weight loss and weight loss maintenance. Resistance exercise should be performed at least 2–3 days per week with a day of rest in between. Stretching can be performed daily *(41)*.

EXERCISE SAFETY – INJURY PREVENTION AND BLOOD GLUCOSE MANAGEMENT

People who exercise at a high intensity, progress quickly with their exercise plan, omit warmups and cooldowns, or avoid stretching exercise may be at high risk for injury. Other causes of injury include inappropriate footwear, faulty biomechanics (high/flat arches, muscle tightness, short leg), and environmental factors, such as icy or slippery surfaces.

Blood glucose checking before, during, and after exercise is strongly recommended, especially for those patients whose treatment regimen places them at risk for hypoglycemia. In order to provide the patient with appropriate guidelines to manage diabetes and lose weight, insulin and oral agents may need regular adjustments as the individual becomes more active and weight loss progresses *(42,43)*. See Table 2 for safety recommendations with exercise.

CONCLUSION – LIFESTYLE APPROACHES IN CLINICAL PRACTICE

Large-scale research trials like the Diabetes Prevention Program and early results from the LookAHEAD study support the positive impact of lifestyle interventions aimed at improving diabetes and cardiac risk factors – by achieving and maintaining modest weight losses over time *(13–15)*. Effective lifestyle programs successfully combine three primary interventions – dietary changes, increased physical activity, and behavioral weight loss strategies. The goal of

Table 2
Safety Recommendations with Exercise

	On insulin alone or in combination with oral agents	Oral diabetes agents
Pre-exercise targets	110 mg/dl or above If below target, eat 15–30 g of carbohydrates prior to exercise	90 mg/dl or above If below target, eat 15–30 g of carbohydrates prior to exercise
During exercise targets	– Maintain adequate hydration – Check BG if at risk for hypoglycemia	– Maintain adequate hydration – Check BG if at risk for hypoglycemia
Managing hyperglycemia	Type 1: check for ketones if BG above 250 mg/dl. Delay exercise if ketones are present	Type 2: If BG is above 400 mg/dl and not feeling well, delay exercise
Hypoglycemia prevention	– Reduce rapid acting insulin/bolus by 30–50% at meal close to exercise time. – Reduce long acting insulin by 20–50% if necessary. – Reduce basal rate by 30–50% between 30 and 60 min pre/postexercise	– Reduce diabetes meds (especially sulfonylurea, Meglinide, Nateglinide) on days of exercise

such a multi-pronged approach is to teach patients the skills they need to maintain a balanced meal plan, a long-term exercise program, and integrate these new habits with cognitive and behavioral principles tailored to their unique potential triggers for relapse. The treatment ideal would consist of a comprehensive and multi-disciplinary diabetes team including a dietician, clinical exercise physiologist, behavioral psychologist, nurse educator, and endocrinologist/diabetologist. However, as the number of patients struggling with diabetes and obesity continues to grow, diabetes educators face increasing pressures to provide lifestyle interventions with less access to such a specialized team. The principles outlined here are intended to provide practical, empirically supported techniques for improving diabetes, and weight-related wellness in this burgeoning patient population.

REFERENCES

1. Mokdad AH, Ford ES, Bowman BA, et al. Diabetes trends in the U.S.: 1990–1998. Diabetes Care 2000;23(9):1278–83.
2. Mokdad AH, Serdula MK, Dietz WH, Bowman BA, Marks JS, Koplan JP. The spread of the obesity epidemic in the United States, 1991–1998. JAMA 1999;282(16):1519–22.

3. King H, Aubert RE, Herman WH. Global burden of diabetes, 1995–2025: prevalence, numerical estimates, and projections. Diabetes Care 1998;21(9):1414–31.
4. Centers for Disease Control and Prevention. National diabetes fact sheet: general information and national estimates on diabetes in the United States, 2005. Atlanta, GA; 2005.
5. Colditz GA, Willett WC, Stampfer MJ, et al. Weight as a risk factor for clinical diabetes in women. American Journal of Epidemiology 1990;132(3):501–13.
6. Tremble J, Donaldson D. Diabetes mellitus type 2, obesity and weight loss. Journal of the Royal Society of Health 1999;119(2):73–5.
7. Hollander P. Anti-Diabetes and Anti-Obesity Medications: Effects on Weight in People With Diabetes. Diabetes Spectrum 2007;20:159–65.
8. Wing RR, Goldstein MG, Acton KJ, et al. Behavioral Science Research in Diabetes: Lifestyle changes related to obesity, eating behavior, and physical activity. Diabetes Care 2001;24(1):117–23.
9. Krentz AJ. UKPDS and beyond: into the next millennium. United Kingdom Prospective Diabetes Study. Diabetes, Obesity & Metabolism 1999;1(1):13–22.
10. UK Prospective Diabetes Study (UKPDS) Group. Intensive blood-glucose control with sulphonylureas or insulin compared with conventional treatment and risk of complications in patients with type 2 diabetes (UKPDS 33). Lancet 1998;352(9131):837–53.
11. UK Prospective Diabetes Study (UKPDS) Group. Effect of intensive blood-glucose control with metformin on complications in overweight patients with type 2 diabetes (UKPDS 34). Lancet 1998;352(9131):854–65.
12. American Diabetes Association position statement: evidence-based nutrition principles and recommendations for the treatment and prevention of diabetes and related complications. Journal of the American Dietetic Association 2002;102(1):109–18.
13. Hamman RF, Wing RR, Edelstein SL, et al. Effect of weight loss with lifestyle intervention on risk of diabetes. Diabetes Care 2006;29(9):2102–7.
14. Lindstrom J, Ilanne-Parikka P, Peltonen M, et al. Sustained reduction in the incidence of type 2 diabetes by lifestyle intervention: follow-up of the Finnish Diabetes Prevention Study. Lancet 2006;368(9548):1673–9.
15. Pi-Sunyer X, Blackburn G, Brancati FL, et al. Reduction in weight and cardiovascular disease risk factors in individuals with type 2 diabetes: one-year results of the look AHEAD trial. Diabetes Care 2007;30(6):1374–83.
16. Wadden TA, West DS, Delahanty L, et al. The Look AHEAD study: a description of the lifestyle intervention and the evidence supporting it. Obesity 2006;14(5):737–52.
17. Puhl RM, Brownell KD. Confronting and coping with weight stigma: an investigation of overweight and obese adults. Obesity 2006;14(10):1802–15.
18. Schwartz MB, Chambliss HO, Brownell KD, Blair SN, Billington C. Weight bias among health professionals specializing in obesity. Obesity Research 2003;11(9):1033–9.
19. DiLillo V, Siegfried NJ, West DS. Incorporating Motivational Interviewing Into Behavioral Obesity Treatment. Cognitive and Behavioral Practice 2003;10:120–30.
20. Powell LH, Calvin JE, 3rd, Calvin JE, Jr. Effective obesity treatments. The American Psychologist 2007;62(3):234–46.
21. Wadden TA, Butryn ML, Byrne KJ. Efficacy of lifestyle modification for long-term weight control. Obesity Research 2004;12 Suppl:151S–62S.
22. Dansinger ML, Gleason JA, Griffith JL, Selker HP, Schaefer EJ. Comparison of the Atkins, Ornish, Weight Watchers, and Zone diets for weight loss and heart disease risk reduction: a randomized trial. JAMA 2005;293(1):43–53.
23. Joslin Diabetes Center. Nutrition Guideline for Overweight and Obese Adults with Type 2 Diabetes, Prediabetes or Those at High Risk for Developing Type 2 Diabetes, (Accessed 2007, at http://www.joslin.org/Files/Nutrition_Guideline_Graded.pdf.

24. Flechtner-Mors M, Ditschuneit HH, Johnson TD, Suchard MA, Adler G. Metabolic and weight loss effects of long-term dietary intervention in obese patients: four-year results. Obesity Research 2000;8(5):399–402.

25. Wansink B, Painter JE, North J. Bottomless bowls: why visual cues of portion size may influence intake. Obesity Research 2005;13(1):93–100.

26. Brownell KD, Horgen KB. Food Fight: The Inside Story of America's Obesity Crisis and What We Can Do About It. Chicago, IL: Contemporary Books; 2003.

27. Rader DJ. Effect of insulin resistance, dyslipidemia, and intra-abdominal adiposity on the development of cardiovascular disease and diabetes mellitus. The American Journal of Medicine 2007;120(3 Suppl 1):S12–8.

28. Kahn BB, Flier JS. Obesity and insulin resistance. The Journal of Clinical Investigation 2000;106(4):473–81.

29. Hamdy O. Lifestyle modification and endothelial function in obese subjects. Expert Review of Cardiovascular Therapy 2005;3(2):231–41.

30. Hamdy O, Goodyear LJ, Horton ES. Diet and exercise in type 2 diabetes mellitus. Endocrinology and Metabolism Clinics of North America 2001;30(4):883–907.

31. Wolpert H. Smart Pumping for People with Diabetes. Alexandria, VA: American Diabetes Association; 2002.

32. Steppel JH, Horton ES. Exercise in Patients with Diabetes Mellitus. In: Kahn CR, Weir GC, King GL, Jacobson AM, Moses AC, Smith RJ, eds. Diabetes Mellitus. Fourteenth ed. Philadelphia: Lippincott, Williams, & Wilkins; 2005.

33. Centers for Disease Control and Prevention. Barriers to Physical Activity Quiz. (Accessed 2007, at http://www.cdc.gov/nccdphp/dnpa/physical/life/barriers_quiz.pdf.)

34. Albright A, Franz M, Hornsby G, et al. American College of Sports Medicine position stand. Exercise and type 2 diabetes. Medicine and Science in Sports and Exercise 2000;32(7): 1345–60.

35. Mullooly CA, Chalmers KH. Diabetes Management Therapies: Physical Activity/Exercise. In: Franz MJ, ed. A CORE Curriculum for Diabetes Education: Diabetes and Complications, Fifth ed. Chicago: American Association of Diabetes Educators; 2003.

36. Eves ND, Plotnikoff RC. Resistance training and type 2 diabetes: Considerations for implementation at the population level. Diabetes Care 2006;29(8):1933–41.

37. Dunstan DW, Daly RM, Owen N, et al. High-intensity resistance training improves glycemic control in older patients with type 2 diabetes. Diabetes Care 2002;25(10):1729–36.

38. Sigal RJ, Kenny GP, Boule NG, et al. Effects of aerobic training, resistance training, or both on glycemic control in type 2 diabetes: a randomized trial. Annals of Internal Medicine 2007;147(6):357–69.

39. Frontera W, Bean J. In: Strength and Power Training: A Guide for Adults of All Ages – A Special Report from Harvard Medical School: Harvard Health Publications; 2005.

40. Persinger R, Foster C, Gibson M, Fater DC, Porcari JP. Consistency of the talk test for exercise prescription. Medicine and Science in Sports and Exercise 2004;36(9):1632–6.

41. Haskell WL, Lee IM, Pate RR, et al. Physical activity and public health: updated recommendation for adults from the American College of Sports Medicine and the American Heart Association. Medicine and Science in Sports and Exercise 2007;39(8): 1423–34.

42. Beaser RS. Joslin's Diabetes Deskbook: A Guide for Primary Care Providers. Revised ed. Boston, MA: Joslin Diabetes Center Publications Department; 2003.

43. Steppel JH, Horton ES. Exercise for the Patient with Type 1 Diabetes Mellitus. In: LeRoith D, Taylor SI, Olefsky JM, eds. Diabetes Mellitus: A Fundamental and Clinical Text. Third ed. Philadelphia: Lippincott, Williams, & Wilkins; 2004.

18 Diabetes Education in Geriatric Populations

Angela Botts, MD and
Medha Munshi, MD

CONTENTS

INTRODUCTION
HEALTH EDUCATION AND LITERACY
    IN GERIATRIC POPULATIONS
COMPREHENSIVE ASSESSMENT AND GOAL SETTING
EXERCISE AND NUTRITION
DIABETES EDUCATION CHALLENGES
    IN GERIATRIC POPULATIONS
DIABETES-RELATED HEALTH LITERACY
COGNITIVE STATUS
DEPRESSION
POLYPHARMACY
PHYSICAL LIMITATIONS
FINANCIAL LIMITATIONS
CONCLUSIONS
REFERENCES

ABSTRACT

The population in the United States, as well as all around the world, is aging rapidly. The management of the chronic diseases in this elderly population is challenging and requires a different approach when compared to younger adults. Diabetes in particular has increasing prevalence in elderly patients. Challenges and

From: *Contemporary Diabetes: Educating Your Patient with Diabetes*
Edited by: K. Weinger and C. A. Carver, DOI 10.1007/978-1-60327-208-7_18,
© Humana Press, a part of Springer Science+Business Media, LLC 2009

barriers to self-care are unique in elderly patients with diabetes. Education that addresses these needs and takes into account the geriatric-specific barriers is important for better control of diabetes and overall quality of life in this population. This chapter focuses on unique challenges faced by elderly patients with diabetes and the importance of customizing education strategies based on such issues.

Key Words: Diabetes education, Geriatric, Elderly, Barriers to self-care.

INTRODUCTION

The challenges specific to the care of older adults with diabetes are becoming increasingly important with the aging of the population and rising prevalence of the disease. Between 2000 and 2020, it is estimated that the US population aged 65 and above will increase by 20% to approximately 55 million and is projected to skyrocket to approximately 87 million by 2050 *(1)*. At this time, people aged 65 and above account for 40% of patients with diabetes in the United States *(2)*. Data from 2005 found that 10.3 million people are aged 60 or above; 20.9% of all people in this age group have diabetes *(3)*. In addition, estimates derived from NHANES data found that 6.9% of adults aged 65 or above have diabetes that is undiagnosed *(4)*. The prevalence of diabetes among the elderly will continue to increase with the aging of the population. Diabetic education tailored to the need of this growing geriatric population is vital in helping them maintain optimal health and quality of life.

HEALTH EDUCATION AND LITERACY IN GERIATRIC POPULATIONS

Over the last century, chronic illnesses such as diabetes have become the most prevalent and costly diseases in the United States affecting more than 90 million Americans *(5)*. About 80% of adults aged 65 or above have at least one chronic condition and 50% suffer from two or more. The most prevalent include heart disease, cancer, stroke, chronic lower respiratory disease, Alzheimer's disease, and diabetes *(6)*. Overall, chronic diseases are responsible for 70% of deaths in the United States and consume more than 75% of the 1.4 trillion dollars spent annually on health care *(5)*. Effective health education is extremely important in decreasing the medical, quality of life, and financial implications of these diseases.

Although there is wide variation among the components of chronic disease self-management education programs, it is generally agreed that the purpose of these programs is to facilitate the patient's role in preventive and therapeutic healthcare activities. The heterogeneous nature of older adults makes it more challenging to attain these goals as the educational intervention must be tailored to the specific needs of each individual. Research focused on the special health education needs of geriatric populations is lacking. Of all the research published in two major health education research journals (*Health Education Quarterly*, now *Health Education and Behavior*, and *Health Education Research*) over a 10-year period, only 15 and 17%, respectively, reported results that included older adults. Older adults who were included in the research were often considered as a homogeneous group instead of differentiating among relatively younger populations (65–85 years) and the oldest old (85 years and above) *(7)*. In addition, geriatric health education research that is available is often lacking in ethnic, racial, and gender diversity.

Despite the paucity of research on chronic disease self-management education programs in the elderly, there is a clear understanding regarding the importance of health literacy among geriatric populations. In *Healthy People 2010*, health literacy is defined as "The degree to which individuals have the capacity to obtain, process, and understand basic health information and services needed to make appropriate health decisions" *(8)*. Health literacy is not simply being able to read but an ability to apply reading, listening, analysis, and decision-making skills to complex health situations. Wolf et al. *(9)* evaluated the understanding of prescription drug warning labels among 74 patients receiving primary care at a major teaching hospital. They found that 58% of subjects correctly interpreted the label "Take with food," 28% understood the instruction "Medication should be taken with plenty of water," and only 4% understood the label stating "You should avoid prolonged or excessive exposure to direct or artificial sunlight while taking this medication." Limited health literacy has been tied to a multitude of issues: delayed diagnosis, problems with use of preventive services, decreased understanding of medical conditions, non-compliance with medical instructions, and poor self-management skills.

A National Assessment of Adult Literacy survey conducted in 2003 found the elderly to be a vulnerable population, with 29% of people aged 65 or above having below-basic health literacy levels and 30% of elders having only basic health literacy skills *(10)*. In comparison, only 10% of people between ages 19 and 39 and 11–13% of people aged 40–64 scored below the basic health literacy level. Lower education and income levels, both more prevalent in geriatric populations than younger adults, place elders at even higher risk of lacking even basic health literacy skills. For example, 81% of patients aged 60 or above at one public hospital could not read or understand basic materials *(11)*. Minority and immigrant populations are also at significantly higher risk for having below-basic health literacy skills. This will have an increasing impact on health education in the elderly as the racial and ethnic diversity of geriatric populations is expected to increase dramatically over the next several decades. Data from the US Census Bureau predict that the proportion of people aged 65 and above will increase across racial and ethnic groups from 1990 to 2050: 13 to

23% for whites; 8 to 14% for blacks; 6 to 13% for American Indians, Eskimos, and Aleuts; 6 to 15% for Asians and Pacific Islanders; and 5 to 14% for Hispanics *(12)*. As the number of US elders with chronic diseases continues to grow, strategies for addressing health literacy disparities will be vital in successful health education for all geriatric populations.

The importance of diabetes education in the successful management has been widely documented. Diabetes education plans include the following components: (1) comprehensive assessment of the patient's knowledge, skills, attitudes, beliefs, psychosocial supports, and physical status; (2) development and prioritization of self-care goals; (3) formulation of an individualized plan to maximize diabetic management; and (4) reassessment and subsequent revision of the plan *(13)*. Several studies have shown that diabetes education programs for older adults have long-lasting benefits on glycemic control, psychosocial functioning, and knowledge *(14,15)*.

COMPREHENSIVE ASSESSMENT AND GOAL SETTING

Geriatric populations with type 2 diabetes are a heterogeneous group, and performing a comprehensive, holistic assessment of each individual patient is an invaluable first step in formulating an appropriate diabetes education program. In addition to traditional assessment, basic assessment in elders should also include evaluation of physical, cognitive, and functional status. Social support systems and availability of caregiver support need to be assessed. Impairments in any of these areas can significantly impact the patient's ability to learn new information and perform certain self-care tasks. The ethnic background of the elderly patient should be considered during formulation of the diabetes education plan as health beliefs, food preferences, and life goals are often significantly impacted (see Chapter 7, which addresses ethnic issues, for further information).

Patient preferences must be taken into account during formulation of a diabetes care plan as healthcare goals and treatment preferences vary widely among elderly individuals. Some patients favor aggressive disease management as recommended by standard diabetes treatment guidelines. However, the overall goal for many elders is to remain as functional and independent as possible. Remaining self-sufficient and managing their illness without assistance may be more important to these individuals than reaching recommended laboratory and treatment goals. For example, elders requiring assistance with insulin administration may choose to take only oral medications even if this results in their hemoglobin A1C remaining elevated. Similarly, a patient with a gait abnormality and history of orthostatic hypotension may decline medication to lower blood pressure for long-term cardiac risk reduction because he or she is concerned that a decrease in blood pressure could contribute to a potentially disastrous fall.

Estimating life expectancy is a very useful component of the comprehensive assessment as there is wide variability in longevity after the age of 65. Walter and Covinsky proposed a framework to guide cancer screening in geriatric populations that included prediction of life expectancy *(16)*. Similar predictions are now being used to tailor treatment in many elders with chronic diseases including diabetes *(17)*. If patients have low estimated life expectancies secondary to multiple morbidities, the focus of diabetes education must be tailored to their specific needs. As approximately 8 years of tight glycemic control is needed to reduce microvascular complications, it may be more beneficial in a patient with a short life expectancy to focus on blood pressure and lipid management which require only 2–3 years to demonstrate a benefit *(17)*. In individuals with a very short life expectancy, a focus on comfort may be most reasonable.

Co-existing medical conditions can act as barriers in patients' ability to learn. Six geriatric syndromes were included in the diabetes mellitus guidelines developed by the American Geriatrics Society Panel on Improving Care for Elders with Diabetes and the California Healthcare Foundation: polypharmacy, depression, cognitive impairment, urinary incontinence, injurious falls, and pain *(18)*. These syndromes were included based on increased prevalence in elders with diabetes and their important role in glycemic control as well as overall quality of life. The presence of these conditions may indicate the need for adjustment in the educational strategy.

Following the initial comprehensive assessment and implementation of the educational plan, frequent reassessment and revision is vital in geriatric populations. As individual patients age, their treatment needs and ability to perform disease self-management tasks change. For example, aggressive therapy aimed at optimal blood glucose management and prevention of complications is appropriate for many elders, but in individuals with a short life expectancy a change in focus to comfort and quality of life may become more appropriate. Caretakers or family members may need to assume a more active role in assisting patients with their diabetes management. Thoughtful reassessment will ensure that each patient's education plan is realistic with achievable goals and provides the most benefit possible to that individual.

EXERCISE AND NUTRITION

Exercise and nutrition are important components of diabetes education programs in elders as in younger adults. Exercise has proven to be beneficial in older adults with a variety of conditions including a history of falls, osteoarthritis, and osteoporosis. It can improve muscle strength, gait and balance, and overall quality of life. In elderly patients with diabetes, certain types of exercise can also result in improved glycemic control and other positive metabolic outcomes. Castaneda et al. evaluated the effect of progressive resistance training (PRT) in 62 Latino elders with type 2 diabetes *(19)*. They found that

Table 1
Issues Pertaining to Management of Diabetes in Elderly Patients

Goal setting	– Aim for best glycemic control (as close to 7% as possible) that can be achieved without hypoglycemic episodes – Change goals for glycemic control based on changes in patient's comorbidities, functional status, or life expectancy
Exercise	– Encourage exercise that is safe for individual patient and reinforce importance of physical activity for better control of blood sugars, blood pressure, cholesterol, and overall health and quality of life – Recommend supervised physical therapy in patients with history of falls or fear of falls
Nutrition	– Evaluate patient's dietary education and understanding as they may have wrong preconceptions – Assess individual food preferences and meal preparation capabilities – Assess for unintended weight loss in frail elderly given increased risk of morbidity and mortality – Evaluate for barriers to adequate nutrition such as decreased appetite or difficulty with chewing/swallowing and recommend appropriate diet counseling
Medications/insulin	– "Start low and go slow" is an excellent principle for all the medications – Consider increased risk of drug-to-drug reactions, hepatotoxicity, nephrotoxicity, and uncommon side effects – Avoid complicated treatment strategies like sliding scale and self-adjustment in patients with cognitive dysfunction or if patient seems overwhelmed
Hypoglycemia	– Educate patients and caregivers that in elderly patients neuroglycopenic symptoms like weakness, confusion, agitation, delirium, or falls can be manifestation of hypoglycemia – Educate regarding risk of even mild hypoglycemia leading to poor outcomes like falls and traumatic injury
Monitoring	– Recommendations for monitoring should take into account patient's cognitive, functional, and socioeconomic limitations

16 weeks of PRT resulted in reduced plasma glycosylated hemoglobin levels, increased muscle glycogen stores, and reduced need for diabetes medications. Daly et al. evaluated the effect of high-intensity resistance training in maintaining bone mass in elderly, overweight diabetics during moderate weight loss *(20)*. Following 6 months of formalized resistance training, weight and fat mass decreased similarly among the control and intervention groups. However, lean mass increased and bone mineral density remained stable among the intervention group compared to decreases in these parameters among the control group. Despite the demonstrated benefits of exercise in patients with diabetes, many do not participate in any regular exercise. In a survey of 260 adults aged 55 or above with type 2 diabetes, 54.6% reported 0 min of physical activity per week *(21)*. Only 23% of subjects reported more than 60 min of physical activity per week. Diabetes education programs should focus on incorporating exercise into the regular routine of elders. Patients should be educated regarding an appropriate exercise program taking into account their individual comorbidities. For example, patients unable to walk long distances may benefit from water therapy or stationary biking. Low-impact exercise can be initiated as tolerated but cardiac clearance should be obtained prior to starting an intensive exercise program. Many older adults, especially those with a history of falls, benefit from exercising in a supervised setting.

Unlike younger people with diabetes, dietary modifications may have a limited role in elders secondary to difficulty changing lifelong eating habits, dependence on others for preparing meals, decreased appetite, concurrent health issues, and financial concerns. Elders who wish to modify their diet to improve glucose control should meet with a nutritionist for additional education. Studies show that participation in a nutrition education program can result in improved metabolic outcomes and nutrition knowledge *(22,23)*. Care should be taken to avoid large fluctuations in blood glucose; significant weight loss which is associated with increased morbidity and mortality in elders; and nutritional deficiency. Please see Table 1 for practical tips regarding diabetes management in elderly patients.

DIABETES EDUCATION CHALLENGES IN GERIATRIC POPULATIONS

Several issues have a significant impact on the ability of geriatric populations to benefit from diabetes education and successfully engage in self-care activities: health literacy, cognitive status, depression, polypharmacy, functional limitations, and financial limitations. These should be addressed in all diabetic elders and adjustments made to the diabetes education plan as needed. Please see Table 2 for practical tips related to these issues.

Table 2
Tips for Educating Older Adults with Co-Existing Medical Conditions

Cognitive dysfunction	– Keep sessions short and slow paced – Always provide written instructions – Include a caregiver in education sessions if possible – Consider individual rather than group lessons – Ask for any symptoms indicating hypoglycemic symptoms as patient may forget to mention it
Depression	– Be aware of signs indicating depression, e.g., disinterest in learning, non-compliance, lack of attention, or memory problems (known as psuedo-dementia)
Physical disability	– Consider glucometers with special features like talking meters, ones with a large display, or ones that do not require coding – Use tools like insulin pens, syringe magnifiers, or prefilled syringes as needed
Polypharmacy	– Encourage patient to always bring all medications to medical visits and keep list updated – Provide understanding of which medication is meant for which disease – Encourage use of memory aids like pill boxes

DIABETES-RELATED HEALTH LITERACY

Below-basic or basic health literacy is common among elders and can have a significant impact on the success of diabetes education programs. Williams et al. evaluated the relationship between functional health literacy levels and ability to answer diabetes-related knowledge questions *(24)*. Among the subjects, of whom 73% had attended diabetes education classes, those with inadequate functional health literacy had significantly less knowledge of their disease. Only 50% of subjects with inadequate functional health literacy knew the symptoms of hypoglycemia compared to 94% of those with adequate functional health literacy. Additionally, only 38% of subjects with below-basic health literacy knew the correct treatment for hypoglycemic symptoms as opposed to 73% of literate subjects. Older subjects were more likely to have inadequate health literacy in this study compared to their younger peers. Schillinger et al. found that subjects with inadequate health literacy were two times more likely to have retinopathy as compared to those with adequate health literacy *(25)*.

Given the significant association between poor health literacy and diabetic knowledge, all elders participating in a diabetes education program should be screened for adequate health literacy. It is important to remember that it is often impossible to determine a patient's health literacy through usual interaction and that many patients go to great lengths to hide their poor health literacy. Two screening questions for which the most validation data are available are "How often do you need to have someone help you when you read instructions, pamphlets, or other written material from your doctor or pharmacy?" and "How confident are you filling out medical forms by yourself?" (8). These questions take less than 1 min to administer and have sensitivities for detecting limited literacy skills ranging from 54 to 83%. Other instruments to assess health literacy include the Newest Vital Sign for which patients review a nutrition label and answer six questions regarding information on the label and the Rapid Estimate of Adult Literacy in Medicine for which patients read a list of 66 words and are scored on correct pronunciation.

If patients are found to have low health literacy, many steps can be taken to make their diabetes education as useful and understandable as possible. The amount of information taught during one session should be limited to one or two important points. It should then be reviewed with patients through the "teach-back" technique (8). Instead of simply asking patients if they have understood, this technique has patients explain or demonstrate what they have been taught to ensure understanding. If the patient is unable to explain correctly, the healthcare provider should assume they have not provided adequate teaching and reteach the information using an alternative technique. Schillinger et al. found that good glycemic control was independently associated with physician application of the "teach-back" technique (26). All written information should be provided in an easy-to-read format. Text should be at or below the 6th grade level, consist of one or two syllable words, and paragraphs should be kept short (8). In addition, although they are not substitutes for verbal and written information, simple diagrams or pictures should be used to enforce important concepts. Video recordings allow patients to review important teaching points at home.

COGNITIVE STATUS

Dementia is a common, devastating condition among geriatric populations affecting between 6 and 10% of all elders (27). The dramatic increase in geriatric populations over the next several decades will lead to a significantly increased prevalence of dementia. Kukull et al. established that incidence rates of dementia increase with age including an increase of 3.5-fold between the age groups of 75–79 years and 80–84 years (28). Multiple epidemiological studies have found a correlation between diabetes and an increased risk of cognitive dysfunction (29–31). In the Rotterdam study, diabetes was found to almost double the risk of dementia (32).

Cognitive impairment in elderly patients with diabetes is associated with functional disability, impaired diabetes self-care, and poor diabetes control. McGuire et al. found that older adults with diabetes and low-normal levels of cognition were approximately 13% more likely to become disabled and 20% more likely to die than diabetic patients with higher levels of cognitive functioning (33). In another study, elders with diabetes and cognitive dysfunction were less likely to manage their diabetes independently, had increased use of health services, and demonstrated a lower functional status as measured by activities of daily living (ADL) scores than those who were cognitively intact (34). In addition, specific impairment on measures of executive function (mediated by the frontal lobe) has been noted in patients with diabetes (35–38). Executive functions include a number of complex behaviors such as problem solving, planning, organization, insight, reasoning, and attention. Given the importance of self-management behaviors in diabetes treatment and the high complexity of diabetes treatment regimens (e.g., blood glucose testing, meal planning, and medication compliance), diabetic patients with such impairments face difficulty performing self-care tasks. Munshi et al. found that cognitive dysfunction is associated with poor glycemic control (39).

All elders participating in a diabetes education program should have a basic cognitive screening as subtle cognitive deficits are often undiagnosed and significantly impact the patient's self-care plan. As complex behaviors are necessary for diabetes self-care, it is especially important to evaluate for deficits in working memory and executive function. Tools such as the clock drawing test and the Mini-Mental State Exam are used commonly to screen for cognitive dysfunction in office settings (40,34). If abnormal, the patient should be referred for further diagnostic testing to evaluate for dementia. It is important to periodically repeat cognitive testing in elders with diabetes as their risk for developing cognitive impairment continues to increase with duration of the disease and advancing age.

If an elderly patient is found to have cognitive impairment, it is absolutely vital to tailor their diabetes education and self-care plan to their level of ability. A patient with mild cognitive impairment may be able to mange a simple, oral regimen independently. However, the same patient may be unable to manage a complex regimen including numerous injections of insulin, adjustment of sliding scale insulin doses, and interpretation of multiple finger sticks per day. Diabetes treatment and self-care plans must be modified to obtain as optimal of disease management as possible while still ensuring the safety of each patient. When possible, caregivers and family members should be included in all education sessions so that they can assist the patient in understanding and implementing the diabetes care plan. Simple written instructions and, when appropriate, diagrams/pictures should be used to reinforce the important educational issues. Patients with known cognitive dysfunction should have frequent reassessment as their ability to understand and implement the diabetes care plan will decline over time and appropriate adjustments will be needed.

DEPRESSION

Depression is a common comorbidity among elderly patients with diabetes and is associated with hyperglycemia, increased risk of diabetic complications, and decreased self-care. Among adults with diabetes, the presence of diabetes doubles the odds of comorbid depression as compared to non-diabetics (41). A recent systematic review and meta-analysis by Ai et al. found the overall prevalence of depression in subjects with type 2 diabetes at 17.6% (42). The prevalence was higher in women at 23.8% compared to men who had a prevalence of 12.8%. Depression occurring at an older age is often chronic and recurrent and is associated with diminished health-related quality of life (43,44).

Several studies have examined the association between diabetes and depression. Brown et al. examined this association in a population-based retrospective cohort study and found that type 2 diabetes, in and of itself, does not increase the risk of depression (45). However, subjects who suffered from comorbid disease and diabetic complications were at increased risk for developing depression. The increased prevalence of depression among diabetics appears to be related to the burden of comorbid chronic diseases and diabetic complications as opposed to a consequence of high blood sugars (45,46). In contrast, depression does appear to be a risk factor for the development of diabetes. A meta-analysis of nine longitudinal studies found that adults with depression or significant depressive symptoms have a 37% increased risk of developing diabetes (47). Engum also determined that symptoms of depression or anxiety are significant risk factors for the development of type 2 diabetes independent of previously established risks including physical inactivity, smoking, increased triglycerides, low HDL cholesterol, and central obesity (48).

Patients with diabetes and concurrent depression have lower adherence with self-care, poorer physical function, and increased risk of hyperglycemia compared to non-depressed patients with diabetes (49–53). Patients with depressive symptoms of medium and high severity have significantly worse adherence with diet and medication than subjects with a low severity of depressive symptoms (49). Park et al. also found an association between higher depressive symptom scores and poor self-care as related to diet and consistent medication use (50). Depressive symptoms were also found to be significantly associated with poor participation in education programs, with depressed subjects being six times more likely to have never participated in a diabetic education program.

The increased prevalence of depression and significant effects on self-care, physical function, and glycemic control make depression screening vital in all elderly diabetics. Screening conducted as part of the patient's diabetic education program must be concise and accurate to be effective in busy clinical practice. Whooley et al. evaluated a concise case-finding instrument consisting of two questions: "During the past month, have you often been bothered by feeling down, depressed, or hopeless?" and "During the past month, have you often been bothered by little interest or pleasure in doing things?" *(54)*. The sensitivity and specificity of the two questions was comparable to the other screening tests. Using such brief screening tools in elderly diabetics presenting for diabetes education is a reasonable first step. If they have a positive response, more comprehensive screening is indicated.

Treatment should be pursued in elders with diabetes diagnosed with depression. A randomized placebo-controlled double-blinded trial evaluating the effects of fluoxetine in depressed patients with diabetes found a significant reduction in depression symptoms among the treatment group *(55)*. In addition, the treatment group demonstrated improvement in glycemic control compared to the control group. However, in other studies, the effect of treatment of depression on glycemic control was not significant *(56)*. Use of other depression treatment modalities such as the use of care managers has also demonstrated improvement in mental and physical function in elderly patients *(57)*. Studies evaluating the cost-effectiveness have shown high clinical benefits of treatment of depression in older adults with diabetes at no greater cost than usual care *(56)*.

POLYPHARMACY

Polypharmacy is a complex, challenging aspect of caring for elderly diabetics who often require multiple medications to optimally manage their diabetes and associated conditions. Polypharmacy has been variably defined in the literature. Traditionally, polypharmacy has been defined as the concurrent use of multiple drugs ranging from two to five or more prescription medications *(58)*. Additional definitions include use of high-risk medications, questionable medication dosing, use of more medications than are clinically indicated, and using two or more drugs from the same chemical class *(58,59)*. Recently, data have emerged regarding the underuse of beneficial medications in medically complex elders such as those with diabetes. Underuse of beneficial medications, or "errors of omission," is more common in elders than in younger patients. Possible reasons for this include insufficient evidence of clinical benefit due to underrepresentation of geriatric patients in clinical trials, fear of polypharmacy, and financial barriers *(60)*. A focus on appropriate prescribing, interventions to increase regimen adherence, and financial feasibility are crucial for successful education of elderly diabetics.

Many studies have found poor adherence to prescribed medication regimens among patients with type 2 diabetes *(61–63)*. In a systematic literature review, adherence rates ranged from 36 to 93% for oral hypoglycemic agents *(61)*. Once-daily and monotherapy regimens had slightly higher compliance rates than more complex treatment regimens. Donnan et al. evaluated adherence (arbitrary cut-off point of 90%) in approximately 3,000 community-dwelling diabetics receiving treatment with a single oral hypoglycemic medication *(62)*. Despite being on a single drug regimen, only 31–34% of subjects were found to be adherent with their treatment regimen. Worse adherence was noted in older subjects and those with a longer duration of diabetes.

Interventions initiated through diabetes education programs can be crucial to increased medication adherence among elderly diabetics. Currently available evidence supports the following interventions: instruction and instructional materials; simplifying the regimen; counseling regarding the regimen; support group sessions; reminders; cuing medications to daily events; reinforcement and rewards; self-monitoring with regular physician review and reinforcement; and involving family members and significant others *(64–66)*. Piette et al. studied bi-weekly automated assessment and self-care education telephone calls with nurse telephone follow-up, a relatively low-cost, time-effective intervention that could be incorporated into diabetes education programs and improve medication adherence *(67)*. Adherence aids are commonly recommended to increase medication adherence. Patients who put their medications in a special place and those who took them in conjunction with a daily event did have better glycemic control than patients without any adherence aid.

Integrating such methods to increase medication adherence in elderly patients with diabetes is crucial to successful treatment of their diabetes and related medical conditions; decreased healthcare cost; and reduced risk of hospitalization. Sokol et al. evaluated the impacts of medication adherence in diabetes and three other chronic disease states *(68)*. In patients with diabetes, high levels of medication adherence were associated with statistically significant reductions in disease-related medical costs. In addition, subjects with 80–100% medication adherence were significantly less likely to require hospitalization as compared to those with lower adherence rates. In another meta-analysis, subjects with good adherence to beneficial drug therapy or placebo had half the mortality risk of subjects with poor adherence *(69)*. Subjects with good adherence to harmful drug therapy had double the risk of mortality as those with poor adherence to these medications.

Diabetes education should include a discussion of standard diabetic treatment guidelines and medication recommendations. This information should then be considered in the context of each patient's health and goals to arrive at an appropriate individual treatment plan. Elderly diabetics who choose aggressive management of their diabetes often require multiple medications to optimally control their blood sugar and achieve recommended goals for risk factor management (e.g., goals for blood pressure and cholesterol control). In addition, they often require several more medications to treat medical comorbidities. Patients should be asked to bring all of their medications to each clinic visit so an accurate list can be ensured and the regimen can be evaluated for possible drug-to-drug interactions.

PHYSICAL LIMITATIONS

Over 50% of elders with diabetes have difficulty performing daily physical tasks *(70)*. Among community-dwelling diabetic elders, 32% of women and 15% of men were unable to walk one-fourth of a mile, climb stairs, or do housework compared to 14% of women and 8% of men without diabetes *(71)*. Patients with diabetes have sighted physical limitations as significant barriers to diabetes education. The most frequently anticipated barriers to successful education are poor vision and hearing difficulties *(72)*. Functional disabilities significantly impact diabetes education and self-management in the elderly.

Given the relatively high frequency of visual and auditory impairments among elderly diabetics and the potential impact on successful diabetes education, visual and auditory assessment should be performed in all patients beginning a diabetes education program. Education in visually impaired patients can be optimized through the use of large print educational materials, auditory educational materials, and a "talking" glucose meter. In addition, using prefilled syringes can prevent unintentional under- or overdosing of insulin. Portable amplifier devices should be available for patients with decreased hearing who do not have hearing aids.

Diabetes and comorbid medical conditions often result in significant impairments in activities of daily living (ADL) and instrumental activities of daily living (IADL) among elderly diabetics. A functional assessment of ADL (bathing, grooming, feeding, dressing, and toileting) and IADL (shopping, housework, finances, telephoning, and transportation) is indicated in all elders with diabetes presenting for diabetes education as education and self-care strategies need to be tailored to account for such impairments. In addition, this assessment should be repeated at regular intervals to ensure there is no decline in overall functional ability.

FINANCIAL LIMITATIONS

Compared with other chronic medical conditions, diabetes can have significant financial implications for elders with high out-of-pocket costs *(73)*. In a cross-sectional survey of 875 community-dwelling adults with diabetes, 19% reported cutting back on medication use in the prior year due to cost and 7% reported cutting back on their diabetes medications at least once per month *(74)*. In addition, 28% of subjects had forgone food or other essentials to pay for their medications. An observational cohort study of diabetic Medicare beneficiaries aged 65 and above found a significant association between household income and use of evidence-based therapies *(75)*. Subjects with an annual household income under $20,000 had significantly lower rates of statin use compared to subjects with a higher annual income. Even with Medicare Part D, co-payments pose a significant financial burden to many low-income diabetic elders.

Patients seldom discuss cost-related medication issues with their physicians and report that they are seldom asked about financial limitations *(76,77)*. Piette et al. surveyed 660 older adults with chronic illnesses who had underused medication within the past year due to cost *(77)*. Two-thirds of subjects did not tell the clinician in advance that they planned to underuse medication due to cost and 35% never discussed the issue. In addition, 66% of subjects reported that they were never asked about their ability to pay for prescriptions. However, when a conversation was held about medication costs, 72% of subjects found it helpful. Asking elderly patients about financial limitations that will impact their ability to adhere to a diabetic treatment regimen is a vital component of diabetes education. Patients with financial limitations should be referred to social work for assistance in applying for free or discounted medications and other medical equipment. Education regarding available Medicare Part D plans and assistance in choosing the best plan for their medication regimen can also be very beneficial in elderly diabetics.

CONCLUSIONS

Effective geriatric diabetes education programs will be increasingly important over the next several decades with the aging of the population and increased prevalence of the disease. To positively impact self-care and quality of life in elderly diabetics, education programs must be tailored to patients' individual needs. A comprehensive assessment should be performed with each patient to understand their individual goals, strengths, and deficits. Many elderly diabetics have issues with health literacy, impaired cognitive status, depression, polypharmacy, physical limitations, and financial limitations. These areas should be screened for in all elders presenting for diabetic education and readdressed on a regular basis as new issues can arise as patients age and their medical conditions progress. Ongoing research in the area of geriatric health education is also vital to customizing education programs to geriatric populations and improving outcomes for all elders.

REFERENCES

1. Interim Projections by Age, Sex, Race, and Hispanic Origin., 2004. (Accessed 17 July 2007, at http://www.census.gov/ipc/www.usinterimproj/.)
2. Engelgau MM, Geiss LS, Saaddine JB, et al. The evolving diabetes burden in the United States. Ann Intern Med 2004;140(11):945–50.

3. National Diabetes Fact Sheet. 2005. (Accessed 17 July 2007, at http://www.cdc.gov/diabetes/pubs/estimates05.htm.)
4. Selvin E, Coresh J, Brancati FL. The burden and treatment of diabetes in elderly individuals in the U.S. Diabetes Care 2006;29(11):2415–9.
5. Chronic Disease Overview. 2005. (Accessed 19 July 2007, at http://0-www.cdc.gov.mill1sjlibrary.org/print/do?url.)
6. Healthy Aging Preserving Function and Improving Quality of Life Among Older Americans. 2007. (Accessed 19 July 2007, at http://0-www.cdc.gov. mill1.sjlibrary.org/print.do?url.)
7. Connell CM. Older adults in health education research: some recommendations. Health Educ Res 1999;14(3):427–31.
8. Health Literacy 2007. 2007. (Accessed 19 July 2007, at http://www.ama-assn.org/amal/pub/upload.mm.367/healthlitclinicians.pdf.)
9. Wolf MS, Davis TC, Tilson HH, Bass PF, 3rd, Parker RM. Misunderstanding of prescription drug warning labels among patients with low literacy. Am J Health Syst Pharm 2006;63(11):1048–55.
10. Health Literacy and Patient Safety: Help Patients Understand. American Medical Association Foundation. (Accessed 23 July 2007, at http://www.ama-assn.org/amal/pub/upload/mm/367/healthlitclinicians.pdf.)
11. Williams MV, Parker RM, Baker DW, et al. Inadequate functional health literacy among patients at two public hospitals. JAMA 1995;274(21):1677–82.
12. The Elderly Population. U.S. Census Bureau, Population Division and Housing and Household Economic Statistics Division, 2001. (Accessed 20 July 2007, at http://www.census.gov/population/www.pop-profile.elderpop.html.)
13. Sitnikov L, Weinger, K. Diabetes Education in Older Adults. New York: Informa Healthcare USA, Inc.; 2007.
14. Gilden JL, Hendryx MS, Clar S, Casia C, Singh SP. Diabetes support groups improve health care of older diabetic patients. J Am Geriatr Soc 1992;40(2):147–50.
15. Gilden JL, Hendryx M, Casia C, Singh SP. The effectiveness of diabetes education programs for older patients and their spouses. J Am Geriatr Soc 1989;37(11):1023–30.
16. Walter LC, Covinsky KE. Cancer screening in elderly patients: a framework for individualized decision making. JAMA 2001;285(21):2750–6.
17. Durso SC. Using clinical guidelines designed for older adults with diabetes mellitus and complex health status. JAMA 2006;295(16):1935–40.
18. Brown AF, Mangione CM, Saliba D, Sarkisian CA. Guidelines for improving the care of the older person with diabetes mellitus. J Am Geriatr Soc 2003;51(5 Suppl Guidelines):S265–80.
19. Castaneda C, Layne JE, Munoz-Orians L, et al. A randomized controlled trial of resistance exercise training to improve glycemic control in older adults with type 2 diabetes. Diabetes Care 2002;25(12):2335–41.
20. Daly RM, Dunstan DW, Owen N, Jolley D, Shaw JE, Zimmet PZ. Does high-intensity resistance training maintain bone mass during moderate weight loss in older overweight adults with type 2 diabetes? Osteoporos Int 2005;16(12):1703–12.
21. Hays LM, Clark DO. Correlates of physical activity in a sample of older adults with type 2 diabetes. Diabetes Care 1999;22(5):706–12.
22. Miller CK, Edwards L, Kissling G, Sanville L. Nutrition education improves metabolic outcomes among older adults with diabetes mellitus: results from a randomized controlled trial. Prev Med 2002;34(2):252–9.
23. Miller CK, Edwards L, Kissling G, Sanville L. Evaluation of a theory-based nutrition intervention for older adults with diabetes mellitus. J Am Diet Assoc 2002;102(8):1069–81.
24. Williams MV, Baker DW, Parker RM, Nurss JR. Relationship of functional health literacy to patients' knowledge of their chronic disease. A study of patients with hypertension and diabetes. Arch Intern Med 1998;158(2):166–72.

25. Schillinger D, Grumbach K, Piette J, et al. Association of health literacy with diabetes outcomes. JAMA 2002;288(4):475–82.
26. Schillinger D, Piette J, Grumbach K, et al. Closing the loop: physician communication with diabetic patients who have low health literacy. Arch Intern Med 2003;163(1):83–90.
27. Bruce DG, Casey GP, Grange V, et al. Cognitive impairment, physical disability and depressive symptoms in older diabetic patients: the Fremantle Cognition in Diabetes Study. Diabetes Res Clin Pract 2003;61(1):59–67.
28. Kukull WA, Higdon R, Bowen JD, et al. Dementia and Alzheimer disease incidence: a prospective cohort study. Arch Neurol 2002;59(11):1737–46.
29. Yaffe K, Blackwell T, Kanaya AM, Davidowitz N, Barrett-Connor E, Krueger K. Diabetes, impaired fasting glucose, and development of cognitive impairment in older women. Neurology 2004;63(4):658–63.
30. Grodstein F, Chen J, Wilson RS, Manson JE. Type 2 diabetes and cognitive function in community-dwelling elderly women. Diabetes Care 2001;24(6):1060–5.
31. Helkala EL, Niskanen L, Viinamaki H, Partanen J, Uusitupa M. Short-term and long-term memory in elderly patients with NIDDM. Diabetes Care 1995;18(5):681–5.
32. Ott A, Stolk RP, van Harskamp F, Pols HA, Hofman A, Breteler MM. Diabetes mellitus and the risk of dementia: The Rotterdam Study. Neurology 1999;53(9):1937–42.
33. McGuire LC, Ford ES, Ajani UA. The impact of cognitive functioning on mortality and the development of functional disability in older adults with diabetes: the second longitudinal study on aging. BMC Geriatr 2006;6:8.
34. Folstein MF, Folstein SE, McHugh PR. "Mini-mental state". A practical method for grading the cognitive state of patients for the clinician. J Psychiatr Res 1975;12(3):189–98.
35. Gold AE, Deary IJ, Frier BM. Hypoglycemia and cognitive function. Diabetes Care 1993;16(6):958–9.
36. Grande L MW, Rudolph J, Gaziano M, McGlinchey R. A Timely Screening for Executive Functions and Memory. J Int Neuropsychol Soc 2005;11:S9–10.
37. Kuo HK, Jones RN, Milberg WP, et al. Effect of blood pressure and diabetes mellitus on cognitive and physical functions in older adults: a longitudinal analysis of the advanced cognitive training for independent and vital elderly cohort. J Am Geriatr Soc 2005;53(7):1154–61.
38. Abbatecola AM, Paolisso G, Lamponi M, et al. Insulin resistance and executive dysfunction in older persons. J Am Geriatr Soc 2004;52(10):1713–8.
39. Munshi M, Grande L, Hayes M, et al. Cognitive dysfunction is associated with poor diabetes control in older adults. Diabetes Care 2006;29(8):1794–9.
40. Nishiwaki Y, Breeze E, Smeeth L, Bulpitt CJ, Peters R, Fletcher AE. Validity of the Clock-Drawing Test as a screening tool for cognitive impairment in the elderly. Am J Epidemiol 2004;160(8):797–807.
41. Anderson RJ, Freedland KE, Clouse RE, Lustman PJ. The prevalence of comorbid depression in adults with diabetes: a meta-analysis. Diabetes Care 2001;24(6):1069–78.
42. Ali S, Stone MA, Peters JL, Davies MJ, Khunti K. The prevalence of co-morbid depression in adults with Type 2 diabetes: a systematic review and meta-analysis. Diabet Med 2006;23(11):1165–73.
43. Schulberg HC, Mulsant B, Schulz R, Rollman BL, Houck PR, Reynolds CF, 3rd. Characteristics and course of major depression in older primary care patients. Int J Psychiatry Med 1998;28(4):421–36.
44. Unutzer J, Patrick DL, Diehr P, Simon G, Grembowski D, Katon W. Quality adjusted life years in older adults with depressive symptoms and chronic medical disorders. Int Psychogeriatr 2000;12(1):15–33.
45. Brown LC, Majumdar SR, Newman SC, Johnson JA. Type 2 diabetes does not increase risk of depression. CMAJ 2006;175(1):42–6.

46. Knol MJ, Heerdink ER, Egberts AC, et al. Depressive symptoms in subjects with diagnosed and undiagnosed type 2 diabetes. Psychosom Med 2007;69(4):300–5.
47. Knol MJ, Twisk JW, Beekman AT, Heine RJ, Snoek FJ, Pouwer F. Depression as a risk factor for the onset of type 2 diabetes mellitus. A meta-analysis. Diabetologia 2006;49(5):837–45.
48. Engum A. The role of depression and anxiety in onset of diabetes in a large population-based study. J Psychosom Res 2007;62(1):31–8.
49. Ciechanowski PS, Katon WJ, Russo JE. Depression and diabetes: impact of depressive symptoms on adherence, function, and costs. Arch Intern Med 2000;160(21):3278–85.
50. Park H, Hong Y, Lee H, Ha E, Sung Y. Individuals with type 2 diabetes and depressive symptoms exhibited lower adherence with self-care. J Clin Epidemiol 2004;57(9):978–84.
51. Ciechanowski PS, Katon WJ, Russo JE, Hirsch IB. The relationship of depressive symptoms to symptom reporting, self-care and glucose control in diabetes. Gen Hosp Psychiatry 2003;25(4):246–52.
52. de Groot M, Anderson R, Freedland KE, Clouse RE, Lustman PJ. Association of depression and diabetes complications: a meta-analysis. Psychosom Med 2001;63(4):619–30.
53. Pouwer F, Snoek FJ. Association between symptoms of depression and glycaemic control may be unstable across gender. Diabet Med 2001;18(7):595–8.
54. Whooley MA, Avins AL, Miranda J, Browner WS. Case-finding instruments for depression. Two questions are as good as many. J Gen Intern Med 1997;12(7):439–45.
55. Lustman PJ, Freedland KE, Griffith LS, Clouse RE. Fluoxetine for depression in diabetes: a randomized double-blind placebo-controlled trial. Diabetes Care 2000;23(5):618–23.
56. Katon W, Unutzer J, Fan MY, et al. Cost-effectiveness and net benefit of enhanced treatment of depression for older adults with diabetes and depression. Diabetes Care 2006;29(2):265–70.
57. Williams JW, Jr., Katon W, Lin EH, et al. The effectiveness of depression care management on diabetes-related outcomes in older patients. Ann Intern Med 2004;140(12):1015–24.
58. Fulton MM, Allen ER. Polypharmacy in the elderly: a literature review. J Am Acad Nurse Pract 2005;17(4):123–32.
59. Viktil KK, Blix HS, Moger TA, Reikvam A. Polypharmacy as commonly defined is an indicator of limited value in the assessment of drug-related problems. Br J Clin Pharmacol 2007;63(2):187–95.
60. Higashi T, Shekelle PG, Solomon DH, et al. The quality of pharmacologic care for vulnerable older patients. Ann Intern Med 2004;140(9):714–20.
61. Cramer JA. A systematic review of adherence with medications for diabetes. Diabetes Care 2004;27(5):1218–24.
62. Donnan PT, MacDonald TM, Morris AD. Adherence to prescribed oral hypoglycaemic medication in a population of patients with Type 2 diabetes: a retrospective cohort study. Diabet Med 2002;19(4):279–84.
63. Kogut SJ, Andrade SE, Willey C, Larrat EP. Nonadherence as a predictor of antidiabetic drug therapy intensification (augmentation). Pharmacoepidemiol Drug Saf 2004;13(9):591–8.
64. McDonald HP, Garg AX, Haynes RB. Interventions to enhance patient adherence to medication prescriptions: scientific review. JAMA 2002;288(22):2868–79.
65. Haynes RB, McDonald HP, Garg AX. Helping patients follow prescribed treatment: clinical applications. JAMA 2002;288(22):2880–3.
66. Bartels D. Adherence to oral therapy for type 2 diabetes: opportunities for enhancing glycemic control. J Am Acad Nurse Pract 2004;16(1):8–16.
67. Piette JD, Weinberger M, McPhee SJ, Mah CA, Kraemer FB, Crapo LM. Do automated calls with nurse follow-up improve self-care and glycemic control among vulnerable patients with diabetes? Am J Med 2000;108(1):20–7.
68. Sokol MC, McGuigan KA, Verbrugge RR, Epstein RS. Impact of medication adherence on hospitalization risk and healthcare cost. Med Care 2005;43(6):521–30.

69. Simpson SH, Eurich DT, Majumdar SR, et al. A meta-analysis of the association between adherence to drug therapy and mortality. BMJ 2006;333(7557):15.
70. Gregg EW, Mangione CM, Cauley JA, et al. Diabetes and incidence of functional disability in older women. Diabetes Care 2002;25(1):61–7.
71. Gregg EW, Beckles GL, Williamson DF, et al. Diabetes and physical disability among older U.S. adults. Diabetes Care 2000;23(9):1272–7.
72. Rhee MK, Cook CB, El-Kebbi I, et al. Barriers to diabetes education in urban patients: perceptions, patterns, and associated factors. Diabetes Educ 2005;31(3):410–7.
73. Bernard DM, Banthin JS, Encinosa WE. Health care expenditure burdens among adults with diabetes in 2001. Med Care 2006;44(3):210–5.
74. Piette JD, Heisler M, Wagner TH. Problems paying out-of-pocket medication costs among older adults with diabetes. Diabetes Care 2004;27(2):384–91.
75. Brown AF, Gross AG, Gutierrez PR, Jiang L, Shapiro MF, Mangione CM. Income-related differences in the use of evidence-based therapies in older persons with diabetes mellitus in for-profit managed care. J Am Geriatr Soc 2003;51(5):665–70.
76. Heisler M, Wagner TH, Piette JD. Clinician identification of chronically ill patients who have problems paying for prescription medications. Am J Med 2004;116(11):753–8.
77. Piette JD, Heisler M, Wagner TH. Cost-related medication underuse: do patients with chronic illnesses tell their doctors? Arch Intern Med 2004;164(16):1749–55.

19 Prevention: Educating Those at Risk for Diabetes

Helena Duffy, APRN-BC, CDE,
Janet O. Brown-Friday, MSN, MPH, RN,
and Elizabeth A. Walker, PhD, RN, CDE

CONTENTS

INTRODUCTION
RATIONALE FOR DIABETES PREVENTION
BACKGROUND OF DIABETES
   PREVENTION RECOMMENDATIONS
IDENTIFICATION OF RISK FACTORS FOR DIABETES
SCREENING FOR DIABETES AND DIABETES RISK
DIABETES PREVENTION PLAN
USE OF PHARMACOLOGIC AGENTS
   FOR DIABETES PREVENTION
CONCLUSION
REFERENCES

ABSTRACT

Many of the therapeutic goals of diabetes care, such as lifestyle changes for weight management and medication adherence, are also effective for diabetes prevention.

The diabetes educator can play a critical role in identifying and educating individuals at high risk for type 2 diabetes. Early detection of high-risk status provides an opportunity for early intervention and long-term health promotion. The diabetes educator is in a unique position to facilitate and support individual's efforts in implementing a diabetes prevention plan. The Diabetes Prevention Program – a national

From: *Contemporary Diabetes: Educating Your Patient with Diabetes*
Edited by: K. Weinger and C. A. Carver, DOI 10.1007/978-1-60327-208-7_19,
© Humana Press, a part of Springer Science+Business Media, LLC 2009

clinical trial sponsored by the National Institute of Diabetes, Digestive, and Kidney Diseases – showed that a lifestyle intervention with the goal of moderate weight loss (5–10% of body weight) and increasing physical activity (150 minutes of moderate intensity exercise per week) are recommended for prevention of type 2 diabetes. The study also showed that pharmacologic treatment with metformin has also shown a degree of effectiveness for diabetes prevention in certain individuals. Prevention of type 2 diabetes can help alleviate the human and economic toll of this chronic disease which has become a worldwide epidemic.

Key Words: Pre-Diabetes, Impaired Glucose Tolerance, Oral Glucose Tolerance Test, Diabetes Prevention Program, Lifestyle Intervention.

INTRODUCTION

The diabetes educator plays a critical role in facilitating and supporting patient's efforts toward monitoring and self-management of diabetes. These skills are also crucial for monitoring and management of diabetes risk for primary prevention of type 2 diabetes. Some of the therapeutic goals of diabetes care, such as lifestyle changes for weight management and medication adherence, are also effective for diabetes prevention. The goal of this chapter is to provide the diabetes educator with an overview of the impact of diabetes, and the role diabetes prevention can play in decreasing the human and economic toll of the disease. The findings of recent research show effective interventions for diabetes prevention. Guidelines for identification and screening of individuals at high risk for type 2 diabetes are an important part of prevention for this disease. The chapter provides a description of the framework for a lifestyle intervention as implemented in the Diabetes Prevention Program, as well as information about pharmacological therapy for diabetes prevention.

RATIONALE FOR DIABETES PREVENTION

The economic and human cost of diabetes remains high despite considerable improvement in diabetes management. Clinical studies such as the Diabetes Control and Complications Trial (1) and the United Kingdom Prospective Diabetes Study (2) revealed that optimizing blood glucose control can decrease the rates of microvascular complications. However, diabetes remains the leading cause of new cases of blindness among adults aged 20–74 years. It is the leading cause of kidney failure and more than 60% of non-traumatic lower limb amputations occur in people with diabetes (3). The long-term impact of diabetes is seen in the increased rates of cardiovascular disease and stroke in this population. Heart disease death rates and risk for stroke are 2–4 times higher among people with diabetes (3). Diabetes was the sixth leading cause of death listed on U.S. death certificates in 2002 and is likely to be underreported as a cause of death.

Overall the risk of death among people with diabetes is twice that of people without diabetes *(3)*. Annual health-care and related costs associated with diabetes are about $132 billion. This accounts for both the direct and the indirect costs of health care. Direct medical costs such as hospitalizations, medical care, and treatment supplies total about $92 billion. Indirect costs such as disability payments, time lost from work, and premature death account for $40 billion *(3)*. In 2002, annual per capita health-care costs for individuals with diabetes were about $13,243 or $10,683 per year more than expenditures for individuals without diabetes *(4)*. Diabetes places an enormous burden on the health-care system and individual patients living with this chronic illness. Costs of direct medical care, education and counseling, glucose monitoring, management and monitoring of complications, patients' out-of-pocket costs, and lost wages due to disability may be diminished through interventions which prevent or delay the onset of diabetes *(5)*. Efforts focused on diabetes prevention may also enhance quality of life *(6,7)*.

BACKGROUND OF DIABETES PREVENTION RECOMMENDATIONS

Recent clinical studies of lifestyle intervention or pharmacological agents have shown varying levels of effectiveness in prevention or delay of type 2 diabetes in people at high risk for the development of the disease *(8–12)*. The results of these trials generate questions and controversy among health-care providers and patients regarding whether study results can or should be translated into the real world. For example, a study of general practitioners' knowledge and perceptions of impaired glucose tolerance, a high-risk pre-diabetes state, identified barriers to screening and intervention *(13)*. Focus groups that were conducted as part of the study identified a low awareness of the prevalence and clinical significance of impaired glucose tolerance. Concern about increased workload, lack of resources, pessimism about the effectiveness of lifestyle intervention, and the belief that screening and treating impaired glucose tolerance places a medical focus on an essentially social problem were also common themes *(13)*.

In 2006, the American Diabetes Association convened a panel of experts in diabetes, endocrinology, and metabolism to address the question of diabetes prevention *(14)*.

The panel acknowledged that, at present, there is little direct data regarding the impact of diabetes prevention on long-term complications. However, possible benefits of prevention include delaying the need for complex treatment;

delaying or preventing microvascular and possibly cardiovascular complications; and the potential preservation of B-cell function. In light of the prospect of these benefits the panel indicated that early intervention is justified. The consensus statement provides background and guidelines for the prevention of type 2 diabetes. Included with the panel's recommendations is a description of the spectrum of glucose tolerance states and associated risk for diabetes, means of identifying patients at high risk, methods of screening, and considerations in the selection of appropriate prevention interventions *(14)*.

IDENTIFICATION OF RISK FACTORS FOR DIABETES

The first step in initiating effective prevention measures is identifying those individuals who are at highest risk. An estimated 54 million American adults, aged 20 years or older, have a pre-diabetes condition called impaired glucose tolerance (IGT) or impaired fasting glucose (IFG). Impaired glucose tolerance and impaired fasting glucose are metabolic states where blood glucose levels are above normal but not as high as the diagnostic level for diabetes. Individuals with blood glucose levels in this range are at increased risk for developing type 2 diabetes, heart disease, and stroke. Over a period of 3–5 years about 25% of patients with impaired glucose tolerance or impaired fasting glucose progress to diabetes, 50% remain in the pre-diabetes glucose range, and 25% revert to normal blood glucose levels *(14–17)*.

There are particular patient characteristics associated with impaired fasting glucose, impaired glucose tolerance, and diabetes. Assessment of these risk factors can assist in targeting screening toward individuals most likely to benefit from prevention or early intervention and treatment.

Risk factors include

- **Age** – over 45 years
- **Body Mass Index** – BMI>24 k/m^2

(Asian Americans increased risk is noted at BMI$\geq$ 23 k/m^2)

- **Family history of type 2 diabetes**
- **Ethnicity**

    African American – Non-Hispanic blacks aged 20 or older are 1.8 times as likely to have diabetes as non-Hispanic whites.
    Hispanic or Latino American – Mexican Americans age 20 or older are 1.7 times as likely to have diabetes as non-Hispanic whites.
    American Indians and **Alaska Natives** age 20 or older are 2.2 times as likely to have diabetes as non-Hispanic whites.

Asian Americans or **Pacific Islanders** are 1.5 times as likely to have diabetes as non-Hispanic whites

- **History of gestational diabetes or having delivered an infant weighing 9 pounds or more** – Women with a history of gestational diabetes have a 20–50% chance of developing diabetes over the next 5–10 years.
- **Hypertension, hyperlipidemia,** and **physical inactivity.** *(3)*
- **Central obesity** – Waist circumference >102 cm for men or >88 cm for women *(18)*

SCREENING FOR DIABETES AND DIABETES RISK

The American Diabetes Association recommends that all individuals aged 45 or older be screened with a fasting plasma glucose and, if the result is within the normal range, repeat screening every 3 years *(19)*. A 2-h oral glucose tolerance test (OGTT) using a 75-g glucose load is also an accepted means of assessing blood glucose and can help determine risk for type 2 diabetes. More frequent and earlier screening is recommended for people with the aforementioned risk factors for type 2 diabetes. The current standard screening for women who have gestational diabetes is to have an assessment of fasting plasma glucose 6–12 weeks after delivery. However, recommendations for post-gestational diabetes screening may soon be extended. A report from the Fifth International Workshop – Conference on Gestational Diabetes Mellitus recommends the use of the oral glucose tolerance test instead of the fasting glucose and notes that repeat testing 1 year after delivery may be warranted *(20)*. In the course of ongoing interaction with patients and their families and through community outreach programs, diabetes educators are in a unique position to increase awareness of diabetes risk factors to promote appropriate screening and preventive intervention.

DIABETES PREVENTION PLAN

Following the identification of pre-diabetes, the health-care provider along with the patient can work together to develop and implement a diabetes prevention plan. In light of the association between obesity and diabetes, the American Diabetes Association consensus statement on management of impaired fasting glucose and impaired glucose tolerance stresses the importance of obesity prevention and maintenance of healthy weight as the first line of intervention in preventing type 2 diabetes. For individuals at high risk, achievement of modest weight loss (5–10% of body weight) and moderate intensity physical activity (approximately 30 minutes each day) is the treatment of choice *(14)*. Lifestyle change which resulted in a moderate weight loss and increased physical activity was the most effective intervention in recent diabetes prevention studies *(8–10)*.

In the Diabetes Prevention Program, which compared lifestyle changes for weight loss and metformin treatment, the lifestyle intervention produced a 58% reduction in the incidence of developing diabetes in individuals at high risk when compared to the placebo group. One case of diabetes was prevented per seven people treated for 3 years. In the program, overweight participants with impaired glucose tolerance and impaired fasting glucose followed a plan to lose and maintain a 7% of body weight and to increase physical activity to 150 minutes per week *(8)*. Promoting healthy lifestyle changes can be difficult for primary care providers, even in the context of type 2 diabetes. Limited team resources and the lack of training in facilitating behavior change create a challenge *(13,21,22)*.

The Diabetes Prevention Program Lifestyle intervention may provide a model or framework for achieving weight loss and activity goals needed for decreasing the risk of developing type 2 diabetes. One of the most important components is a collaborative approach in which the individual's strengths and limitations are considered in order to develop an individualized, feasible plan with realistic goals. The Diabetes Prevention Program was a multi-center clinical study, and the lifestyle intervention team varied from center to center. Physicians, nurses, behavioral scientists, exercise physiologists, and registered dietitians contributed to the development of the lifestyle intervention protocol. During the study intervention, dietitians played a vital role. Diabetes Prevention Program lifestyle participants met with their case manager 16 times over the first 6 months of the program as they completed a core curriculum *(23)*.

Diabetes Prevention Program Dietary Recommendations

Initially a low-fat (<25% of total calories) diet was recommended. If goals were not achieved with a reduction in fat, then calorie restriction was recommended. Recommendations for fat and calorie goals were based on the patient's baseline weight as described in Table 1 *(23)*.

Table 1
Diabetes Prevention Program Lifestyle Intervention Meal Plan Recommendations

Baseline weight	Fat g/day (<25% of total calories)	kcal/day
120–174 lbs (54–78 kg)	33 g fat	1,200 kcal/day
175–219 lbs (79–99 kg)	42 g fat	1,500 kcal/day
220–249 lbs (100–113 kg)	50 gm fat	1,800 kcal/day
250 lbs or more (≥ 114 kg)	55 g fat	2,000 kcal/day

At 1 year, participants in the lifestyle intervention group had reduced daily intake by a mean of 450 ± 26 k/cal (p<0.001). Average fat intake, which was 34.1% of total calories at baseline, decreased by $6.6\pm 0.2\%$ in the lifestyle intervention group (p<0.001) *(8)*.

Increasing physical activity was another important component of the Diabetes Prevention Program lifestyle intervention. Prior to starting the activity intervention, individuals with underlying coronary artery disease underwent an exercise tolerance test *(24)*. Participants were encouraged to increase their activity slowly and to exercise at least three times per week for at least 10 minutes per session. Brisk walking was the exercise of choice, and volunteers participated in individual or group walks using pedometers and activity records in order to track progress and increase motivation. Alternative activities such as dancing or following aerobic exercise videos, and so forth were recommended based on participants' interests. No more than 75 minutes per week of strength training could be applied to the activity goal of 150 minutes per week *(23)*. At the end of the 16-session core curriculum (at 24 weeks), 50% of the participants in the lifestyle intervention group had achieved the goal weight loss of 7% or more and 74% of participants met the goal of at least 150 minutes of physical activity per week.

Many components of the Diabetes Prevention Program Lifestyle intervention helped participants achieve diet and exercise goals. Individual case managers or "lifestyle coaches" helped set clearly defined weight loss and physical activity goals. Participants made decisions regarding which part of the intervention, diet, or increasing activity, they desired to initiate first. Volunteers participated in an intensive ongoing intervention with supervised exercise sessions, flexible scheduling, supplemental group classes on motivation, relapse prevention, and restart opportunities. A "tool box" approach was used and materials were available and provided as they were relevant to individual's specific needs. Program materials and strategies, which were developed by collaboration of local and national expertise, considered the needs of the ethnically diverse participant population. Training, feedback, and clinical support were also provided by this network *(23)*. The Diabetes Prevention Program lifestyle intervention objectives and materials are available via the internet *(25)*.

The importance of an individualized, culturally sensitive approach is also recognized in materials offered by the National Diabetes Education Program (NDEP). The "Small Steps. Big Rewards Prevent Type 2 Diabetes" is jointly sponsored by the National Institutes of Health and the Centers for Disease Control and Prevention. The NDEP developed the handouts based on the results of the Diabetes Prevention Program. The program materials which specifically address the needs of an ethnically diverse, at risk population are available on line at www.ndep.nih.gov *(26)*. All materials on the NDEP website can be downloaded free of charge and are free of copyright restrictions (any organization can add their logo to the educational materials for community use).

In reviewing aspects of the lifestyle intervention which promoted success in reaching long-term weight loss and activity goals, the Diabetes Prevention Program study group stressed the importance of the "jump start." In the program, early success at achieving weight loss goals predicted later success. Participants who achieved weight loss goals at the end of the core curriculum were three times more likely to achieve the goal at the end of the study. Participants who achieved the activity goal at the end of the core curriculum were 1.5 times more likely to achieve the goal at the final intervention visit. Record keeping or self-monitoring of diet and activity was also related to meeting weight loss and activity goals (27). These findings suggest the importance of initiating a formalized program which provides support through frequent contacts and follow-up.

The core curriculum which was covered with each Diabetes Prevention Program participant focused first on practical measures for weight loss during the initial sessions. Later sessions focused more on behavioral aspects of weight loss and maintenance of weight loss. Maintaining a collaborative approach and facilitating motivation were important goals of the Diabetes Prevention Program Lifestyle coach. To foster this goal, coaches were trained and encouraged to develop skills in the use of motivational interviewing (MI). Motivational interviewing is a technique in which the clinician interacts with the patient as a guide to explore ambivalence about setting goals and making lifestyle changes (28). The provider's role in the process of motivational interviewing is to act as a coach instead of an advisor. The approach recognizes the patient as an expert in his own life and focus is on realistic short-term goals as chosen by the patient. Additional information on motivational interviewing is available on the Internet at www.motivationalinterview.org/training/mint.htm. Materials for the Diabetes Prevention Program Lifestyle sessions (23) are available on the Internet at www.bsc.gwu.edu/dpp/manuals.htmlvdoc.

Limited resources, associated costs, and concerns about potential adverse effects may be barriers for practitioners initiating and supporting a lifestyle intervention. A group intervention may provide an effective means of implementing a plan with limited resources (5). The Diabetes Prevention Program Lifestyle Intervention was developed as a structured program for individuals or groups. A recent study of a behavioral weight loss program showed that intervention with a small group of 8–12 participants was more effective than an intervention with individuals (29). The effectiveness of lifestyle intervention coaches outside the health-care provider realm is now under investigation. In an ongoing study, the Indiana University Diabetes Translational Research Center has collaborated with local YMCA to adapt the DPP Lifestyle Intervention in a community setting. The pilot study showed a 6% weight loss after 6 months with maintenance after 12 months. The emerging results of this study indicate that a lifestyle intervention in a group setting, facilitated by trained YMCA staff, achieved results similar to those seen in the Diabetes Prevention Program *(30)*. Health-care providers may also be concerned about the feasibility and safety of lifestyle intervention in patients over 60 years of age. Increasing age is a risk factor for diabetes, and in the Diabetes Prevention Program the lifestyle intervention was most effective in preventing diabetes in older participants, with a 71% reduction in the development of diabetes *(8)*.

Studies of lifestyle change to promote weight loss and increase activity indicate that interventions are safe and may provide other beneficial health effects. For example, in the Diabetes Prevention Program participants in the lifestyle intervention showed an improvement in cardiovascular disease risk factors compared to participants in medication or placebo groups. At baseline 30% of Diabetes Prevention Program participants had hypertension. Rates increased in the metformin and placebo groups and decreased in the lifestyle intervention group. At 3 years of follow-up, the use of medications to achieve hypertension control was 27–28% less in the lifestyle intervention group compared with placebo and metformin groups. Twenty-five percent less of lifestyle intervention participants were on pharmacological agents for hyperlipidemia treatment. Over the course of the 3 year intervention there was no difference in number of cardiovascular disease events between treatment groups; however, decreasing risk factors for cardiovascular disease over a more extended period of time may reduce cardiovascular disease events *(31)*.

USE OF PHARMACOLOGIC AGENTS FOR DIABETES PREVENTION

In the United States there are currently no medications approved for diabetes prevention. Some recent studies which looked at medications presently used for diabetes treatment indicate that these agents may play a role for diabetes prevention in individuals at high risk. However, when considering medication use for prevention, health-care providers and patients must consider risks and benefits.

Insulin-sensitizing agents, troglitazone and rosiglitazone, in the thiazolidinedione class were assessed in the TRIPOD *(32)* and DREAM *(12)* studies and showed effectiveness for diabetes prevention in patients with a high body mass index and markers of insulin resistance such as high waist circumference. Cost, increased rates of congestive heart failure, and increased rate of fractures in women on rosiglitazone where noted in the consensus panels discussion on potential risks of this intervention. Troglitazone was removed from the market due to liver damage in some patients on the medication.

Metformin, a biguanide, and Acarbose *(11)*, an alpha glucosidase inhibitor, were also studied for use in diabetes prevention. In the Diabetes Prevention Program, metformin reduced the incidence of diabetes by 31% compared to placebo *(8)*. The greatest effect was seen in younger individuals with a higher body mass index. Based on this finding the American Diabetes Association consensus panel for prevention recommends consideration of metformin treatment for individuals younger than 60 years with a body mass index greater than or equal to $35\,kg/m^2$ and at highest risk, with combined impaired fasting glucose and impaired glucose tolerance, as determined by an oral glucose tolerance test. During the Diabetes Prevention Program, metformin was well tolerated. Potential gastrointestinal side effects such as stomach upset and risk of lactic acidosis need to be addressed for patients on this medication. Acarbose may be as effective as metformin for diabetes prevention, but the panel indicates that cost and common gastrointestinal side effects should be a consideration *(14)*.

In treating patients with diabetes, the diabetes educator addresses concerns regarding medication use with the goal of optimizing effectiveness while controlling for potentially adverse effects. These concerns are also a focus in the use of medication for diabetes prevention. Adherence to medication for prevention can be a challenge because no immediate effect, such as symptom control, is noted by patients. The benefit of the effect is seen over time.

Monitoring and promoting adherence to preventive medication was an issue addressed by the Diabetes Prevention Program *(33)*. In the Diabetes Prevention Program, a brief structured interview was initiated with participants every 3 months. The goal of the interview was to identify barriers to adherence to taking the study medication and to collaborate with the patient to develop strategies for overcoming these barriers. In addition, the interview included a request for feedback on previously implemented adherence strategies. The Diabetes Prevention Program medication adherence "tool box" provided recommendations for managing individual barriers to medication adherence including various reminder devices. Detailed information regarding Diabetes Prevention Program Medication "tool box" guidelines is available on the Internet at http://www.bsc.gwu.edu/dpp/index.htmlvdoc.

CONCLUSION

The role of the diabetes educator is expanding. Luckily, the tools available for use by the educator are also expanding and taking into account diverse populations. Recent studies, along with programs such as the National Diabetes Education Program (NDEP) and organizations such as the American Diabetes Association, the American Dietetic Association, and the American Association of Diabetes Educators, are working to provide additional educational materials to supplement the knowledge and skills of the educator in order to address the needs of the multifaceted populations they serve. This information can only strengthen the role of the diabetes educator in both institutional (hospital or outpatient care) and community settings. Successful prevention also requires a focus on behavioral intervention that supports lifestyle changes. Because of their orientation to cognitive, emotional, and behavioral aspects of the individual at risk, the diabetes educator is the ideal "preventionist" for type 2 diabetes.

REFERENCES

1. The Diabetes Control and Complications Trial Research Group. The effect of intensive treatment of diabetes on the development and progression of long-term complication in insulin-dependent diabetes mellitus. N Engl J Med 1993;329:977–986.
2. UK Prospective Diabetes Study (UKPDS) Group. Intensive blood glucose control with sulphonylureas or insulin compared with conventional treatment and risk of complication in patients with type 2 diabetes (UKPDS 33). Lancet 1998;352:837–853.
3. CDC: National Diabetes Fact Sheet, 2005 available from http://www.cdc.gov/diabetes/pubs/factsheet05.htm Accessed 29 October 2007.
4. American Diabetes Association: Direct and Indirect Costs of Diabetes in the United States On the internet at: http://www.diabetes.org/diabetes-statistics/cost-of-diabetes-in-us.jsp Accessed 29 October 2007.
5. The Diabetes Prevention Program Research Group: Within-trial cost effectiveness of lifestyle intervention or metformin for the primary prevention of type 2 diabetes. Diabetes Care 26:2518–2523,2003.
6. Tapp RJ, Dunstan DW, Phillips P, Tonkin A, Zimmet PZ, Shaw JE for the Aus Diab study group. Association between impaired glucose metabolism and quality of life: results from the Australian Diabetes Obesity and Lifestyle Study. Diabetes Res Clin Pract 2006;74:154–161.
7. Banegas JR, Lopez-Garcia E, Graciani A, et al.: Relationship between obesity, hypertension and diabetes, and health-related quality of life among the elderly. Eur J Cardiovac Prev Rehabil 2007;14(3):456–462.
8. The Diabetes Prevention Program Research Group: Reduction in the incidence of type 2 diabetes with lifestyle intervention or metformin. N Engl J Med 2002;346:393–403.
9. Pan XR, Li GW, Hu YH, et al. Effects of diet and exercise in preventing NIDDM in people with impaired glucose tolerance: the DaQing IGT and Diabetes Study. Diabetes Care 1997;20:537–544.
10. Tuomilehto J, Lindstrom J, Eriksson JG, et al. Prevention of type 2 diabetes mellitus by changes in lifestyle among subjects with impaired glucose tolerance. N Engl J Med 2001;344:1342–1350.
11. Chiasson JL, Josse RG, Gomis R, Hanefetd M, Karasik A, Laakso M, the STOP-NIDDM Trial Research Group: Acarbose for prevention of type 2 diabetes mellitus: the STOP-NODDM randomized trial. Lancet 2002;359:2072–2077.
12. Gerstein HC, Yusuf S, Borch J, Pogue J, Sheridan P, Dinccag N, Hanefetd M, Hoogwerf B, Lasskso M, Mohan V, Shaw J, Zinman B, Holman RR: Dream (Diabetes Reduction Assessment with Ramipril and Rosiglitazone Medication) Trial Investigators: Effect of rosiglitazone on the frequency of diabetes in patients with impaired glucose tolerance or impaired fasting glucose: a randomized controlled trial. Lancet 2006;368:1096–1100.
13. Wylie G, Hungin AP, Neely J: Impaired glucose tolerance: qualitative and quantitative study of general practitioner's knowledge and perceptions. BMJ 2002;324:1190.

14. Nathan D, Davidson M, DeFronzo RA, Heine RJ, Henry RR, Pratley R, Zinman B: Impaired fasting glucose and impaired glucose tolerance. Diabetes Care 2007;30:753–759.

15. Shaw JE, Zimmet PZ, de Courten M, Dowse GK, Chtson P, Gareeboo H, Hemraj F, Fareed D, Tuomilehto J, Alberti KG: Impaired fasting glucose or impaired glucose tolerance: what best predicts future diabetes in Mauritius: Diabetes Care 1999;22:399–402.

16. Nichols GA, Hillier TA, Brown JB:Progression from newly acquired impaired fasting glucose to type 2 diabetes. Diabetes Care 2007;30:228–233.

17. Stern MP, Williams K, Haffner SM: Identification of persons at high risk for type 2 diabetes mellitus: do we need the oral glucose tolerance test? Ann Intern Med 2002;136:575–581.

18. National Heart, Lung, and Blood Institute. Clinical Guidelines on the Identification, Evaluation, and Treatment of Overweight and Obesity in Adults. Bethesda, Md: National Heart, Lung and Blood Institute: 1998.

19. American Diabetes Association: Standard of care for diabetes-2006.Diabetes Care 2006;29 (Suppl.):S4–S42.

20. Metzger BE, Buchanan TA, Coustan DR, et al.:Summary and recommendations of the Fifth International Workshop-conference on Gestational Diabetes Mellitus. Diabetes Care 2007;30:S251–S260.

21. Lawler DA, Keen S, Neal RD. Can general practitioners influence the nation's health through a population approach to provision of lifestyle advice?. Br J Gen Pract 2000;50:455–459.

22. Pill R, Stott NCH, rollnick SR, Rees M. A randomized controlled trial of an intervention designed to improve the care given in general practice to type 2 diabetic patients: patient outcomes and professional ability to change behavior. Fam Pract 1998;15:229–35.

23. The Diabetes Prevention Program Research Group: The Diabetes Prevention Program description of lifestyle intervention. Diabetes Care 2002;25:2163–2171.

24. American College of Sports Medicine, ACSM's Guidelines for Exercise Testing and Prescription, 7th ed, Baltimore, MD: Lippincott Williams & Wilkins, 2006.

25. Diabetes Prevention Program Study Repository. For further information regarding the Diabetes Prevention Program Lifestyle session, materials, learning objectives. On the internet: www.bsc.gwu.edu/dpp/manuals.htmlvdoc Accessed 29 October 2007.

26. National Diabetes Education Program. For further information regarding the "Small Steps. Big Rewards. Prevent type 2 Diabetes" materials On the internet: http//www.ndep.nih.gov Accessed 29 October 2007.

27. The Diabetes Prevention Program Research Group: Achieving weight and activity goals among Diabetes Prevention Program lifestyle participants. Obes Res 2004;12:1426–1434.

28. West DS, DiLillo V, Bursac Z, et al.: Motivational interviewing improves weight loss in women with type 2 diabetes. Diabetes Care 2007;30:1081–1087.

29. Renjilian DA, Perri MG, Nezu AM, McKelvey WF, Shermer RL, Anton SD: Individual versus group therapy for obesity: effects of matching participants to their treatment preferences. J Consult Clin Psychol 2001;69:717–721.

30. Marrero D, Ackermann R: Providing long-term support for lifestyle changes: a key to success in diabetes prevention. Diabetes Spectrum 2007;20:205–209.

31. The Diabetes Prevention Program Research Group: Impact of intensive lifestyle and metformin therapy on cardiovascular disease risk factors in the Diabetes Prevention Program. Diabetes Care 2005;28:888–894.

32. Buchanan TA, Xiang AH, Peters Rk, Kjos Sl, Maroquin A, Goico J, et al. Preservation of pancreatic beta-call function and prevention of type 2 diabetes by pharmacological treatment of insulin resistance in high risk Hispanic women. Diabetes 2002;51:2796–803.

33. Walker E, Molitch M, Kramer MK, Kahn S, Yong M, Edelstein S, et al. Adherence to preventive medications predictors and outcomes in the Diabetes Prevention Program. Diabetes Care 2006;29:1997–2002.

INDEX

A

AADE-7 Self-Care Behaviors, 58, 100, 147
Acanthosis nigricans, 20
Acarbose, 318
Acculturation and DSME, 117–118
ACE inhibitors, 216, 244
Adolescence, 252
    diabetes education for, 263–265
Aerobic exercise, 282, 284
Aging, 98
Alpha-glucosidase inhibitors, review in outpatient diabetes, 73
Alprostadil, 220
Alternative coping, in weight loss and diabetes management, 277
Alternative medicine and DSME, 126
American Association of Diabetes Educators (AADE), 6, 78, 155, 165, 180–181, 185, 318
American Diabetes Association (ADA) Education Recognition Program, 161, 163, 180–181
American Diabetes Association (ADA) Provider Recognition Program, 160
American Diabetes Association Clinical Standards for Diabetes Care, 165
American Urological Association Guidelines on the Pharmacologic Management of Premature Ejaculation, 225
Anxiety, 201–202
Arthritis, 98, 110–111

Assessment
    components, 47–48
    of diabetes education, 46–49
    and goal setting for geriatric populations, 292–293
Asthma, 160
Autonomic neuropathy, 109–110, 282

B

Basal insulin therapy, 74
Behavioral Risk Factor Surveillance System (BRFSS), 123, 127
Behavioral strategies, for weight loss and diabetes management, 274, 276–277
Bladder dysfunction, 109
Blood glucose
    data gathering, 146–149
    guidelines and targets, 145–146
    in inpatient diabetes education, 88
    management, 284–285
    monitoring results, 88, 150, 258
    pattern management, 146–149
    in pediatric diabetes education, 258
Blood ketone testing, 68
Body image, 128
Bolus therapy, 74
Breastfeeding, for women with preexisting or gestational diabetes, 247–248
Brief test of functional health literacy in adults (Brief-TOHFLA), 121

C

Calcium channel blockers, 243
    diabetes camps, 252, 262–263
Cancer, 98–99, 110, 222, 290, 293
Carbohydrate counting, 90
Cardiovascular autonomic
    neuropathy, 109
Cardiovascular disease, 21, 216, 237,
    247, 274, 317
Cerebrovascular disease, 18, 103
Challenging patients
    active problem-oriented coping
        style, 208–209
    co-morbid conditions and,
        205–207
    definition, 200
    in diabetes treatment, 197–209
    encounters, 198–200
    psychosocial problems and,
        200–205
        hyperglycemia fear, 202–204
        hypoglycemia fear, 201–202
        weight gain fear, 204–205
    working alliance, 198–200
        patients' beliefs and
            behaviors, 199, 208
        professional self-awareness,
            198–199, 207–208
        support treatment
            environment, 208
Children and adolescents with diabetes
    development patterns of, 253,
        255
    education of, 259 (*See also*
        Pediatric diabetes
        education)
    treatment goals for, 255–257
Chronic care model, 37–38
Chronic obstructive pulmonary
    disease, 99
Clinical information systems, 38
Clinical practice
    lifestyle approach in, 284–285
    weight and diabetes
        management in, 274–285
Clinician–patient interaction, and
    language, 119

Cognitive restructuring, in weight loss
    and diabetes management, 277
Cognitive status, of geriatric
    populations, 296–298
Communication, among providers of
    inpatient diabetes education,
    91–93
    diabetes educator role, 92
    educating staff to be diabetes
        educator, 92
    quality improvement projects,
        92–93
Community pharmacists, 55
Co-morbid conditions, and challenging
    diabetes patients, 205–207
Comorbidities
    arthritis, 111
    depression, 111
    impact on self-care, 98–100
    medication strategies, 101
    polypharmacy with, 100–101
Congestive obstructive pulmonary
    disease, 160
Continuous glucose monitoring (CGM),
    136, 138–141
Continuous quality improvement (CQI)
    process 190–193
Continuous subcutaneous insulin
    infusion (CSII), 136
Cultural competence and DSME, 118
Culture, and health-care practice,
    116–117

D

Daily calorie consumption, in weight
    loss and diabetes management,
    279
DASH meal plan, 103
Dawn phenomenon, 136
Dementia, 297
Depression, 110–111, 205–207, 264
    and diabetes mellitus, 22–23
    and DSME, 129
    in geriatric populations, 296,
        299–300
Diabetes action plan, 64
Diabetes care at school, 259–262

Diabetes complications, 9, 18, 97–112
    autonomic neuropathy,
        109–110
    cerebrovascular disease, 103
    diabetic eye disease, 105
    diabetic neuropathies, 107–110
    group education, 112
    impact on self-care, 98–100
    macrovascular complications,
        101–103
    medication strategies, 101
    nephropathy, 105–107
    and optimum self-care, 97–112
    peripheral arterial disease,
        104–105
    peripheral neuropathies,
        107–109
    polypharmacy with, 100–101
Diabetes Control and Complications
    Trial (DCCT), 12, 23,
    251–253, 259
Diabetes discharge checklist, 94
Diabetes education
    effectiveness of, 9–12, 30
    focus on self-care, 5–6
    in geriatric populations,
        289–303
    history of, 4–5
    implications for, 135–141
    plan, 50–51, 53–54
    for prevention of diabetes,
        309–318
    process, 45–59
        assessment, 47–49
        documentation and
            informatics, 56–59
        follow up, 54–55
        goal setting, 51–53
        open-ended assessment
            questions, 49–50
    role in diabetes, 3–12
    technology in self-care,
        135–141
    theoretical models, 32–33
Diabetes education program
    CQI process, 190–193
    evaluation of, 177–193
        effectiveness, 178–179

rationale for, 178–179
reach, 177
resources allocation, 179
risk, 179
growth in, 187–189
operational metrics, 180–184
other customer groups,
    189–190
patient satisfaction, 189
program operations, 184–187
Diabetes educators
    patient's readiness to learn, 49
    professional performance, 51
    role in men's sexual health,
        230–231
Diabetes medical management plan
    (DMMP), 261–262
Diabetes mellitus
    barriers to self management,
        6–7
    behavioral interventions, 8, 11
    behavior change and outcomes
        measurement, 171–172
    burnout, 9
    β cells autoimmune
        destruction, 16–17
    certifications for practice
        settings, 162–163
    classification of, 17–19
    complications, 9, 18, 97–112
    cost of, 17
    day-to-day management, 46
    depression and, 22–23,
        110–111, 129, 205–207,
        264, 296, 299–300
    diagnosis, 7–8, 19–20
    diagnostic criteria, 19
    effectiveness of educational
        interventions, 9–12
    gestational diabetes, 18–19
    health related literacy and,
        296–297
    health system models, 36–39
    hypoglycemia risk and, 18, 23
    lifestyle changes, 23–24
    living with, 7–9
    measurement sets for practice
        settings, 162–163

model, 5–6, 29–40
outpatient visit, 61–78
patient–educator interaction
    models, 31–34
poverty, 124
practice level models, 34–36
pregnancy, 20, 235–244
prevalence, 16
prevention, 8–9, 309–319
    dietary recommendations
        for, 314
    pharmacological agents used
        for, 317–318
    plan, 313–317
    rationale for, 310–311
    recommendations for,
        311–312
psychological interventions, 11
related health education,
    296–297
resources for people with, 111
risk factors, 312–313
role of diabetes education, 3–12
screening for, 313
self-care model, 5–6
self-management, 24–25, 30
severe complications, 9
sexual health, 213–231
symptoms, 17, 19
treatment, 20–22
type 1, 7, 12, 16–17
type 2, 8, 11, 16–18
weight gain, 23 (*See also*
    Weight and diabetes
    management)
Diabetes Physician Recognition Program
    (DPRP), 162
Diabetes Prevention and Control
    Programs (DCPC), 160, 163
Diabetes Prevention Program, 10, 284,
    309–310, 314–318
Diabetes Problem-Solving Interview
    (DSPI), 164
Diabetes resources, 78
Diabetes self-care behavior, science of
    measuring, 164–165

Diabetes self-management education
    (DSME), 30, 34, 36–37, 46, 57,
    81–84, 91–92, 95, 116–131, 144
    acculturation and, 117
    alternative medicine, 126
    body image, 128
    cultural competence, 117–118
    depression, 129
    educational level, 123
    family integration and support,
        130
    fears, 124–125
    health literacy, 119–122
        alternative ways to deliver
            messages, 122
        measures, 121
        scope of, 119–122
        vocabulary and
            understanding, 120,
            122
    individual and social
        interaction, 131
    judgment and belief about
        disease, 124
    knowledge about disease, 123
    language, 118–119
    myths, 124
    national standards for, 161, 165,
        170, 178, 180, 190
    nutritional preferences,
        126–127
    outcome standards, 161
    physical inactivity, 127–128
    quality of life, 130
    religion and faith, 129–130
    socioeconomic status of patient,
        124
    teach-back technique, 297
    work environment, 128–129
Diabetes Self-Management Education
    Outcome Standards, 161
Diabetes self-management skills, 89
Diabetes-specific communication, 95
Diabetes support groups, 55
Diabetes technology, 136–141
Diabetic eye disease, 105
Diabetic ketoacidosis (DKA), 137, 264

in women with preexisting
diabetes, 242
Diabetic kidney disease, 98
Diabetic nephropathy, 100, 107–110
Dietary supplements, 126
Dipeptidyl peptidase IV (DPP-IV)
inhibitors, 20–21, 72
Distal symmetric polyneuropathy
(DPN), 107
Documentation
components, 57
consumers, 56
in diabetes education process,
56–58
model records, 58–59
purpose, 56
Dyslipidemia, 102, 104
Dyspareunia (painful intercourse), 226

E

Education, *See* Diabetes education
Educational level, and DSME, 123
Education plan, 50–51, 53–54
Educator considerations
for patient self-care behaviors
after heart failure, 102
with kidney disease, 107
with peripheral
neuropathies, 108
with visual impairment, 106
Empowerment model, of diabetes
education, 32
Elderly patients with diabetes, *See*
Geriatric populations
Electronic medical records (EMRs), 58
Epidemiology of Diabetes Interventions
and Complications (EDIC) study,
12, 252
Erectile dysfunction
anatomy and physiology,
215–216
first-line therapies for, 218–219
risk factors, 216–217
second-line therapies for,
220–221
treatment options, 217–221
Erythrocytosis, 241
Euglycemia, 244

Exenatide, 21, 23, 72, 275
Exercise
facilities, 55
in gestational diabetes, 245
and nutrition in geriatric
populations, 293–295
for pregnant women with
preexisting diabetes,
240–241
safety recommendations with
exercise, 285
for weight loss and diabetes
management, 282–285

F

Faith and DSME, 129–130
Family integration, and DSME, 130
Family management, of diabetes, 255
Fatigue, 17
Fears, and DSME, 125
Fetal risks, for pregnant women with
preexisting diabetes, 241–242
Five A's model of self-management
support, 33–35
Flexibility exercise, 283
Food preferences, 102, 126

G

Gangrene, 18
Gastroparesis, 109
Geriatric populations
assessment and goal setting,
292–293
challenges of diabetes
education in, 295–296
cognitive status, 296–298
depression, 296, 299–300
diabetes education in, 289–303
exercise and nutrition, 293–295
financial limitations, 302–303
health education and literacy in,
290–292, 296–297
physical limitations, 296, 302
polypharmacy, 296, 300–302
Gestational diabetes, 18–19, 244–248
Glargine insulin, 239
Glinides, 21

Glucose management
    in gestational diabetes,
        245–246
    in pregnant women with
        preexisting diabetes,
        238–239
Glucose toxicity, 16
α-glucosidase inhibitors, 20–21
Glycemic management,
Glycosuria, 275
Goal setting
        for inpatient diabetes education,
            84–85
        technique, 51–53
        in weight loss and diabetes
            management, 276
Group assessment, 49

H

Harris–Benedict formula, for daily
    calorie consumption, 278–279
Health belief model, of diabetes
    education, 32
Health care outcomes continuum, 166
Health-care systems, 30, 34, 37, 38
Health Effectiveness Data and
    Information Set (HEDIS), 160,
    162
Health literacy
        alternative ways to deliver
            messages, 122
        and DSME, 119–123
        in geriatric populations,
            290–292, 295–296
        measures, 48, 121
        scope of, 119–120
        vocabulary and understanding,
            120, 122
Heart failure, 98
        patient self-care behaviors after,
            102
Height and weight monitoring, in
    outpatient diabetes, 69
HELLP syndrome, 243
Hyperbilirubinemia, 241, 245
Hyperglycemia, 81–83, 92, 95, 102,
    104–106, 109–110, 137–138, 157,
    241, 247, 254, 274

fear in challenging diabetes
    patients, 202–204
Hyperlipidemia, 104, 229, 274, 317
Hypertension, 100, 102–103, 105, 109,
    160, 205, 229, 238, 243, 246–247,
    274, 317
    gestational, 250
    transient, 250
Hypertensive disorders, in pregnant
    women with preexisting
    diabetes, 243
Hypertrophic cardiomyopathy, 241
Hypocalcemia, 245
Hypoglycemia, 51, 55, 70, 73, 83,
    85, 89, 138–140, 146, 157, 239,
    245, 253–255, 258, 275, 278,
    281, 285
        fear in challenging diabetes
            patients, 201–202
        risk and diabetes mellitus, 18,
            23

I

Impaired fasting glucose (IFG),
    311–314, 318
Impaired glucose tolerance (IGT),
    311–314, 318
Incretins, review in outpatient diabetes,
    72–73
Indian Health Service (IHS), 161, 163
Individual education program (IEP),
    261–262
Individual health care plan (IHP),
    261–262
Individualized exercise plan, for weight
    loss and diabetes management,
    281–282
Influenza, 110
Injury prevention, in exercise for weight
    loss and diabetes management,
    284–285
Inpatient diabetes education
        assessment, 83
        communication among
            providers, 91–93
        certified diabetes educator
            role, 92

educating staff to be diabetes educator, 92
quality improvement projects, 92–93
components, 83
diabetes discharge checklist, 94
discharge, 93–95
educational delivery, 89–91
carbohydrate counting, 90
documentation, 91
education material for, 89
making hospitals diabetes friendly, 89–91
goal setting, 84–85
key topics of content
additional education, 88
blood glucose monitoring, 88
meal planning, 86
medications, 86–88
potential barriers and advantages, 84
self-management education process, 82–96
transition from inpatient to outpatient, 93–95
Insulin, 4, 70
on board, 137
glargine, 21
in gestational diabetes, 246
mismanagement patients, 205
pump therapy, 136–137
resistance, 7, 16–17, 20, 23
review in outpatient diabetes, 72, 75–76
self-administration, 87
therapy, 21–22, 87, 275
Intrauterine growth restriction, in pregnant women with preexisting diabetes, 242

J

JCAHO Disease Specific Certification for Inpatient Diabetes, 162
Joslin Diabetes Center Affiliated program, 178, 183
Judgment and belief about disease, and DSME, 124

K

Ketones production control, in pregnant women with preexisting diabetes, 241, 245
Ketone testing, in outpatient diabetes, 68
Kidney disease, self-care behaviors for patients with, 105, 107
Knowledge about disease, and DSME, 123

L

Labetolol, 243
Language and DSME, 118–119
Latino Diabetes Initiative, 125
Lifestyle approach
in clinical practice, 284–285
and diabetes mellitus, 23–24
LookAHEAD trial, 275–276

M

Macrovascular complications
coronary artery disease, 101–102
in diabetes, 101–103
education consideration for, 101–103
Macrovascular diseases, 98
Malformation risks, for pregnant women with preexisting diabetes, 241
Maternal risks, for pregnant women with preexisting diabetes, 242–243
Maternal surveillance, in gestational diabetes, 246
Meal planning, for inpatient diabetes education, 86
Medical assessment, 47
of pregnant women with preexisting diabetes, 238
Medical nutrition therapy (MNT), 257
Medication
for inpatient diabetes education, 86–88
in pediatric diabetes education, 257
for pregnant women with preexisting diabetes, 239
strategies, 101
taking behavior, 172

Meglitinides, 73
Men's sexual health, 214–225
    diabetes educator role, 230–231
    erectile dysfunction, 214–221
    premature ejaculation, 225
    testosterone deficiency,
        222–225
    testosterone replacement
        therapies, 223–224
    therapies for erectile
        dysfunction, 218–221
Mental health providers, 55
Metformin, 23, 239, 275, 317–318
    review in outpatient diabetes,
        70–72
Methyldopa, 243
Microvascular diseases, 98
Mifflin–St. Jeor equations, for daily
    calorie consumption, 278–279
Minority groups, health-care disparities,
    116, 129
Monitoring, of outpatient diabetes,
    67–68
Motivational interviewing technique, 50,
    316
Myocardial infarction, 98
    patient self-care behaviors after,
        102
Myths and DSME, 124

N

National Committee on Quality
    Assurance (NCQA) Provider
    Recognition Program, 160, 162
National Diabetes Education Program
    (NDEP), 259, 261–262, 315, 318
National Standards for Diabetes
    Self-Management Education, 16,
    56, 161, 165, 170, 178, 180, 190
Neonatal hypoglycemia, 241, 244
Nephropathy, 18, 100, 105–107, 205,
    238
Neuropathy, 18, 98–99, 107–108, 205,
    226, 282
Newest vital sign (NVS), 48, 121
Nocturnal diarrhea, 109
Nursing care plan, 261

Nutrition
    in geriatric populations,
        293–295
    in pregnant women with
        preexisting diabetes,
        239–240
    for weight loss and diabetes
        management, 277–280
Nutritional preferences and DSME,
    126–127

O

Obesity, 102, 111, 247
    and diabetes management (*See*
        Weight and diabetes
        management)
    lifestyle interventions for,
        275–276, 284–285
Obstetric considerations, in gestational
    diabetes, 246–247
Older adults with co-existing medical
    conditions, education for, 296
Operational metrics, 180–184
    business plan and pro forma,
        182–183
    marketing plan, 183–184
    mission statement, 181–182
    programme goals and
        objectives, 182
    staff productivity goals, 183
Oral diabetes medications, in gestational
    diabetes, 246
Oral glucose tolerance test (OGTT),
    19–20, 247, 313, 318
Organogenesis, 241
Osteoarthritis, 99
Outpatient diabetes
    commonly asked questions,
        75–77
    diabetes resources, 78
    diabetes team role, 62–66
    healthy eating, 66–67
    height and weight monitoring,
        69
    instruction for, 66–67
    ketone testing, 68
    management, 61–62, 77–78
    medication management, 70–72

medication review by type and
action
alpha-glucosidase inhibitors,
73
incretins, 72
insulin, 72, 74–75
metformin, 70–72
oral agents, 71
secretagogues, 72–73
thiazolidinediones, 73
monitoring, 67–68
office flow for, 65–66
physical activity, 69–70

P

Parent management, of diabetes, 254
Paroxetine, 225
Patient
centered diabetes treatment,
197
centered education method, 50
educator interaction models
of diabetes mellitus, 31–33
teaching–learning process,
31
provider interactions, 198
provider relationship and
cultural competence, 118,
131
self-care behaviors and
educator considerations,
102, 106–107
socioeconomic status and
DSME, 123–124
Pattern management
PDCA cycle (plan–do–check–act), 190
Pediatric diabetes education, 253–259
transition in, 259–266
adolescence, 263–265
diabetes camps, 262–263
diabetes care at school,
259–262
young adulthood, 265–266
Penile implants, 221
Peripheral arterial disease, 104–105
Peripheral neuropathies, 98, 107–109
Peripheral vascular disease, 18

Physical inactivity
and DSME, 127–128
Pioglitazone, 20–21, 73
Placental hormones, 236
Plan–do–study act (PDSA) cycle, 36
Polycystic ovarian disease, 229
Polydipsia, 17
Polyphagia, 17
Polypharmacy
with comorbidities and diabetes
complications, 100–101
in geriatric populations, 296,
300–302
Polyuria, 17
Post-partum management
in gestational diabetes, 246–247
in pregnant women with
preexisting diabetes, 244
Practice level models, of diabetes
mellitus education, 34–36
Pramlintide, 20–21, 23, 275
Pre-diabetes, identification of, 312–313
Preeclampsia, 243, 245
Pregnancy
diabetes and, 235–244
gestational diabetes and,
244–248
metabolic changes during, 236
women with preexisting
diabetes, 236–244
contraception, 237
delivery, 243–244
DKA risks, 242
exercise, 240–241
fetal risks, 241–242
glucose management,
238–239
hypertensive disorders, 243
intrauterine growth
restriction, 242
ketones production control,
241
malformation risks, 241
maternal risks, 242–243
medical assessment, 238
medications, 239

nutrition, 239–240
  nutritional
    recommendations, 253
  post-partum management,
    244
  preconception evaluation
    and counseling,
    236–238
  renal function, 243
  retinopathy risks, 242
  weight gain
    recommendations, 245
Premature ejaculation, 225
Primary care providers, 62
Problem Areas in Diabetes (PAID)
  Tool, 47
Program evaluation
  diabetes education
    ensure effectiveness,
      178–179
    rationale for, 178–179
    reach, 179
    resources allocation, 179
    risk, 179
  operational metrics, 180–184
  types of, 180
Program operations
  assessment, 185–186
  for diabetes education, 184–187
  geographic reach, 188
  impact on other services, 188
  marketing efforts analysis, 188
  patient volume and productivity
    metrics, 187–188
  satisfaction, 189–190
  staff time-study assessment,
    188–189
Progressive resistance training (PRT),
  294–295
Psychosocial problems
  in challenging diabetes patients,
    200–205
    hyperglycemia fear, 202–204
    hypoglycemia fear, 201–202
    weight gain fear, 204–205
Pump, See continuous subcutaneous
  insulin infusion

Q

Quality of life, and DSME, 130–131

R

Rapid estimate of adult literacy in
  medicine (REALM), 121
RE-AIM framework model, 39
Real-time continuous glucose
  monitoring (RT-CGM), 138–141
Relapse prevention, in weight loss and
  diabetes management, 277
Religion and DSME, 129–130
Resistance exercise, 283, 284
Resources, for people with diabetes, 111
Respiratory distress, 241
Retinopathy, 18, 205, 238, 282
  risks in pregnant women with
    preexisting diabetes, 242
Rosiglitazone, 73, 317

S

Secretagogues, review in outpatient
  diabetes, 72–73
Sedentary lifestyle, 102, 111
Selective serotonin reuptake inhibitor
  (SSRI) medications, 225–226
Self-care behaviors, 48, 102, 106–107
  application of, 169–170
  assessment and measurement,
    165–169
  change and outcomes, 171–172
  and diabetes management, 206
  for patients
    after heart failure, 102
    with kidney disease, 107
    with peripheral
      neuropathies, 108
    with visual impairment, 106
Self-Care Inventory-Revised
  (SCI-R), 164
Self-care model, of diabetes
  management, 5–6
Self-care technology
  in diabetes education, 135–141
    insulin pump therapy,
      136–137
    real-time continuous glucose
      monitoring, 138–141

Self-efficacy model, of diabetes
    education, 32
Self-management, 24, 30
    behaviors, 123, 125
    core concepts of, 35
    diabetes education, 30, 34,
        36–37
    education process for inpatient
        diabetes, 82–96
    skills, 84
    support, 30–31, 34, 36–38
Self-monitoring
    in outpatient diabetes, 67–68
    in weight loss and diabetes
        management, 277
Self-monitoring of blood glucose
    (SMBG), 145–157
Sertraline, 225
Sexual dysfunction, 109, 205
    in women with diabetes,
        227–228
Sexual health
    and diabetes, 213–231
    diabetes educator role,
        230–231
    of men, 214–225
    of women, 225–230
Short test of functional health literacy in
    adults (S-TOHFLA), 121
Sildenafil, 219, 230
Sitagliptin, 72, 275
Smoking, 102, 104, 111
Social cognitive theory model, of
    diabetes education, 32
Social interaction, and DSME, 131
Socioeconomic status, of patient and
    DSME, 124
Standard of Professional Performance
    for Diabetes Educators, 51
Stress management, in weight loss and
    diabetes management, 277
Substance abuse, 83
Sudomotor dysfunction, 109
Sulfonylureas, 20, 23
Survival skills, 63, 84–86

T

Tadalafil, 219
Test of functional health literacy in
    adults (TOHFLA), 48, 121
Testosterone
    deficiency, 222–225
    replacement therapies, 223–224
Thiazolidinediones (TZDs), 20–21, 23,
    70, 73
Thyroid disease, 98
Transtheoretical model, of diabetes
    education, 32–33, 49
Tricyclic antidepressant
    clomipramine, 225
Troglitazone, 317
Type 1 diabetes mellitus, 7, 12, 16–17
Type 2 diabetes mellitus, 8, 11,
    16–18, 90

U

Urinary tract infections, 17
Urine ketone testing, 68

V

Vaginal infections, 17, 226
Vardenafil HCl, 219
Vascular impairment, 226
Visual impairment, 98, 105
    self-care behaviors for patients
        with, 106

W

Walking clubs, 55
Weight and diabetes management, See
    also Weight loss and diabetes
    management
    in clinical practice, 274–285
Weight-bearing activities, 282
Weight gain, fear in challenging diabetes
    patients, 204–205
Weight loss and diabetes management
    behavioral strategies, 274,
        276–277
        cognitive restructuring, 277
        provider stance and
            approach, 276
        realistic goal setting, 276
        relapse prevention, 277

self-monitoring and stimulus
control, 277
stress management and
alternative coping, 277
daily calorie consumption, 279
exercise, 282–285
nutrition recommendations for,
277–280
Weight Watchers, 55
Women's sexual health
common sexual problems, 226
depression and, 226
and diabetes, 225–230
diabetes educator role, 230–231
glucose control and, 229
hormones fluctuations and, 229

mind–body connection and,
226, 229
treatment, 229–230
Work environment and DSME, 128–129
Working alliance
with challenging diabetes
patients, 198–200
patients' beliefs and
behaviors, 199, 208
professional self-awareness,
198–199, 207–208
support treatment
environment, 208

Y

Young adulthood, diabetes education for,
265–266